Child and Adolescent Obesity

This book addresses the ever-increasing problem of obesity in children and adolescents, the long-term health and social problems that arise from this, and approaches to prevention and management. This comprehensive survey of an important and growing medical problem will help inform, influence and educate those charged with tackling this crisis. It covers all aspects of obesity from epidemiology and prevention to recent developments in biochemistry and genetics, and to the varied approaches to management which are influenced by social and clinical need. A Foreword by William Dietz and a forward-looking 'future perspectives' conclusion by Philip James embrace an international team of authors, all with first-hand experience of the issues posed by obesity in the young. Aimed at doctors, and all health-care professionals, it will be of interest to all those concerned about the increasing prevalence of obesity in children and adolescents.

'The epidemic of obesity is not yet viewed with the urgency that it demands… The questions and challenges that the epidemic provokes provide us with an exciting and unique opportunity to shape a new field.'
William H. Dietz
From the Foreword

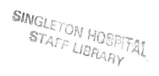

Child and Adolescent
Obesity

Causes and Consequences,
Prevention and Management

Edited by

Walter Burniat
University Hospital for Children 'Queen Fabiola', Free University of Brussels

Tim J. Cole
Institute of Child Health, London

Inge Lissau
National Institute of Public Health, Copenhagen

Elizabeth M. E. Poskitt
International Nutrition Group, London School of Hygiene and Tropical Medicine

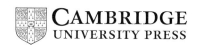
CAMBRIDGE
UNIVERSITY PRESS

PUBLISHED BY THE PRESS SYNDICATE OF THE UNIVERSITY OF CAMBRIDGE
The Pitt Building, Trumpington Street, Cambridge, United Kingdom

CAMBRIDGE UNIVERSITY PRESS
The Edinburgh Building, Cambridge CB2 2RU, UK
40 West 20th Street, New York, NY 10011-4211, USA
477 Williamstown Road, Port Melbourne, VIC 3207, Australia
Ruiz de Alarcón 13, 28014 Madrid, Spain
Dock House, The Waterfront, Cape Town 8001, South Africa

http://www.cambridge.org

First published 2002
Reprinted 2003

Printed in the United Kingdom at the University Press, Cambridge

Typeface Minion 10.5/14pt   *System* Poltype® [V N]

A catalogue record for this book is available from the British Library

Library of Congress Cataloguing in Publication data

Child and adolescent obesity: causes and consequences, prevention and management /
edited by Walter Burniat . . . [et al.].
    p.   cm.
Includes bibliographical references and index.
ISBN 0 521 65237 5
1. Obesity in children.   2. Obesity in adolescence.   3. Children – Nutrition.
4. Teenagers – Nutrition.   5. Reducing diets.   I. Burniat, Walter, 1949–
RJ399.C6 C46 2002
618.92'398–dc21   2001043920

ISBN 0 521 65237 5 hardback

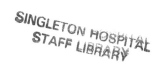

Contents

List of contributors   xi

Foreword   William H. Dietz   xv

Preface   xix

Part I   **Causes**   1

1   Measurement and definition   3
       Tim J. Cole and Marie Françoise Rolland-Cachera
       1.1 Introduction   3
       1.2 Natural history of adiposity   4
       1.3 Measurement of body fat   4
       1.4 Adiposity as proxy for later adiposity, morbidity and mortality   14
       1.5 Definition of childhood obesity   15
       1.6 Conclusions   22
       1.7 References   22

2   Epidemiology   28
       Michèle Guillaume and Inge Lissau
       2.1 Introduction   28
       2.2 Epidemiology and methods   28
       2.3 The scale of the problem   34
       2.4 Conclusions   44
       2.5 References   45

3   Molecular and biological factors with emphasis on adipose tissue   50
       development
       Martin Wabitsch
       3.1 Introduction   50
       3.2 Regulation of body weight   51
       3.3 Single gene defects   52
       3.4 Regulation of body energy stores at adipose tissue level   55
       3.5 Changes of body fat stores during development   55

3.6 Changes at cellular level related to changes in body fat　　57

3.7 Lipid storage in adipose tissue (lipogenesis)　　58

3.8 Lipid mobilization (lipolysis)　　59

3.9 Preadipocytes in human adipose tissue　　60

3.10 Proliferation and differentiation of preadipocytes　　60

3.11 Adipogenic activity of human serum　　60

3.12 Hormonal and nutritional factors regulating adipose differentiation　　62

3.13 Human adipocytes are secretory cells　　65

3.14 Conclusions　　66

3.15 References　　66

4　　Nutrition　　69

Marie Françoise Rolland-Cachera and France Bellisle

4.1 Introduction　　69

4.2 Secular trends of nutrition and obesity　　69

4.3 Relationship between nutrition and adiposity　　74

4.4 Qualitative assessment of intake behaviour　　79

4.5 Lifestyle　　83

4.6 Conclusions　　85

4.7 References　　86

5　　Physical Activity　　93

Yves Schutz and Claudio Maffeis

5.1 Introduction　　93

5.2 Energy expenditure assessment　　93

5.3 Energy intake vs. energy expenditure　　94

5.4 Components of total energy expenditure　　95

5.5 Excess energy intake vs. low energy expenditure　　98

5.6 Aerobic capacity ($VO_{2\,max}$) in obesity　　101

5.7 Substrate oxidation and substrate balance　　102

5.8 Conclusions　　104

5.9 References　　105

6　　Psychosocial factors　　109

Andrew J. Hill and Inge Lissau

6.1 Children's social background　　109

6.2 Attitudes to obesity　　111

6.3 Children's self-worth　　115

6.4 Parents and peers　　118

6.5 Conclusions　　122

6.6 References　　123

Part II	**Consequences**	129
7	Clinical features, adverse effects and outcome	131
	Karl F.M. Zwiauer, Margherita Caroli, Ewa Malecka-Tendera and Elizabeth M.E. Poskitt	
	7.1 Clinical findings and immediate adverse effects	131
	7.2 Intermediate medical consequences	142
	7.3 Long-term consequences	145
	7.4 References	147
8	The obese adolescent	154
	Marie-Laure Frelut and Carl-Erik Flodmark	
	8.1 Biophysical factors	154
	8.2 Psychological aspects	160
	8.3 References	166
9	Prader–Willi and other syndromes	171
	Giuseppe Chiumello and Elizabeth M.E. Poskitt	
	9.1 Introduction	171
	9.2 Endocrine problems	171
	9.3 Prader–Willi syndrome (PWS)	174
	9.4 Other obesity syndromes	180
	9.5 References	184
10	Hormonal and metabolic changes	189
	Ewa Malecka-Tendera and Dénes Molnár	
	10.1 Pituitary-adrenal axis	190
	10.2 Pituitary–gonadal axis	192
	10.3 Pituitary–thyroid axis	194
	10.4 Growth hormone and insulin-like growth factors	195
	10.5 Hyperinsulinaemia and insulin resistance	198
	10.6 Leptin	203
	10.7 References	209
11	Risk of cardiovascular complications	221
	David S. Freedman, Sathanur R. Srinivasan and Gerald S. Berenson	
	11.1 Introduction	221
	11.2 Secular trends	223
	11.3 Associations with risk factors	224
	11.4 Body fat patterning	230
	11.5 Longitudinal analyses	234
	11.6 Conclusions	235
	11.7 References	235

Part III	**Prevention and management**	**241**

12	Prevention	243
	Inge Lissau, Walter Burniat, Elizabeth M.E. Poskitt and Tim J. Cole	
	12.1 Prevention before management	243
	12.2 Why prevention?	243
	12.3 Prevention strategy	245
	12.4 Responsibilities for prevention	248
	12.5 Reduce sedentary activity	252
	12.6 Reduce poor dietary habits	257
	12.7 Prevention programmes	263
	12.8 Monitoring and evaluation	264
	12.9 Conclusions	264
	12.10 References	265
13	Home-based management	270
	Elizabeth M.E. Poskitt	
	13.1 Introduction	270
	13.2 Principles of modifying lifestyles to encourage slimming in obese children	273
	13.3 What can be recommended?	275
	13.4 Eating and diet	277
	13.5 Conclusions	280
	13.6 References	280
14	Dietary management	282
	Margherita Caroli and Walter Burniat	
	14.1 Introduction	282
	14.2 History of dietary therapy	282
	14.3 Aims of dietary treatment	283
	14.4 Types of diet	284
	14.5 Consequences of dieting	290
	14.6 Guidelines for weight goals and dietetic treatments	299
	14.7 Conclusions	301
	14.8 References	302
15	Management through activity	307
	Jana Parizkova, Claudio Maffeis and Elizabeth M.E. Poskitt	
	15.1 Introduction	307
	15.2 Aims of the programmes	308
	15.3 Efficacy of exercise in lowering fat mass	310
	15.4 General principles	313

15.5 Physical activity and exercise programmes   314

15.6 How to improve compliance   320

15.7 The role of the family   321

15.8 Conclusions   322

15.9 References   323

16   Psychotherapy   327

Carl-Erik Flodmark and Inge Lissau

16.1 Obesity – a disease put into perspective   327

16.2 The treatment of obesity   328

16.3 Conclusions   340

16.4 References   341

17   Drug therapy   345

Dénes Molnár and Ewa Malecka-Tendera

17.1 Appetite suppressants   345

17.2 Thermogenic agents   348

17.3 Digestive inhibitors   349

17.4 Hormone analogues and antagonists   350

17.5 References   352

18   Surgical treatment   355

Alessandro Salvatoni

18.1 Introduction   355

18.2 Surgical techniques and their complications   355

18.3 Bariatric surgery in adolescence   357

18.4 Conclusions   358

18.5 References   358

19   Interdisciplinary outpatient management   361

Beatrice Bauer and Claudio Maffeis

19.1. Goal and general philosophy   361

19.2 Multifaceted treatment programmes   364

19.3 Organizing team work   370

19.4 Acknowledgements   374

19.5 References   374

20   Interdisciplinary residential management   377

Marie-Laure Frelut

20.1 Historical background and implementation   377

20.2 A comprehensive approach   378

20.3 Results and outcome   385

20.4   Conclusions   386

20.5   References   386

21   The future   389

W. Philip T. James

21.1   Introduction   389

21.2   Assessment of childhood obesity   389

21.3   Ethnic differences in children's anthropometry   391

21.4   The Thrifty Genotype   393

21.5   The prevalence of childhood obesity   394

21.6   Weaning practices and early eating habits   395

21.7   The 'obesogenic' environment   396

21.8   Can policy initiatives work?   397

21.9   Devising and implementing new policies   399

21.10   References   401

Index   403

Contributors

Beatrice Bauer
Centre for Eating Disorders
(DIDASCO), via C. Abba 17, 37126
Verona, Italy.
E-mail: bbauer@didascodca.com

France Bellisle
Hotel Dieu – Unité Inserm 341, Place du
Parvis Notre Dame, 1, 75181 Paris Cedex
04, France.
E-mail: bellisle@imaginet.fr

Gerald S. Berenson
Tulane Center for Cardiovascular
Health, Tulane University School of
Public Health and Tropical Medicine,
1440 Canal Street, Suite 2140, New
Orleans LA 70112-2715 USA.
E-mail:
berenson@mailhost.tcs.tulane.edu

Walter Burniat
Department of Pediatrics, University
Hospital for Children 'Reine Fabiola',
Free University of Brussels, Av. J.J.
Crocq, 15, 1020 Brussels, Belgium.
E-mail: wburniat@ulb.ac.be

Margherita Caroli
Nutrition Unit, Department of
Prevention AUSL BR1
(Brindisi) Italy.
E-mail: caroli@mail.clio.it

Giuseppe Chiumello
Clinica Paediatrica III, Universita degli
Studi di Milano, Via Olgettina 60, 20132
Milano, Italy.
E-mail: chiumello.giuseppe@hsr.it

Tim J. Cole
Department of Paediatric Epidemiology
& Biostatistics, Institute of Child Health,
London WC1N 1EH, UK.
E-mail: tim.cole@ich.ucl.ac.uk

William H. Dietz
Division of Nutrition and Physical
Activity, Center for Disease Control and
Prevention, 4770 Buford Hwy NE
Mailstop K-24, Atlanta GA 30341 USA,
E-mail: wcd4@cdc.gov

Carl-Erik Flodmark
Department of Paediatrics, University
Hospital in Malmö, Sweden.
E-mail:
carl-erik.flodmark@pediatrik.mas.lu.se

David S. Freedman
Division of Nutrition and Physical
Activity, Centers for Disease Control and
Prevention, CDC Mailstop K-26, 4770
Buford Highway, Atlanta GA
30341-3724, USA.
E-mail: dxf1@cdc.gov

Marie-Laure Frelut
Robert Debré University Hospital Paris
and Centre Thérapeutique Pédiatrique
95580 Margency, France.
E-mail: frelut@club-internet.fr

Michèle Guillaume
Department of Preventive Medicine,
Province of Luxembourg, Chaussée
d'Houffalize, 1 bis, 6600 Bastogne,
Belgium.
E-mail: dir.prevention.sante@province.
luxembourg.be

Andrew J. Hill
Academic Unit of Psychiatry and
Behavioural Sciences, School of
Medicine, University of Leeds, Leeds
LS2 9LT, UK.
E-Mail: a.j.hill@leeds.ac.uk

W. Philip T. James
International Obesity TaskForce, 231–3
North Gower Street, London NW1 2NS,
UK.
E-Mail: jeanhjames@aol.com

Inge Lissau
National Institute of Public Health, 25
Svanemøllervej, 2100 Copenhagen OE,
Denmark.
E-mail: INL@niph.dk

Claudio Maffeis
Department of Paediatrics, University
Hospital, Largo AL Scuro 34, Verona,
Italy.
E-mail: maffeis@borgoroma.univr.it

Ewa Malecka-Tendera
Department of Pathophysiology, Silesian
School of Medicine, Medykow 18, 40 752
Katowice, Poland.
E-mail: ewt@box43.gnet

Dénes Molnár
Department of Paediatrics, Medical
Faculty, University of Pécs, József A. u.7,
7623 Pécs, Hungary.
E-mail: dmolnar@apacs.pote.hu

Jana Parizkova
Centre for the Management of Obesity,
3rd. Med. Dept., U Nemocnice 2, Prague
2, 12806 Czech Republic.
E-mail: parizek@mbox.cesnet.cz

Elizabeth M.E. Poskitt
International Nutrition Group, London
School of Hygiene and Tropical
Medicine, 49-51 Bedford Square,
London WC1B 3DP, UK.
E-mail: mopsa@emep.freeserve.co.uk

Marie Françoise Rolland-Cachera
Institut Scientifique et Technique de la
Nutrition et de l'Alimentation (ISTNA)
– Conservatoire National des Arts et
Métiers (CNAM) 2 rue Conté, 75003
Paris, France.
E-mail: cachera@cnam.fr

Alessandro Salvatoni
Paediatric Department, University of
Insubria, Via F. del Ponte, 19, 21100
Varese, Italy.
E-mail: clipedva@tin.it

Yves Schutz
Institute of Physiology, University of
Lausanne, Lausanne, Switzerland.
E-mail: yves.schutz@iphysiol.unil.ch

Sathanur R. Srinivasan
Tulane Center for Cardiovascular
Health, Tulane University School of
Public Health and Tropical Medicine,
1440 Canal Street, Suite 2140, New
Orleans LA 70112-2715 USA.
E-mail: ssriniv1@tulane.edu

Martin Wabitsch
Department of Paediatrics, University of
Ulm, Prittwitzstr. 43, D-89075 Ulm,
Germany.
E-mail:
martin.wabitsch@medizin.uni-ulm.de

Karl F.M. Zwiauer
Department of Paediatrics, General
Hospital Saint Poelten, A-3100 Saint
Poelten, Propst-Fuehrer Str. 4 – Austria.
E-mail: k.zwiauer@kh-st-poelten.at

Foreword

Childhood obesity has now become the most prevalent nutritional disease in developed countries. For example, the prevalence of obesity, defined as a body mass index (BMI) equal to or above the 95th centile for children of the same age and sex, now affects 10–15% of children and adolescents in the United States (Flegal et al., 1998). When the prevalence of obesity in the United States is compared across nationally representative surveys conducted over the last 30 years, the most rapid increases in prevalence occurred between 1980 and 1994. The greatest increases in body weight have occurred in children and adolescents in the upper half of the BMI distribution (Troiano & Flegal, 1998). Stated another way, the mean BMI for children of the same age and sex has increased more than the median. These observations suggest at least two possibilities. They may suggest that the genes that predispose to obesity occur in approximately 50% of the population. Alternatively, these observations suggest that the factors that influence the development of obesity are discrete, and act only on half of the population.

Elsewhere in the world, obesity is also increasing rapidly. Nevertheless, the world-wide prevalence of obesity is generally lower than the prevalence observed among children and adolescents in the United States.

The factors that account for the rapid changes in prevalence remain unclear. The rapidity of the changes in prevalence clearly excludes a genetic basis for the changes, because the gene pool remained unchanged between 1980 and 1994. Because obesity can only result from an imbalance of energy intake and expenditure, it may be useful to review the changes in diet and activity that occurred synchronously with the changes in prevalence. It should be clear throughout this discussion that no data yet exist that link obesity to any of the following behaviours. Nevertheless, these behavioural shifts offer reasonable and testable hypotheses. For example, in the 1970s, the advent of the microwave oven made it possible for children to select and prepare their own meals without parental oversight. Likewise, substantial increases have occurred in food consumption outside the home. Currently, 35% of a family's food expenditure in the United States is spent on food consumed outside the home. Between 7% and 12% of children and adolescents skip breakfast. Few children consume a dietary pattern consistent with the food guide pyramid. The consumption of soft drinks has almost doubled in the last 15 years. Over 12 000 new food products are introduced annually in the United States. All of these dietary factors may increase the difficulty associated with the establishment and maintenance of a healthy body weight.

Activity deserves equal attention. Marked declines in vigorous physical activity occur in adolescent girls, at a time when susceptibility to obesity is heightened (Heath et al., 1994). In the United States, the number of schools that offer daily physical education has declined by almost 30% over the past decade. In addition, the percentage of children who watch five or more hours of television daily has increased to 30%. Increased numbers of working mothers and a perceived lack of neighbourhood safety may contribute further to increased levels of inactivity.

Until quite recently, obesity in children was viewed as a cosmetic problem. The major risks associated with obesity in children and adolescents were those consequences that resulted when obesity persisted into adulthood. However, more recent experience indicates that significant health risks are associated with obesity in childhood. For example, we have recently shown that 65% of overweight 5- to 10-year-olds have at least one cardiovascular disease risk factor, such as elevated blood pressure or lipid levels, and 25% have two or more risk factors (Freedman et al., 1999). Furthermore, type II diabetes mellitus now accounts for up to 30% of new diabetes cases in some paediatric clinics, and up to 3% of some paediatric populations, such as Native Americans, now suffer from this problem. The overwhelming majority of type II paediatric diabetic cases occur in obese patients.

To summarize, obesity is prevalent, it appears to be increasing and significant effects are demonstrable in childhood. Effective treatment of affected children, and prevention of obesity in children who are susceptible must become a priority. The challenge is how to accomplish both goals. Care for mildly to moderately overweight patients will require the service of primary care practitioners, and guidelines now exist to enhance these services (Barlow & Dietz, 1998). Effective treatment for severely obese children is essential and will probably require care in speciality clinics. However, effective prevention of obesity in nonoverweight children may also help reduce body weight in children who are already overweight. As with nutritional deficiency diseases, where the addition of iodine to salt reduces goitre, or the addition of fluoride to water reduces dental decay, environmental modification may represent the most durable, effective and cheapest intervention. Nevertheless, until the causes of obesity are better understood, the target of the environmental dietary intervention must be based on logic rather than science.

In contrast to dietary interventions, efforts that increase physical activity or reduce inactivity appear warranted. Although we lack data to demonstrate that such measures effectively reduce the incidence of obesity in the population, increased physical activity has demonstrated benefit for the comorbidities of obesity, such as hypertension, diabetes and hyperlipidaemia.

Prevention presents additional challenges. The epidemic of obesity is not yet viewed with the urgency that it demands. Paediatricians are poorly equipped to treat obesity, and methods that help primary-care providers target specific behaviours, like computer-based interactive questionnaires, are still in a developmental phase. Effective means to maintain weight in those who are gaining weight too rapidly or to reduce weight in those who are overweight must be established. Finally, the environmental infrastructure necessary to promote physical activity in the many settings that affect children must be developed and evaluated.

Rarely have we had the opportunity to observe an epidemic of chronic disease occur before our eyes. The questions and challenges that the epidemic provokes provide us with an exciting and unique opportunity to shape a new field. As Winston Churchill once said:

Now this is not the end. It is not even the beginning of the end. But it is, perhaps, the end of the beginning.

REFERENCES

Barlow, S.E. & Dietz, W.H. (1998). Obesity evaluation and treatment: expert committee recommendations. *Pediatrics*, **102**, e29.

Flegal, K.M., Carroll, M.D., Kuczmarski, R.J. & Johnson, C.L. (1998). Overweight and obesity in the United States: prevalence and trends, 1960–1994. *International Journal of Obesity*, **22**, 39–47.

Freedman, D.S., Dietz, W.H., Srinivasan, S.R. & Berenson, G.S. (1999). The relation of overweight to cardiovascular risk factors among children and adolescents: the Bogalusa Heart Study. *Pediatrics*, **103**, 1175–82.

Heath, G.W., Pratt, M., Warren, C.W. & Kann, L. (1994). Physical activity patterns in American high school students: results from the 1990 Youth Risk Behavior Survey. *Archives of Pediatric and Adolescent Medicine*, **148**, 1131–6.

Troiano, R.P. & Flegal, K.M. (1998). Overweight children and adolescents: description, epidemiology, and demographics. *Pediatrics*, **101**, 497–504.

William H. Dietz

Preface

Overnutrition in the form of unusual fatness has been recognized over the ages and in all societies. In the past, fatness was usually seen as a sign of health, opulence and/or fertility. Today we know that obesity tends to be accompanied by a number of adverse health risks, and obese individuals are too often viewed as figures either of fun or of dislike. Yet, for all the health disadvantages and social opprobrium, obesity and overweight are developing in epidemic proportions in the westernized developed world. We recognize this epidemic in the need to enlarge and reinforce seats in theatres and aeroplanes and in the need for change in clothing styles and sizes, for example. Even in less affluent countries, the fat 'little Emperors' of small families amongst the urban well-to-do are becoming legendary.

The extent to which the high prevalence of adult obesity has its origins in childhood obesity is widely debated. The question remains unanswered but it is clear that, along with increasing obesity in adults, there is increasing obesity in children at all ages. We are not short of theories for the development of obesity in children but we seem powerless to control the increase – leading to great concerns for future adult health.

Two of us met in 1988 because of a shared concern that too few of those speaking for obesity in childhood were clinically involved with children and their health. From this meeting arose the European Childhood Obesity Group, perhaps still the only international group of paediatric health professionals working with obese children. Many of our authors are members of this group and relate their varied clinical experiences, making the book not only a source of research information but also an emporium of practical expertise.

In the book we attempt to examine the epidemiology, sociology and pathology behind childhood obesity. Having presented the current situation regarding childhood obesity, we go on to discuss approaches to prevention and management. Throughout, we have tried to be practical and realistic whilst recognizing that there are no simple answers nor easy treatments for obesity, whether in children or adults.

As we compiled the book we were conscious that there were common issues and themes running through many chapters. We have tried to avoid unnecessary repetition by frequent textual references to other chapters but we recognize the book is not likely to be read at one sitting. Each chapter should 'stand by itself' and be complete in itself. Thus some topics do feature in several sections of the book, albeit in relation to different aspects of childhood obesity and overweight.

It is our belief that Society needs to have more sympathy and understanding for the problems of the obese. However, Society also needs to create communal environments that facilitate lifestyles which discourage the development of obesity. Unless we can achieve changes at national and community as well as at individual levels, the present epidemic of obesity and overweight seems likely to continue until overweight is the norm. The complications of excess weight will then become the accepted consequences of a lifetime of inappropriate nutrition and inactivity. It is our hope that this book will go some way to raising the issue of child obesity to a wider circle than the health workers and research workers for whom it is primarily written.

The Editors
Cambridge, January 2002

Walter Burniat
Tim J. Cole
Inge Lissau
Elizabeth M.E. Poskitt

Part I

Causes

Measurement and definition

Tim J. Cole[1] and Marie Françoise Rolland-Cachera[2]

[1]Department of Paediatric Epidemiology and Biostatistics, Institute of Child Health, London. [2]ISTNA-CNAM, Paris

1.1 Introduction

A simple definition of obesity is an excess of body fat. However, as a definition it immediately raises questions – how is body fat measured and what cut-off is used to define 'excess'? The two questions are addressed in this chapter.

If obesity is an excess of body fat, a more neutral term is needed for the amount of body fat in the body, and here it is called adiposity. Adiposity is the amount of body fat expressed either as the absolute fat mass (in units of kilograms) or, alternatively, as the percentage of total body mass. Fat mass is highly correlated with body mass, while per cent fat mass is relatively uncorrelated with body size.

It is not only the amount but also the distribution of body fat within the body that is important in adults. The distribution or patterning of body fat is associated with later disease risk, independent of the level of obesity (Vague, 1956). Adults with central, trunk or android fat patterning, who are at greater risk (Björntorp, 1985), deposit fat preferentially around the waist, while with gynoid patterning fat is found more towards the extremes of the body.

Some obese adults were fat as children, so child fatness may be a risk factor in its own right for later disease (Power et al., 1997). This is relevant for setting a fatness cut-off. However, in assessing fatness an important distinction needs to be made between childhood and adulthood – children grow in size, so that anthropometric cut-offs for fatness have to be adjusted for age and in adolescence for maturation as well. For this reason, the assessment of adiposity in childhood and adolescence differs from its assessment in adults.

So, obesity is excess adiposity, which requires a suitable measure of body fat and a suitable cut-off. In adults, adiposity is commonly assessed using the body mass index (BMI; weight/height^2; also known as Quetelet's index), and obesity cut-offs based on mortality risk are defined in body mass index units of kilograms per metre squared (kg/m^2).

The rest of the chapter is concerned with these issues in children: Section 1.2

describes briefly the natural history of child adiposity, Section 1.3 addresses the question of how to measure adiposity in children, Section 1.4 describes the predictive value of child adiposity for later obesity, morbidity and mortality, and Section 1.5 considers the references and cut-offs needed for the definition of child obesity.

1.2 Natural history of adiposity

Body fat is made up of fat cells or adipocytes. The changes in fat mass that occur in the growing child arise in two separate ways, through changes in the number and in the mean size of adipocytes. In infancy adipocyte enlargement contributes most to the increasing fat mass, while after infancy fat mass gain arises mainly through cell proliferation (Knittle et al., 1979). As a result, fat mass rises steeply during the first year and then falls again, with a second rise in later childhood. Figure 1.1 illustrates the pattern and also shows how anthropometric indices, like the body mass index or subscapular skinfold, follow the same age-related trends. Section 3.5 gives a more detailed description of the underlying processes.

1.3 Measurement of body fat

An ideal measure of body fat should be accurate, precise, accessible, acceptable and well documented. Accuracy and precision mean that the measure should be unbiased and repeatable; accessibility relates to the simplicity, cost and ease of use of the method; acceptability refers in the broadest sense to the invasiveness of the measurement and documentation concerns the existence of age-related reference values of the measurement for clinical assessment.

No existing measure satisfies all these criteria. Highly accurate reference methods like deuterium dilution or underwater weighing are expensive, and more accessible, cheaper methods based on anthropometry are not very accurate.

1.3.1 Research methods

Several accurate and direct measures of total body fat are now available, for example underwater weighing, dual energy X-ray absorptiometry (DEXA), computer tomography or magnetic resonance imaging (MRI) (see the review by Davies & Cole (1995) for more details). They are generally noninvasive, except for the water bath in underwater weighing. As research tools they are very valuable, and are particularly useful to validate other measures based on anthropometric measurements (Ashwell et al., 1985). However, they are inappropriate for routine clinical practice because of their high cost, slow response time and limited access (the equipment is found mostly in research or tertiary referral centres).

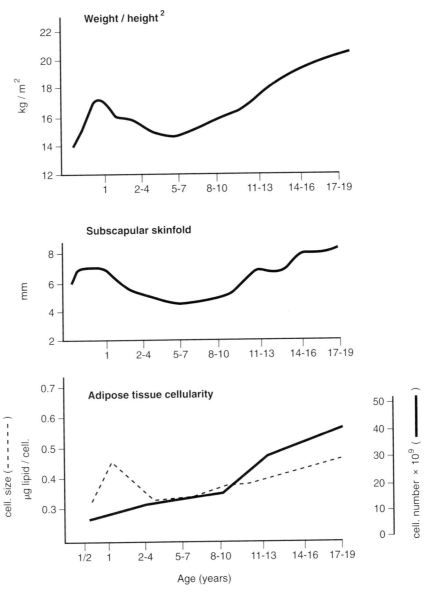

Figure 1.1   Trends in body mass index and subscapular skinfold thickness through childhood and the corresponding trends in adipose tissue cellularity (Rolland-Cachera et al., 1982; Sempé et al., 1979; Knittle, 1979).

Bioelectrical impedance analysis (BIA) is an indirect method that has become popular due to its relatively low cost (Davies & Cole, 1995). It works on the principle that body fat contains no water and, therefore, is of high electrical resistance (or impedance). Electrodes are attached to the extremities of the body, usually the hands and feet, and a small current is passed to measure the impedance between the electrodes.

The impedance is strongly correlated with body size and needs to be adjusted accordingly, usually by dividing by the square of height. There is some uncertainty as to just how much extra information BIA provides over and above simple anthropometry, but it is sufficiently popular for the latest forms of weighing scales to incorporate an impedance measurement (Jebb et al., 2000).

1.3.2 Anthropometry

Anthropometry is the single universally applicable, inexpensive and noninvasive method available to assess the size, shape and composition of the human body. It reflects both health and nutrition and predicts performance, risk factors and survival (de Onis & Habicht, 1996). The most widely used measurements to predict fatness are weight and height, skinfolds and circumferences.

Measurement technique

A common misconception with anthropometry is that it is easy to do and that no special training or supervision are required to obtain accurate and precise measurements. This is not the case if the measurements are to be of any value. For detailed information on measurement technique see, for example, Cameron (1986). Some general pointers are given here.

Children should be weighed in their underwear and for infants an adjustment should be made for any clothing. The instrument should ideally be digital or, failing that, a beam balance or, failing that, a high quality spring balance.

To measure length, at least two measurers are needed, one at the infant's head, to ensure proper contact with the headboard, and the other at the feet, to make the measurement. Use a good quality length board. For height there are several good stadiometers on the market and they should be checked and calibrated before each session. The child's head should be held in the Frankfort plane, that is with the line of vision perpendicular to the body, and the child requested to stand straight with heels, buttocks and shoulders touching the wall. There is no need to stretch the child.

Height is not as easy to measure as weight. In particular, to measure height velocity over time it needs highly trained observers and continuous quality control to ensure high precision. For single measurements to assess adiposity it is less critical but, even so, training is important to minimize interobserver variation.

In large-scale epidemiological studies, self-reported values of weight and height are used, but in adolescence and later they tend to be biased in opposite directions, with weight underestimated and height exaggerated, and the weight error is larger in heavier subjects.

Skinfolds are the most difficult of all measurements to make. An experienced trainer and continuous quality control are essential, as even experienced measurers disagree systematically in their skinfold measurements.

Circumferences are easier than skinfolds to measure, but the placing and tension of the tape are important. Again, quality control is recommended to minimize inter- and intraobserver variation.

Percent of median, centiles and Z-scores

Anthropometry changes with age during childhood. To assess individual children, measurements need to be adjusted to compare them with those of other children of the same age. In addition, weight may need to be adjusted for height. The adjustment is made by comparing the child's measurement with a suitable reference value, obtained either from a chart or table, though computers are now simplifying the process.

There are three different ways of expressing the adjusted anthropometry value: as a percentage of the median, as a centile and as a Z-score. The per cent of median is 100 times the measurement divided by the median or mean reference value for the child's age (or in the case of weight-for-height, weight divided by the median for the child's height). For centiles, the measurement is plotted on a growth centile chart and the child's centile interpolated from the growth curves. Z-scores are closely related to centiles and indicate the number of standard deviations the child's measurement lies above or below the mean or median reference value.

As an example, three proposed cut-offs to define overweight based on age-adjusted weight are 120% of the median, the 97th centile and +2 Z-scores respectively. These cut-offs are all similar to each other, identifying 2–3% of the reference population as being overweight.

Per cent of the median is the simplest of the three forms to calculate, and has been in use the longest (Gomez et al., 1956). Centiles are easy to read off the chart and are well understood by parents. If the measurement is normally distributed, centiles and Z-scores are interchangeable. However, often there is no known distribution by which to convert the centiles on the chart to Z-scores. This applies particularly to skew data like weight and skinfold thickness.

Recently, it has become possible to construct charts that convert between centiles and Z-scores when the data are not normally distributed, for example weight (Cole et al., 1998) and triceps skinfold (Hughes et al., 1997). For the purposes of epidemiological analysis, Z-scores are more appropriate than centiles – it is not correct for example to average centiles, as they are on a nonlinear scale. Calculations such as these should always be done on the Z-score scale.

Weight

We now turn to anthropometric measures of adiposity. Weight is the simplest and most direct index of body size, easy to measure, cheap and reproducible. It is also reasonably highly correlated with body fat (Cole, 1991). Weight-for-age tables and charts were originally used to assess undernutrition (Waterlow, 1972), and weight-for-age is currently recommended by the World Health Organization (WHO, 1995) to assess nutritional status.

However, weight is highly correlated with height, and height is only weakly correlated with body fat (Himes & Roche, 1986). So, by adjusting weight for height the relationship between weight and body fat can be strengthened, leading to a more sensitive and specific index of adiposity. Note, though, that weight–height indices do not measure fatness as such, only overweight.

Weight-for-height

There are many different forms of index based on weight and height, dating back over 150 years (Cole, 1991). One of the simplest is relative weight. It requires a table or chart of expected weight for the child's height and sex (and sometimes age and maturation as well), and the child's weight is expressed as a percentage of their expected weight (per cent of median). If the expected weight is based on just height and sex, then the index is known as weight-for-height. Weight-for-height, because it takes no account of the child's age, is useful in parts of the world where dates of birth are not recorded, but for children who are particularly tall or short for age it leads to a biased assessment in infancy and adolescence (Cole, 1985).

The World Health Organization's international growth reference weight-for-height chart (Dibley et al., 1987) is truncated at the age of 10 years for girls and 11.5 years for boys. The reason is that, past this age, weight-for-height cannot be adjusted for, although it remains age-dependent. As a result, weight-for-height is of no use at all for assessing adiposity during adolescence.

The need to adjust weight for both height and age is now widely accepted (Cole, 1979; Rolland-Cachera et al., 1982), and it has led to the study of power indices like weight/height^2 and weight/height^3.

Weight/height^p uncorrelated with height

The rationale for adjusting weight for height is to strengthen the relationship between weight and adiposity (see above). However, this has not always been the intention – weight was originally adjusted for height to give an index that was uncorrelated with height, irrespective of adiposity. These two alternative approaches lead to slightly different forms of weight–height index, one uncorrelated with height and the other maximally correlated with adiposity.

Relative weight is weight adjusted for height and so is, by definition, uncorrelated with height. The same principle applies to indices like weight/height^p – the power of height, p, can be chosen to make the index uncorrelated with height. If the adjustment is done ignoring the age of the individual child, the optimal whole-number value for p throughout childhood is 2 (Cole, 1991).

However, it is important to adjust for age and, to achieve this, the calculation to optimize p is done in narrow age groups (Rolland-Cachera et al., 1982) or else weight and height are adjusted for age first (Cole, 1979). In early childhood p is near 2, so the best index is weight/height^2 (Cole et al., 1981; Gasser et al., 1995). The value of p increases during childhood and peaks during adolescence, reaching a value of 3 or more (i.e. weight/height^3), and then drops back to 2 in adulthood (Rolland-Cachera et al., 1982; Cole, 1986). So, earlier in childhood the body mass index (or BMI), weight/height^2, is optimal, while during adolescence Rohrer's index, weight/height^3, is better.

Weight/height^p highly correlated with adiposity

An alternative is to choose the index weight/height^p explicitly for maximal correlation with body fat, rather than zero correlation with height. The two criteria lead to the same index only if, after adjusting for age, height and body fat are uncorrelated.

In practice, body fat, like the body mass index, is weakly positively associated with height in adolescence (Himes & Roche, 1986; Lazarus et al., 1996), and the two correlations tend to cancel out. This means that in adolescence, though body mass index is correlated with height, it is also more strongly correlated with adiposity than alternative indices like Rohrer's index. For this reason, body mass index is generally accepted as the optimal weight–height index of child and adolescent adiposity.

Body mass index

The interdependence between weight, height, body mass index and body fat is often insufficiently well understood. The body mass index is sometimes criticized because of its association with height (O'Dea & Abraham, 1995; Lazarus et al., 1996), yet this is only a flaw if the index is required to be uncorrelated with height. From a broader perspective the association is actually an advantage, as it flags the greater fatness of tall children during adolescence. Recent studies (Daniels et al., 1997; Pietrobelli et al., 1998) have shown high correlations between BMI and per cent body fat measured by DEXA.

Equally it is important to realize that the body mass index cannot be used to demonstrate an association between adiposity and height in adolescence – body mass index does not measure adiposity directly. To investigate the correlation

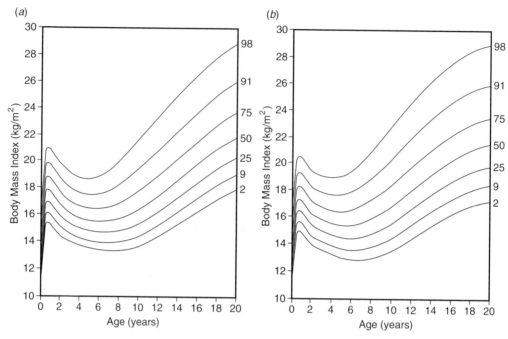

Figure 1.2   Centiles of body mass index for British boys (*a*) and girls (*b*) in 1990. The seven centiles are spaced two-thirds of a Z-score apart, i.e. the 2nd, 9th, 25th, 50th, 75th, 91st and 98th centiles.

between adiposity and height a direct measure of body fat, for example by DEXA, should be used.

The natural history of body mass index is similar to that for body fat, a steep rise during infancy with a peak at 9 months of age, followed by a fall until age 6 years and then a second rise, which lasts until adulthood. The earliest published charts of body mass index were for French children (Rolland-Cachera et al., 1982), and more recently charts have appeared for North American, British, Swedish, Hong Kong and Dutch populations (Hammer et al., 1991; Must et al., 1991; Rolland-Cachera et al., 1991; Cole et al., 1995; Lindgren et al., 1995; Leung et al., 1998; Cole & Roede, 1999; He et al., 2000; Kuczmarski et al., 2000). Figure 1.2 shows the British centiles for body mass index (Cole et al., 1995). It shows broadly the same age and sex trends as other national centile charts, with body mass index rising more steeply in boys than girls during puberty.

Indices based on weight centile and height centile

It has long been standard practice to plot children's weights and heights on centile charts, and some have treated the difference between the two centiles as a measure of over- or underweight. Hulse & Schilg (1996), for example, have suggested that a

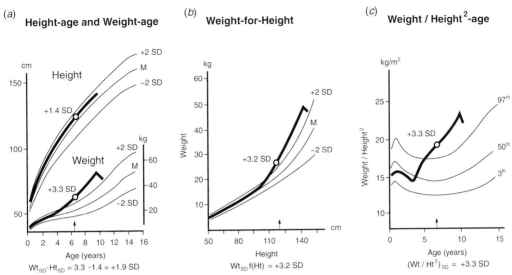

Figure 1.3   Comparison of three methods for assessing weight adjusted for height : weight centile compared to height centile (*a*), weight-for-height Z-score (*b*) and body mass index Z-score (*c*).

weight centile more than three centile channels above the height centile is an indicator of obesity. This is a simple but crude index, which is biased for children who are fairly tall or short for their age (Cole, 1997). Mulligan & Voss (1999) have shown that in obese children, the difference between their weight and height centiles depends on their age and height.

Figure 1.3 compares the index with two alternative indices, weight-for-height and the body mass index centile. In the example, a tall and very heavy child appears only marginally overweight with the weight centile–height centile index (Z-score = 1.9), whereas weight-for-height and BMI rate the child as obese, with a Z-score exceeding 3.

Because of the link between centiles and Z-scores, the centile–centile index is equivalent to the difference between weight Z-score and height Z-score. A better index is weight Z-score *adjusted* for height Z-score, which depends on the correlation between weight and height, typically 0.7 (Cole, 1997). This leads to the index (1.4 × weight Z-score − height Z-score) which has a standard deviation of 1, and is a Z-score of weight-centile-adjusted-for-height-centile. So, the correct way to compare weight and height centiles is to convert them to Z-scores, multiply the weight Z-score by 1.4 and subtract the height Z-score (Cole, 1994). Applying this formula to the example in Fig. 1.3 gives a Z-score of 3.2, agreeing closely with the other two indices.

Generally this form of Z-score is similar to the body mass index Z-score, which is easily obtained by plotting on a body mass index chart. The availability of such charts makes this alternative centile-based approach largely redundant, but it shows the basis of the connection between weight, height and body mass index centiles.

Skinfold thickness

Skinfold thickness measures subcutaneous fat at various sites of the body, most commonly the triceps and subscapular sites. Skinfold thickness is cheap and fairly simple to measure but the need to partially undress may put some subjects off, leading to bias. It is difficult to measure reproducibly, with appreciable inter- and intraobserver variation, particularly if the subject is fat. For this reason, strict quality control is necessary, which increases the overall cost.

Skinfold measurements also predict total and percentage body fat (Parizkova, 1961; Rolland-Cachera, 1993). In children, the triceps skinfold correlates more highly than the subscapular with per cent body fat, while the reverse is true for total body fat (Roche et al., 1981). Body fatness can be predicted from regression equations based on skinfolds, for example those first established for adults and adapted for children (Lohman, 1986). However, they are population specific and may not apply to all individuals, especially those with abnormal growth.

Body fat distribution can be assessed by comparing trunk (e.g. subscapular) and extremity (e.g. triceps) skinfolds. The relationship between skinfolds and intra-abdominal fat as assessed by DEXA has been examined in children by Goran et al. (1998). Skinfolds, particularly trunk skinfolds, are better predictors of intra-abdominal fat than the ratio of trunk and extremity skinfolds. Similarly, trunk skinfold is better than the trunk/extremity skinfold ratio for predicting cardiovascular risk factors in adolescence (Sangi & Mueller, 1991). Body fat distribution is known to relate to future health in adults, but it has not yet been established in children and needs to be treated with caution.

Centile charts for triceps and subscapular skinfold have been published for several countries including Britain, France and the USA (Tanner & Whitehouse, 1975; Sempé et al., 1979; Must et al., 1991), though the British charts are now outdated (Savage et al., 1999). The age trend in subscapular skinfold thickness is similar to that for the body mass index, with its rise, fall and second rise, and this is another argument in favour of the body mass index over alternative weight–height indices.

There are currently no growth charts for skinfold ratios. The large measurement error of skinfold thickness is compounded in skinfold ratios, which substantially reduces their predictive power.

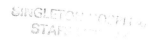

Circumferences and diameters

Circumferences are simple and cheap to measure, and with suitable training are adequately reproducible. Mid-upper arm circumference is widely used to monitor underweight in preschool children, either alone or adjusted for height (Briend & Zimicki, 1986). It may also be a useful proxy for fatness during later childhood, although its value could lie in measuring changes in muscle as much as fat.

Formulae based on mid-upper arm circumference and arm skinfolds were developed by Gurney and Jelliffe (1973), who calculated arm areas assuming the arm and its constituents to be cylindrical. Arm fat areas are no better than the corresponding skinfolds for estimating percentage body fat, but they are better for estimating body fat mass (Himes et al., 1980). The advantage of arm areas is that they assess both lean and fat compartments. The formula used tends to underestimate the amount of fat (Forbes et al., 1988), but an improved formula has been developed (Rolland-Cachera et al., 1997).

Only relatively recently have circumferences at the waist, hip and thigh been used to predict body fat distribution in children (Weststrate et al., 1989; Rolland-Cachera, 1993). Both waist and hip circumference are good predictors of intra-abdominal fat (Goran et al., 1998), which may explain why the waist/hip circumference ratio predicts intra-abdominal fat only poorly. Waist and hip circumferences are also better than their ratio at predicting cardiovascular risk factors (Sangi & Mueller, 1991). The trunk/extremity skinfold ratio correlates better than the waist/hip ratio with cardiovascular risk factors (Freedman et al., 1987; Sangi & Mueller, 1991) and the insulin response to a glucose load (Caprio et al., 1996). Abdominal skinfolds and waist circumference are better than BMI for predicting intra-abdominal fat (Goran et al., 1998).

Working with circumference ratios can mask the fact that either circumference on its own, or their average, is more predictive than the ratio. For this reason, circumferences should always be analysed as separate entities to start with, and should only be combined as ratios subsequently. Circumferences have the advantage over skinfolds of a smaller measurement error, and the same is true for circumference ratios compared to skinfold ratios (Mueller & Kaplowitz, 1994).

Diameters are sometimes used instead of circumferences when somatotype photographs are available (Casey et al., 1994), or when measurement with an anthropometer is felt to be more convenient than with a tape. In terms of acceptability, photographs are likely to be less acceptable than anthropometer or tape.

Centile charts for arm and head circumference have existed for many years, but so far there are few waist or hip circumference charts (e.g. Zannolli & Morgese, 1996).

Summary

Anthropometry is by far the cheapest way to assess adiposity clinically and for large-scale screening anthropometry is essential. The main contenders are the body mass index and selected skinfolds. Body mass index is more acceptable and reproducible than skinfolds, but its correlation with body fat is weaker. In addition, to assess body fat distribution two or more skinfolds or possibly body circumferences are required. Suitable charts exist for body mass index, but those for skinfolds are mainly out-of-date and there are few charts for waist or hip circumference.

1.4 Adiposity as proxy for later adiposity, morbidity and mortality

1.4.1 Tracking

Many studies have examined the persistence (tracking) of adiposity from childhood to adulthood, and the literature has recently been reviewed (Parsons et al., 1999). The magnitude of tracking is important when considering treatment or prevention strategies. The chance of childhood obesity persisting into adulthood depends on the measure of adiposity used, the cut-off used to define obesity and the age of initial assessment. However, it is a consistent finding that fatter children are more likely than thin children to be obese later in life (Power et al., 1997).

There is relatively low tracking from early childhood to adulthood, while fat adolescents have a high risk of obesity as adults (Rolland-Cachera et al., 1987; Whitaker et al., 1997). BMI tracks more strongly than skinfolds (Rolland-Cachera et al., 1989; Clarke & Lauer, 1993; Gasser et al., 1995), and waist/hip ratio tracks more than skinfolds though less than BMI (Casey et al., 1994).

The point of minimal BMI on the centile chart at about age 6 years (see Fig. 1.2) is known as the adiposity rebound (Rolland-Cachera et al., 1984). As a rule, age at adiposity rebound (when the BMI begins to rise again from the minimal level) predicts adult BMI (Rolland-Cachera et al., 1987; Siervogel et al., 1989; Prokopec & Bellisle, 1993; Whitaker et al., 1998) but it is probably not as good a predictor as the child's BMI at that age (Gasser et al., 1995).

Overall, prediction of adult obesity from child adiposity is only moderate.

1.4.2 Morbidity and mortality

It is important to know if adiposity is associated with current and future morbidity and mortality. There have been several studies relating weight–height indices to subsequent mortality in children (Cole, 1991) but only one has tested whether or not the index used was optimal. The weight/height^p index was used to assess the risk of death in a group of malnourished children (Prudhon et al., 1995). The optimal height power p was found to be close to 2, that is BMI, and the BMI was a better predictor of early death than the weight-for-height Z-score.

Relatively few data are available relating BMI to morbidity and mortality in children and adolescents, but associations have been found between BMI or change in BMI, and increased blood pressure, adverse lipoprotein profile, non-insulin-dependent diabetes mellitus and early atherosclerosis lesions (Dietz & Robinson, 1998). Two follow-up studies have examined the association between child BMI and adult outcome. In the Harvard Growth Study, overweight girls and boys had an increased risk of later obesity-associated morbidity as compared to their lean adolescent peers (Must et al., 1992). In another study based on the Boyd Orr cohort, subjects who as children were above the 75th centile for BMI had a higher risk of ischaemic heart disease mortality than those whose BMI as a child was between the 25th and 49th centiles (Gunnell et al., 1998). The study also found that those who were underweight in childhood had a higher all-cause mortality rate than those of average weight. This is consistent with the increased mortality in adults associated with both low and high BMI (Seltzer & Mayer, 1966).

1.5 Definition of childhood obesity

1.5.1 Associated outcome measure

Criteria for overweight or obesity are levels of adiposity exceeding some prespecified cut-off. Ideally, such cut-offs should be based on an outcome measure for which obesity is a risk factor, such as current morbidity, later morbidity or later mortality.

Whichever outcome measure is used, the strength of its association with child or adolescent obesity should be used to set the cut-off. Unfortunately, such a point cannot be identified with any precision, for three reasons: (a) children have less obesity-related disease than adults, (b) the link between child obesity and adult health risk is mediated through adult obesity, which is associated with both child obesity and adult disease, and (c) the dose–response curve linking obesity and outcome is essentially linear over a broad spectrum of adiposity, so that no obvious cut-off point exists. This makes the setting of a cut-off essentially arbitrary.

Anthropometry is used not only at the individual level, as a clinical screening aid, but also at the population level to assess the health of groups. As a screening aid the assessment of obesity should be sensitive and specific (Himes & Bouchard, 1989; Robinson, 1993), while as a public-health tool it should detect differences between groups concurrently or over time. In the epidemiological situation there is less need for a cut-off, since the degree of obesity can be handled satisfactorily as a continuously varying quantity (Flegal, 1993). This reflects the nature of the association between fatness and later outcome. However, even in the public-health context a cut-off is important for classification purposes.

1.5.2 Defining the cut-off

In adults, a cut-off of 25 kg/m^2 for body mass index is used to define overweight, and 30 kg/m^2 is the cut-off for obesity (Garrow & Webster, 1985). If a fixed cut-off like this were applied to children it would screen in different proportions of children at different ages, and differences in maturation would complicate the issue further. This is apparent from the shape of the body mass index chart (Fig. 1.2). Artificial age trends in the pick-up rate need to be avoided, particularly when they reflect physiological rather than pathological differences. For this reason an age-related cut-off is essential.

The body mass index centile chart can be used to provide the cut-off, but it introduces the difficulty of deciding which chart to use. Which reference population is appropriate to act as the 'gold standard' for obesity? There are two relevant criteria, medical and political. Should the reference population be chosen on the basis of its health (e.g. because the data were collected before the current obesity epidemic started) or because it is in some sense internationally representative? Or both? Such considerations rule out most available samples, though Cole & Roede (1999) have argued that their charts of body mass index for Dutch children in 1980 predate the rise in obesity. Even so, the Dutch 1980 charts are not internationally representative in any sense, which probably rules them out. Section 1.5.4 describes an alternative way of identifying the reference population.

Once a suitable chart has been identified, the simplest choice of cut-off is some fixed percentage, say 120% of the median. However, this, like a fixed cut-off, screens in different proportions of the population at different ages, unless the coefficient of variation of body mass index is constant over age, which, in general, it is not (Cole et al., 1998).

The other alternative is some predetermined age–sex centile of the measurement, say the 85th centile for body mass index or triceps skinfold (Must et al., 1991). Alternatively, Himes & Dietz (1994) have proposed the 95th centile body mass index to define obesity and the 85th centile for overweight. In Britain, other body mass index centiles are available (Cole et al., 1995), for example the 91st, 98th and 99.6th, which are based on centiles spaced two-thirds of a Z-score apart, and correspond to Z-scores of $+1.33$, $+2$ and $+2.67$, respectively (see Fig. 1.2).

The provision of a cut-off based on a centile defines what resources are required to treat all the subjects who exceed the cut-off. For example, the 85th centile implies that 15% of the population need treatment. Conversely if the cut-off is raised to the 98th centile this reduces the prevalence of obesity to 2%, less by a factor of 7. At the same time, if obesity (as assessed by these two definitions) is related to later outcome, the risk is likely to appear greater using the more extreme definition. So the choice of cut-off defines both the prevalence of obesity and also the strength of its association with later outcome.

It is important to emphasize that using a centile as cut-off sets the prevalence of obesity, at all ages in both sexes, to the proportion of the reference population above the chosen centile, that is 15% for the 85th centile. The *true* level of obesity is very unlikely to be independent of age and sex, but in the absence of a 'gold standard' to assess it, this unsatisfactory statistical assumption has to be made.

Even the choice of the 85th or the 95th or 91st or 99.6th centile is entirely arbitrary. There is no objective criterion available to decide which centile to use, and this is a further fundamental problem with the definition of child obesity. Section 1.5.4 shows how the cut-off can be defined by linking it to a widely accepted cut-off used for adults.

At a time when the prevalence of obesity is increasing steeply in adults (Gulliford et al., 1992; Bennett et al., 1995) and children (Troiano et al., 1995), it may be counterproductive to update centile charts for body mass index and skinfolds on a regular basis. If they were to be updated regularly, as for height and weight (Freeman et al., 1995), the prevalence of obesity would not appear to change at all. A better strategy is to 'freeze' the charts at a particular moment in time, and then use them to quantify subsequent changes in obesity prevalence over time.

1.5.3 WHO definition

For international use in children, WHO (1995) recommends that overweight be expressed as weight-for-age or weight-for-height greater than $+2$ Z-scores based on the National Center for Health Statistics (NCHS)/WHO reference. For adolescents, the recommended anthropometric indices are BMI, triceps and subscapular skinfold adjusted for age, and WHO (1995) gives reference BMI for 9–24 years and skinfolds for 9–18 years.

There are several practical problems with these definitions. First, the NCHS/WHO reference is old and has technical problems in infancy; second, the weight-for-height, BMI and skinfold reference data are limited in age; third, the reference data are in no sense internationally representative, being based on US children; fourth, the proposed cut-offs have no objective justification.

A separate problem is that BMI and triceps skinfold assess obesity in different ways and can disagree about obesity prevalence. Flegal (1993) described two studies of obesity trends based on the same three national surveys of US adolescents, where the conclusions were diametrically opposed due to the studies using different definitions of obesity, body mass index in one and triceps skinfold in the other. The proportion of subjects exceeding the 85th centile of body mass index

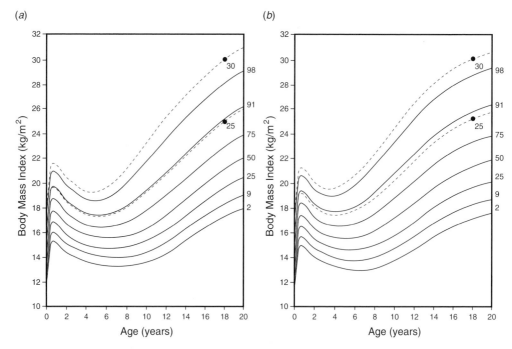

Figure 1.4   The British BMI chart with extra 'centiles' added passing through BMI 25 kg/m² and 30 kg/m² at age 18 years. (*a*) boys, (*b*) girls.

remained fairly constant across the three surveys over time, whereas with the 85th centile for triceps skinfold the proportion increased sharply.

This highlights the arbitrariness of any definition of obesity. Body fat is more closely associated with triceps skinfold than with body mass index, which suggests that in Flegal's example body fat actually increased over time. The lack of a time trend in body mass index may have arisen because the increase in body fat was compensated for by a decrease in muscle mass. This cautionary tale reminds us that body mass index, though correlated with body fat, does not measure it directly.

1.5.4 IOTF definition

There is a broad consensus that BMI is the most suitable adiposity index for children, as supported by the European Childhood Obesity Group (Poskitt, 2000), the NCHS and the WHO (WHO, 1995). However, to provide an acceptable definition of overweight and obesity two further questions remain, the reference population for BMI to be used and the reference BMI centile to act as cut-off.

Recently, the International Obesity TaskForce (IOTF) agreed on a novel approach to answer these questions, using a sample of pooled nationally representative data on BMI from six different countries, and child BMI centiles linked to the

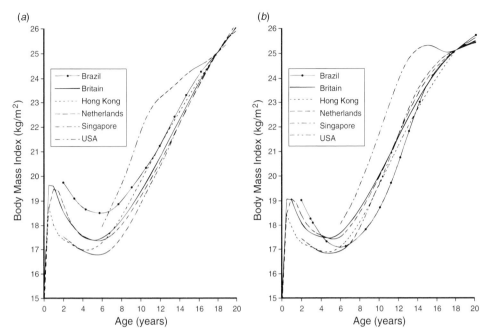

Figure 1.5   National cut-offs for overweight for (a) boys and (b) girls. Centiles passing through BMI 25 kg/m² for data from Brazil, Britain, Hong Kong, the Netherlands, Singapore and the USA.

widely accepted adult BMI cut-offs of 25 kg/m² and 30 kg/m² (Dietz & Robinson, 1998; Cole et al., 2000).

The key to this approach is the statistical analysis known as the LMS method (Cole & Green, 1992). It has been used to construct several of the published BMI centile charts (Rolland-Cachera et al., 1991; Cole et al., 1995; Lindgren et al., 1995; Leung et al., 1998; Cole & Roede, 1999; Kuczmarski et al., 2000). The shapes of the centile curves depend on three underlying curves known as the L, M and S curves (hence the name of the method), and once these curves have been estimated they can be used to draw *any* centile curve. The M curve is the median, the S curve is the coefficient of variation and the L curve is the power transformation needed to bring the data close to Normality. The three curves show how the relevant parameter changes with age.

So it is simple to draw extra 'centile' curves passing through particular values of BMI at particular ages. As an example, Fig. 1.4 shows two extra centile curves drawn to pass through BMI 25 and 30 at age 18 years on the British BMI chart. These points are chosen as they are well accepted as overweight and obesity cut-offs in adults, and the age of 18 years acts as a boundary between child and adult.

The curves for the two sexes passing through BMI 25 are near the British 91st

(a)   (b)

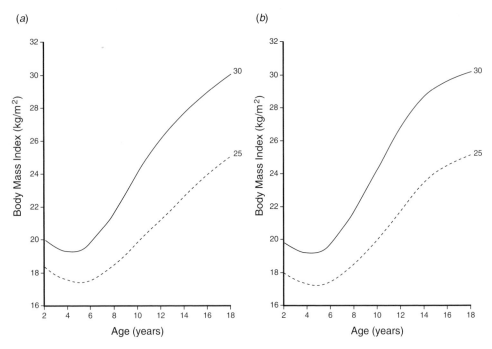

Figure 1.6   IOTF cut-offs for child overweight and obesity for (a) boys and (b) girls, obtained by averaging the national curves passing through BMI 25 kg/m² and 30 kg/m² respectively at age 18 years.

centile, while those crossing BMI 30 are similar to the 99th centile. On the principle that a centile is a consistent cut-off for all ages, these curves represent overweight/obesity in young adults, and by extension throughout childhood as well. Thus we have a child cut-off for overweight which links directly to the corresponding adult cut-off, and the same for obesity.

This principle provides the basis for politically acceptable child overweight and obesity cut-offs, but the British reference in Fig. 1.4 is not suitable for international use. Instead, the reference population was obtained by using data from several countries that are sufficiently homogeneous. Large, nationally representative samples of child BMI data were identified from Brazil, Britain, Hong Kong, the Netherlands, Singapore and the USA, then BMI centiles were fitted to each using the LMS method (Cole et al., 2000). Centile curves passing through BMI 25 and 30 at age 18 years, similar to those in Fig. 1.4, were constructed for each national sample, and the resulting curves were averaged across countries. Figure 1.5 shows the overweight curves for the six countries, and they show reasonable agreement across the age range 2–18 years. By definition the curves all pass through BMI 25 at age 18.

Finally, Fig. 1.6 gives the mean curves by sex for overweight and obesity, averaged across the six countries. Table 1.1 gives the same data in tabular form.

Table 1.1. International body mass index cut-offs for overweight and obesity by sex between 2 and 18 years, defined to pass through body mass index 25 and 30 at age 18 years

Age (years)	Body mass index 25		Body mass index 30	
	Boys	Girls	Boys	Girls
2	18.4	18.0	20.1	19.8
2.5	18.1	17.8	19.8	19.5
3	17.9	17.6	19.6	19.4
3.5	17.7	17.4	19.4	19.2
4	17.6	17.3	19.3	19.1
4.5	17.5	17.2	19.3	19.1
5	17.4	17.1	19.3	19.2
5.5	17.5	17.2	19.5	19.3
6	17.6	17.3	19.8	19.7
6.5	17.7	17.5	20.2	20.1
7	17.9	17.8	20.6	20.5
7.5	18.2	18.0	21.1	21.0
8	18.4	18.3	21.6	21.6
8.5	18.8	18.7	22.2	22.2
9	19.1	19.1	22.8	22.8
9.5	19.5	19.5	23.4	23.5
10	19.8	19.9	24.0	24.1
10.5	20.2	20.3	24.6	24.8
11	20.6	20.7	25.1	25.4
11.5	20.9	21.2	25.6	26.1
12	21.2	21.7	26.0	26.7
12.5	21.6	22.1	26.4	27.2
13	21.9	22.6	26.8	27.8
13.5	22.3	23.0	27.2	28.2
14	22.6	23.3	27.6	28.6
14.5	23.0	23.7	28.0	28.9
15	23.3	23.9	28.3	29.1
15.5	23.6	24.2	28.6	29.3
16	23.9	24.4	28.9	29.4
16.5	24.2	24.5	29.1	29.6
17	24.5	24.7	29.4	29.7
17.5	24.7	24.8	29.7	29.8
18	25	25	30	30

This new approach provides a statistical solution to the joint problems of finding a reference and a cut-off point that are internationally acceptable. It ensures continuity in both measurement and cut-off between child and adult definitions of obesity.

The first results based on the IOTF cut-offs, obesity prevalence and trends in British children over 20 years, have recently been published (Chinn & Rona, 2001). The next few years will show whether the cut-offs are adopted sufficiently widely to unify the definition of child obesity.

1.6 Conclusions

BMI is the optimal single measure for assessing overweight, and the IOTF cut-off for BMI offers an internationally acceptable definition of overweight and obesity. As such it should make interstudy comparisons more valid, and may help identify factors responsible for the recent steep rise in child obesity. However, BMI does not distinguish between body fat and lean body mass, and the correlation of BMI with body fat is weaker than for skinfolds. If body fat distribution is of particular concern then skinfold or circumference data should be collected as well as weight and height, though they are less reliable and adequate reference data are lacking.

1.7 REFERENCES

Ashwell, M., Cole, T.J. & Dixon, A.K. (1985). Obesity: new insight into the anthropometric classification of fat distribution shown by computer tomography. *British Medical Journal,* **290**, 1692–4.

Bennett, N., Dodd, T., Flatley, J., Freeth, S. & Bolling, K. (1995). Obesity and other anthropometric measures. In *The Health of the Nation Survey for England 1993: a survey carried out by the Social Survey Division of OPCS on behalf of the DoH,* ed. Anonymous, pp. 31–43. London: OPCS.

Björntorp, P. (1985). Regional patterns of fat distribution. *Annals of Internal Medicine,* **103**, 994–5.

Briend, A. & Zimicki, S. (1986). Validation of arm circumference as an indicator of risk of death in one to four year old children. *Nutrition Research,* **6**, 249–61.

Cameron, N. (1986). The methods of auxological anthropometry. In *Human Growth: A Comprehensive Treatise,* eds. F. Falkner & J.M. Tanner, pp. 3–46. New York: Plenum Press.

Caprio, S., Hyman, L.D., McCarthy, S., Lange, R., Bronson, M. & Tamborlane, W.V. (1996). Fat distribution and cardiovascular risk factors in obese adolescent girls: importance of intra abdominal fat depots. *American Journal of Clinical Nutrition,* **64**, 2–7.

Casey, V.A., Dwyer, J.T., Berkey, C.S., Bailey, S.M., Coleman, K.A. & Valadian, I. (1994). The distribution of body fat from childhood to adulthood in a longitudinal study population. *Annals of Human Biology,* **21**, 39–55.

Chinn, S. & Rona, R. J. (2001). Prevalence and trends in overweight and obesity in three cross sectional studies of British children, 1974–94. *BMJ*, **322**, 24–6.

Clarke, W.R. & Lauer, R.M. (1993). Does childhood obesity track into adulthood? *Critical Reviews in Food Science and Nutrition*, **33**, 423–30.

Cole, T.J. (1979). A method for assessing age-standardized weight-for-height in children seen cross-sectionally. *Annals of Human Biology*, **6**, 249–68.

Cole, T.J. (1985). A critique of the NCHS weight for height standard. *Human Biology*, **57**, 183–96.

Cole, T.J. (1986). Weight/height^p compared to weight/height^2 for assessing adiposity in childhood: influence of age and bone age on p during puberty. *Annals of Human Biology*, **13**, 433–51.

Cole, T.J. (1991). Weight–stature indices to measure underweight, overweight and obesity. In *Anthropometric Assessment of Nutritional Status*, ed. J.H. Himes, p. 83. New York: Alan R Liss.

Cole, T.J. (1994). A new index of child weight-for-height based on weight and height Z-scores (abstract). *Annals of Human Biology*, **21**, 96.

Cole, T.J. (1997). Growth monitoring with the British 1990 growth reference. *Archives of Disease in Childhood*, **76**, 1–3.

Cole, T.J. & Green, P.J. (1992). Smoothing reference centile curves: the LMS method and penalized likelihood. *Statistics in Medicine*, **11**, 1305–19.

Cole, T.J. & Roede, M.J. (1999). Centiles of body mass index for Dutch children aged 0–20 years in 1980 – a baseline to assess recent trends in obesity. *Annals of Human Biology*, **26**, 303–8.

Cole, T.J., Donnet, M.L. & Stanfield, J.P. (1981). Weight-for-height indices to assess nutritional status – a new index on a slide-rule. *American Journal of Clinical Nutrition*, **34**, 1935–43.

Cole, T.J., Freeman, J.V. & Preece, M.A. (1995). Body mass index reference curves for the UK, 1990. *Archives of Disease in Childhood*, **73**, 25–9.

Cole, T.J., Freeman, J.V. & Preece, M.A. (1998). British 1990 growth reference centiles for weight, height, body mass index and head circumference fitted by maximum penalized likelihood. *Statistics in Medicine*, **17**, 407–29.

Cole, T.J., Bellizzi, M.C., Flegal, K.M. & Dietz, W.H. (2000). Establishing a standard definition for child overweight and obesity: international survey. *British Medical Journal*, **320**, 1240–3.

Daniels, S.R., Khoury, P.R. & Morrison, J.A. (1997). The utility of body mass index as a measure of body fatness in children and adolescents: differences by age, gender. *Pediatrics*, **99**, 804–7.

Davies, P.S.W. & Cole, T.J. (eds.) (1995). *Body Composition Techniques in Health and Disease*. Society for the Study of Human Biology Symposium 36. Cambridge: Cambridge University Press.

de Onis, M. & Habicht, J.P. (1996). Anthropometric reference data for international use: recommendations from a World Health Organisation expert committee. *American Journal of Clinical Nutrition*, **64**, 650–8.

Dibley, M.J., Goldsby, J.B., Staehling, N.W. & Trowbridge, F.L. (1987). Development of normalized curves for the international growth reference: historical and technical considerations. *American Journal of Clinical Nutrition*, **46**, 736–48.

Dietz, W.H. & Robinson, T.N. (1998). Use of the body mass index (BMI) as a measure of overweight in children and adolescents. *Journal of Pediatrics*, **132**, 191–3.

Flegal, K.M. (1993). Defining obesity in children and adolescents: epidemiologic approaches. *Critical Reviews in Food Science and Nutrition*, **33**, 307–12.

Forbes, G.B., Brown, M.R. & Griffiths, H.J.L. (1988). Arm muscle plus bone area: anthropometry and CAT scan compared. *American Journal of Clinical Nutrition*, **47**, 929–31.

Freedman, D.S., Srinivasan, S.R., Burke, G.L., Shear, C.L., Smoak, C.G., Harsha, D.W., Webber, L.S. & Berenson, G.S. (1987). Relation of body fat distribution to hyperinsulinemia in children and adolescents: the Bogalusa heart study. *American Journal of Clinical Nutrition*, **46**, 403–10.

Freeman, J.V., Cole, T.J., Chinn, S., Jones, P.R.M., White, E.M. & Preece, M.A. (1995). Cross sectional stature and weight reference curves for the UK, 1990. *Archives of Disease in Childhood*, **73**, 17–24.

Garrow, J.S. & Webster, J. (1985). Quetelet's index (W/H^2) as a measure of fatness. *International Journal of Obesity*, **9**, 147–53.

Gasser, T., Ziegler, P., Molinari, L., Largo, R.H. & Prader, A. (1995). Prediction of adult skinfolds and body mass from infancy through adolescence. *Annals of Human Biology*, **22**, 217–33.

Gomez, F., Ramos-Galvan, R., Frenk, S., Cravioto, J.M., Chavez, R. & Vasquez, J. (1956). Mortality in second and third degree malnutrition. *Journal of Tropical Paediatrics*, **2**, 77–83.

Goran, M.I., Gower, B.A., Treuth, M. & Nagy, T.R. (1998). Prediction of intra-abdominal and subcutaneous abdominal adipose tissue in healthy pre-pubertal children. *International Journal of Obesity*, **22**, 549–58.

Gulliford, M.C., Rona, R.J. & Chinn, S. (1992). Trends in body mass index in young adults in England and Scotland from 1973 to 1988. *Journal of Epidemiology and Community Health*, **46**, 187–90.

Gunnell, D.J., Frankel, S.J., Nanchahal, K., Peters, T.J. & Davey Smith, G. (1998). Childhood obesity and cardiovascular mortality: a 57-y follow-up study based on the Boyd Orr cohort. *American Journal of Clinical Nutrition*, **67**, 1111–18.

Gurney, J.M. & Jelliffe, D.B. (1973). Arm anthropometry in nutritional assessment: nomogram for rapid calculation of muscle circumference and cross sectional muscle and fat areas. *American Journal of Clinical Nutrition*, **26**, 912–15.

Hammer, L.D., Kraemer, H.C., Wilson, D.M., Ritter, P.L. & Dornbusch, S.M. (1991). Standardized percentile curves of body mass index for children and adolescents. *American Journal of Diseases in Childhood*, **145**, 259–63.

He, Q., Albertsson-Wikland, K. & Karlberg, J. (2000). Population-based body mass index reference values from Göteborg, Sweden: birth to 18 years of age. *Acta Paediatrica*, **89**, 582–92.

Himes, J. & Bouchard, C. (1989). Validity of anthropometry in classifying youths as obese *International Journal of Obesity*, **13**, 183–93.

Himes, J.H. & Dietz, W.H. (1994). Guidelines for overweight in adolescent preventative services: recommendations from an expert committee. *American Journal of Clinical Nutrition*, **59**, 307–16.

Himes, J.H. & Roche, A.F. (1986). Subcutaneous fatness and stature – relationship from infancy to adulthood. *Human Biology*, **58**, 737–50.

Himes, J.H., Roche, A.F. & Webb, P. (1980). Fat areas as estimates of total body fat. *American Journal of Clinical Nutrition*, **33**, 2093–100.

Hughes, J.M., Li, L., Chinn, S. & Rona, R.J. (1997). Trends in growth in England and Scotland, 1972 to 1994. *Archives of Disease in Children*, **76**, 182–9.

Hulse, J.A. & Schilg, S. (1996). Monitoring children's growth (letter). *British Medical Journal*, **312**, 122.

Jebb, S.A., Cole, T.J., Doman, D., Murgatroyd, P.R. & Prentice, A.M. (2000). Evaluation of the novel Tanita body-fat analyser to measure body composition by comparison with a four-compartment model. *British Journal of Nutrition*, **83**, 115–22.

Knittle, J.L., Timmers, K., Ginsberg-Fellner, F., Brown, R.E. & Katz, D.P. (1979). The growth of adipose tissue in children and adolescents. Cross sectional and longitudinal studies of adipose cell number and size. *Journal of Clinical Investigation*, **63**, 239–46.

Kuczmarski, R.J., Ogden, C.L., Grummer-Strawn, L.M., Flegal, K.M., Guo, S.S., Wei, R., Mei, Z., Curtin, L.R., Roche, A.F. & Johnson, C.L. (2000). *CDC Growth Charts: United States.* Hyattsville, Maryland: National Center for Health Statistics. Advance data from Vital and Health Statistics: no. 314.

Lazarus, R., Baur, L., Webb, K. & Blyth, F. (1996). Adiposity and body mass indices in children: Benn's index and other weight for height indices as measures of relative adiposity. *International Journal of Obesity*, **20**, 406–12.

Leung, S.S.F., Cole, T.J., Tse, L.Y. & Lau, J.T.F. (1998). Body mass index reference curves for Chinese children. *Annals of Human Biology*, **25**, 169–74.

Lindgren, G., Strandell, A., Cole, T.J., Healy, M.J.R. & Tanner, J.M. (1995). Swedish population reference standards for height, weight and body mass index attained at 6 to 16 years (girls) or 19 years (boys). *Acta Paediatrica*, **84**, 1019–28.

Lohman, T.G. (1986). The applicability of body composition techniques and constants for children and youths. *Exercise Sports Science Review*, **14**, 325–7.

Mueller, W.H. & Kaplowitz, H.J. (1994). The precision of anthropometric assessment of body fat distribution in children. *Annals of Human Biology*, **21**, 267–74.

Mulligan, J. & Voss, L.D. (1999). Identifying very fat and very thin children: test of criterion standards for screening test. *British Medical Journal*, **319**, 1103–4.

Must, A., Dallal, G.E. & Dietz, W.H. (1991). Reference data for obesity: 85th and 95th percentiles of body mass index (wt/ht^2) and triceps skinfold thickness. *American Journal of Clinical Nutrition*, **53**, 839–46.

Must, A., Jacques, P.F., Dallal, G.E., Bajema, C.J. & Dietz, W.H. (1992). Long-term morbidity and mortality of overweight adolescents: a follow-up of the Harvard Growth Study of 1922 to 1935. *New England Journal of Medicine*, **327**, 1350–5.

O'Dea, J. & Abraham, S. (1995). Should body-mass index be used in young adolescents? *Lancet*, **345**, 657.

Oppert, J.M. & Rolland-Cachera, M.F. (1998). Prevalence, évolution dans le temps et conséquences économiques de l'obésité. *Médecine/sciences*, **14**, 939–43.

Parizkova, J. (1961). Total body fat and skinfold thickness in children. *Metabolic and Clinical Experimentation*, **10**, 794–807.

Parsons, T.J., Power, C., Logan, S. & Summerbell, C.D. (1999). Childhood predictors of adult obesity. *International Journal of Obesity*, **23** (Suppl. 8), S1–S107.

Pietrobelli, A., Faith, M.S., Allison, D.B., Gallagher, D., Chiumello, G. & Heymsfield, S.B. (1998). Body mass index as a measure of adiposity among children and adolescents: a validation study. *Journal of Pediatrics*, **132**, 204–10.

Poskitt, E.M.E. (2000). Body mass index and childhood obesity: are we nearing a solution? *Acta Paediatrica*, **89**, 507–9.

Power, C., Lake, J.K. & Cole, T.J. (1997). Measurement and long-term health risks of child and adolescent fatness. *International Journal of Obesity*, **21**, 507–26.

Prokopec, M. & Bellisle, F. (1993). Adiposity of Czech children followed from 1 month of age to adulthood: analysis of individual BMI patterns. *Annals of Human Biology*, **20**, 517–25.

Prudhon, C., Briend, A., Laurier, D., Golden, M.H.N. & Mary J.Y. (1995). Comparison of weight- and height-based indices for assessing the risk of death in severely malnourished children. *American Journal of Epidemiology*, **116**, 116–23.

Robinson, T.N. (1993). Defining obesity in children and adolescents: clinical approaches. *Critical Reviews in Food Science and Nutrition*, **33**, 313–20.

Roche, A.F., Siervogel, R.M., Chumlea, W.B. & Webb, P. (1981). Grading body fatness from limited anthropometric data. *American Journal of Clinical Nutrition*, **34**, 2831–8.

Rolland-Cachera, M.F. (1993). Body composition during adolescence: methods, limitations and determinants. *Hormone Research*, **39** (suppl.), 25–40.

Rolland-Cachera, M.F., Sempé, M., Guilloud-Bataille, M., Patois, E., Pequignot-Guggenbuhl, F. & Fautrad, V. (1982). Adiposity indices in children. *American Journal of Clinical Nutrition*, **36**, 178–84.

Rolland-Cachera, M.F., Deheeger, M., Bellisle, F., Sempé, M., Guilloud-Bataille, M. & Patois, E. (1984). Adiposity rebound in children: a simple indicator for predicting obesity. *American Journal of Clinical Nutrition*, **39**, 129–35.

Rolland-Cachera, M.F., Deheeger, M., Guilloud-Bataille, M., Avons, P., Patois, E. & Sempé, M. (1987). Tracking the development of adiposity from one month of age to adulthood. *Annals of Human Biology*, **14**, 219–29.

Rolland-Cachera, M.F., Bellisle, F. & Sempé, M. (1989). The prediction in boys and girls of the weight/height^2 index and various skinfold measurements in adults: a two decade follow-up study. *International Journal of Obesity*, **13**, 305–11.

Rolland-Cachera, M.F., Cole, T.J., Sempé, M., Tichet, J., Rossignol, C. & Charraud, A. (1991). Body mass index variations – centiles from birth to 87 years. *European Journal of Clinical Nutrition*, **45**, 13–21.

Rolland-Cachera, M.F., Brambilla, P., Manzoni, P., Akrout, M., Del Maschio, A. & Chiumello, G. (1997). A new anthropometric index, validated by Magnetic Resonance Imaging (MRI), to assess body composition. *American Journal of Clinical Nutrition*, **65**, 1709–13.

Sangi, H. & Mueller, W.H. (1991). Which measure of body fat distribution is best for epidemiologic research among adolescents? *American Journal of Epidemiology*, **133**, 870–83.

Savage, S.A.H., Reilly, J.J., Edwards, C.A. & Durnin, J.V.G.A. (1999). Adequacy of standards for assessment of growth and nutritional status in infancy and early childhood. *Archives of Disease in Childhood*, **80**, 121–4.

Seltzer, C.C. & Mayer, J. (1966). Some re-evaluations of the build and blood pressure study 1959 as related to ponderal index, somatotype and mortality. *New England Journal of Medicine*, **274**, 254–9.

Sempé, M., Pédron, G. & Roy-Pernot, M.P. (1979). *Auxologie*. Paris: Théraplix.

Siervogel, R.M., Roche, A.F., Guo, S., Mukherjee, D. & Chumlea, W.C. (1989). Patterns of change in weight/stature from 2 to 18 years: findings from long-term serial data for children in the Fels longitudinal growth study. *International Journal of Obesity*, **15**, 479–85.

Tanner, J.M. & Whitehouse, R.H. (1975). Revised standards for triceps and subscapular skinfolds in British children. *Archives of Disease in Childhood*, **50**, 142–5.

Troiano, R.P., Flegal, K.M., Kuczmarski, R.J., Campbell, S.M. & Johnson, C.L. (1995). Overweight prevalence and trends for children and adolescents. *Archives of Pediatric and Adolescent Medicine*, **149**, 1085–91.

Vague, J. (1956). The degree of masculine differentiation of obesities: a factor determining predisposition to diabetes, atherosclerosis, gout, and uric calculus disease. *American Journal of Nutrition*, **4**, 20–34.

Waterlow, J.C. (1972). Classification and definition of protein-calorie malnutrition. *British Medical Journal*, **3**, 566–9.

Weststrate, J.A., Deurenberg, P. & van Tintern, H. (1989). Indices of body fat distribution and adiposity in Dutch children from birth to 18 years of age. *International Journal of Obesity*, **13**, 465–77.

Whitaker, R.C., Wright, J.A., Pepe, M.S., Seidel, K.D. & Dietz, W.H. (1997). Predicting obesity in young adulthood from childhood and parental obesity. *New England Journal of Medicine*, **337**, 869–73.

Whitaker, R.C., Pepe, M.S., Wright, J.A., Seidel, K.D. & Dietz, W.H. (1998). Early adiposity rebound and the risk of adult obesity. *Pediatrics*, **101**, e5.

WHO (1995). Physical status: the use and interpretation of anthropometry. Report of a WHO Expert Committee. (Technical report series, No 854), 452p. Geneva: World Health Organization.

Zannolli, R. & Morgese, G. (1996). Waist percentiles: a simple test for atherogenic disease? *Acta Paediatrica*, **85**, 1368–9.

Epidemiology

Michèle Guillaume[1] and Inge Lissau[2]

[1]Department of Preventive Medicine, Province of Luxembourg. [2]Senior Researcher, National Institute of Public Health, Copenhagen

2.1 Introduction

The epidemiology of obesity is concerned with the frequency, distribution and determinants of obesity in populations. Although it includes studies of the association of obesity in childhood with obesity in adult life, with heart disease and diabetes, and with the prevention of obesity, these aspects of epidemiology are discussed extensively in Chapters 6, 8 and 12 and are not discussed further here.

Epidemiological data aid understanding of the complex natural history of obesity in childhood and adolescence, providing information on general patterns of obesity, geographic, ethnic and social class differences and differences in prevalence over time. Epidemiological studies may help predict the likelihood of obesity persisting into adulthood and the consequent risks for morbidity and mortality. Populations at high risk of obesity can then be identified – something which could be of major interest in the development of prevention programmes.

This chapter discusses the current prevalence of obesity world-wide; how fatness is associated with ethnicity, socioeconomic group, and school performance; what can be learnt from trends in obesity over time and across geographic areas; and whether it is possible to identify groups at higher risk of obesity or at risk of persistent obesity.

2.2 Epidemiology and methods

2.2.1 Definition

The advantages and disadvantages of relative body mass index (BMI) for the diagnosis of overweight and obesity and the choices for reference populations and cut-off points have been reviewed in Chapter 1. Standardization of methodology, cut-off points and reference populations is important to determine the prevalence of obesity in children and adolescents world-wide and to facilitate analysis of secular trends in disease pattern and prevalence internationally.

Table 2.1. Methodological differences in prevalence studies of overweight and obesity

Definition of overweight/obesity
    Criteria
    Cut-off points
    Reference populations

Selection of children
    Random
    Not random

Representativeness
    Local
    National

Population studied
    Sample size
    Age group
    Sex

Year of the study

2.2.2 Current practice

Table 2.1 illustrates the variety of methods for assessing and defining obesity (cut-off points, use of reference tables), the varied selection of children (random, not random), and the representativeness (region, nationality) of sample size, age-group, and sex (Lissau, 1997).

Guillaume (1999) has reviewed data from 26 countries in order to evaluate methods, cut-off points and reference materials used in defining obesity in childhood and adolescence. She concluded that three elements were required to define obesity:

- a method of measuring adiposity;
- a reference population;
- cut-off points above which individuals would be considered as overweight or obese.

What is done in practice?

The information now available suggests that the obesity index used most frequently, particularly in Europe, is the BMI. Prior to 1990, BMI was used less frequently (Frelut et al., 1995). The European Childhood Obesity Group (ECOG) has helped to accomplish these changes (Poskitt, 1995). However, weight-for-height and weight/ideal weight are also still used. A few studies report the use of skinfold measurements and weight/height[3]. On the American continent, several indices have been used in national surveys of obesity, reflecting a lack of consensus in methodology. In Latin America and Asia, weight-for-height is often used, although BMI is recorded in Japan. Cut-off points for overweight and obesity vary between countries. When BMI is used, selected cut-off points vary from above the 85th to above the 97th centile. Nomenclature also varies. Above the 97th centile BMI is *obesity* in the Netherlands (Spee van der Wekke et al., 1994; Brugman et al., 1995) and *super-obesity* in France (Rolland-Cachera et al., 1987). For weight/ideal weight and skinfold measurements, a cut-off limit for obesity at greater than 120% of 'mean', 'average' or 'expected' values is often used.

The reference populations used in different studies also vary widely. Many countries compile their own reference data and rely on these local references. In other countries, American (Must et al., 1991), British (Cole et al., 1995) and French (Rolland-Cachera et al., 1987) references as well as the Tanner standards (Tanner et al., 1966a,b) have been used. Little information has been provided on sample size, sample selection, representation or refusal rates in these studies. Yet, even small differences between reference populations or in cut-off points may produce widely different estimates of the prevalence of obesity when applied to various populations. Using different criteria for definition of obesity exacerbates these differences. For example, the 85th centile at different ages from Australia (Lazarus et al., 1995) and the US (Must et al., 1991) overlap whereas British data (Cole et al., 1995) are slightly lower. Such apparently small differences may be important. When data from six countries were analysed using the 85th BMI centile for the US (Must et al., 1991) and Britain (Cole et al., 1995), the youngest children (6–8 years) with the British reference had 0–4% lower prevalence than with the US reference. From 9 years on, the differences reversed with 3–13% higher obesity prevalence using the British instead of the US reference. These differences increased with age (Guillaume, 1999).

Discrepancies in the prevalence of obesity may be even greater if different indices are used. The prevalence of obesity more than doubled in Argentina when the 85th BMI centile of the US (Must et al., 1991) was used instead of greater than 120% weight-for-height of a local reference population (Carmuega et al., 1996).

The data presented here are far from complete, and represent only the responses to a limited inquiry. However, they make it clear that international comparisons of the prevalence of childhood obesity are currently of limited value. International consensus on definition is needed. Cole et al. (2000) have proposed age-specific definitions for overweight and obesity in children by determining age related BMI values equivalent to BMI centiles achieving greater than $25 \, \text{kg/m}^2$ and BMI greater than $30 \, \text{kg/m}^2$ in 18-year-olds (definitions for adult overweight and obesity respectively) (see Chapter 1).

Table 2.2. Mean BMI (kg/m^2) in children and adolescents in several European countries

Country and year of study	6 years		9 years		12 years		15 years	
	Boys	Girls	Boys	Girls	Boys	Girls	Boys	Girls
Finland 1980 (Dahlstrom et al., 1985)	15.6	16.6	16.6	16.5	17.9	18.4	19.9	20.1
Greece 1982 (Mamalakis & Kafatos, 1996)	17.1	17.1	17.8	17.5	18.5	20.4	20.2	22.4
Italy – Verona 1987 (Pinelli et al., 1987)	16.2	16.1	17.5	17.3	18.9	19.2	20.7	21.2
Czech Republic 1990 (Blaha, 1991)	15.4	15.3	16.2	16.1	17.7	17.6	19.8	19.9
Middle Italy 1991 (Zannolli & Morgese, unpublished data)	16.2	16.7	18.5	17.8	19.7	20.1	—	—
Belgium 1992 (Guillaume et al., 1996)	16.0	16.0	17.0	17.0	18.0	18.0	—	—

Table 2.3. Prevalence (%) of obesity in children and adolescents

Region	Country and reference	Year	Definition	Age range (years)	Prevalence (%)		
					Boys	Both sexes	Girls
Europe	Hungary	1993–94	BMI ⩾ 90th centile Local reference	6–18		13.2	
	Netherlands (Brugman et al., 1995)	1993–94	BMI ⩾ 97th centile French reference	4–13		10.0	
	UK		BMI ⩾ 85th centile English reference	6–8		15.0	
				9–11		15.1	
				12–14		13.2	
				15–18		13.6	
	Belgium – Brussels (De Spiegelaere et al., 1998a)	1990	BMI ⩾ 120% median BMI ⩾ 140% median French reference	12	20 5		19 5
	France (Rolland-Cachera et al., 1992)	1990	BMI ⩾ 90th centile French reference	4–17		14.9	
	Italy – North-East (Maffeis et al., 1993)	1992	Weight for height > 120% Tanner reference	7–8	10		
				9–11	18		
				11–13	17		
Americas	USA NHANES III (Troiano & Flegal, 1998)	1988/94	BMI > 85th centile US reference	6–11 (white)	11.2		9.1
				12–17 (white)	12.2		9.4
	Argentina (Carmuega et al., 1996)	1995	BMI > 85th centile US reference	Schoolchildren		33	
				Adolescents		21	

Asia	Japan (Kotani, 1997)	1993	SBW 120%	6–14	12
	Singapore (Rajan, 1994)	1995	Weight-for-height > 120% Local reference	6–16	12.1
	Thailand (Mo-Suwan & Geater, 1996)	1991/92	Weight-for-height > 120% 110–120% Bangkok reference	6–13	14.1 11.6
Middle East	Saudi Arabia (Al-Nuaim et al., 1996)	1994/95	BMI 110–120% NCHS reference	6 9 12 15	15.2 11.4 12.2 11.9

2.3 The scale of the problem

Current data on the prevalence of obesity in children and adolescents should be interpreted cautiously for the reasons outlined above. Frelut et al. (1995) reviewed the literature within Europe and found prevalence rates which varied from 0.5% in The Netherlands to 21% in Berlin. Nevertheless, all methods used to classify obesity report increasing prevalences.

2.3.1 Current prevalence

In Europe, only the Netherlands has specific, nationally representative, surveys where children's heights and weights are measured at regular intervals and which are comparable to the USA's successive National Health and Nutrition Examination Surveys (NHANES) which have illustrated the prevalence and secular trends for obesity in US youth since 1960. Table 2.2 summarizes European data on mean BMI at different ages for boys and girls. The BMIs are similar for boys and girls before the age of 12 years. After that age, values are higher for girls. Italian and Greek children have higher BMIs than other cohorts for whom national differences are not very marked. Table 2.2 also illustrates the North–South gradient in BMI for both sexes in all age-groups. The increasing trend from North to South is well recognized in adult surveys. US values are in the middle.

Table 2.3 summarizes data available on prevalence recorded as percentage of obesity in different local or national populations. The variety of methods used to obtain the data makes valid comparison difficult. In France (Lorraine), overweight and obesity, defined as BMI above the 90th centile of the French standard, was 14.9% of 4- to 17-year-old children and adolescents in 1990 (Rolland-Cachera et al., 1992). In Italy, prevalence assessed in several different areas was usually greater than 11%, with more than 20% obesity in boys aged 10 years in the North East (Maffeis et al., 1993). In Singapore, 12–13% of schoolchildren and 10.7% of adolescents were diagnosed as obese in comparison with a local reference population (Rajan, 1994). Japan had 12% obesity in 6- to 14-year age-groups (Kotani, 1997). In the USA, 13.8% of 6- to 8-year-old white boys, 17% of 9- to 11-year-olds and 17.9% of 12- to 14-year-olds had BMI over the 85th centile of an American reference population (Troiano & Flegal, 1998). Prevalence fell to 14.5% in the oldest (15- to 18-year) age-group.

Childhood obesity is not confined to industrialized countries. High rates of overweight and obesity are already evident in some developing countries. The prevalence of obesity (weight-for-height > 120% of the Bangkok reference) amongst schoolchildren 6–12 years old in Thailand rose from 12.2% in 1991 to 15.6% in 1993 (Mo-Suwan & Geater, 1996). A recent study of 6- to 18-year-old schoolboys in Saudi Arabia found a prevalence of 15.8% obesity (Al-Nuaim et al., 1996).

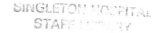

2.3.2 Trends in obesity and overweight prevalence

Whatever method is used to define obesity in children and adolescents, the increasing prevalence seems universal. Table 2.4 depicts trends in changing prevalence reported as obesity or mean BMI values.

In the USA, nationally representative surveys using comparable methods showed significant increases in the prevalence of overweight (Troiano & Flegal, 1998). Data from other US studies confirm these observations. The prevalence of overweight (above the 85th centile of weight-for-height) amongst 5- to 24-year-olds from a biracial community in Louisiana increased approximately two-fold between 1973 and 1994. Furthermore, the yearly increases in relative weight and obesity during the latter part of the study period (1983–94) were approximately 50% greater than those between 1973 and 1982 (Freedman et al., 1997). Similar trends have been observed in Japan (Table 2.5). The frequency of obese schoolchildren (> 120% expected body weight; EBW) aged 6–14 years increased from 5% to 10%, and that of extremely obese children (> 140% EBW) from 1% to 2% in the 20 years from 1974 to 1993. The increase was most prominent in male students aged 9–11 years (Kotani, 1997).

In Belgium, Van Meerbeeck (1988) showed that between 1968 and 1988, the number of young men enrolled into compulsory military service weighing more than 100 kg increased four-fold.

2.3.3 What can we learn from the BMI distribution?

Changes in the prevalence of obesity could reflect either a general increase in fatness of the whole population, or an expression of increased obesity in subgroups of presumably susceptible individuals. Consequently, using the average BMI as a measurement of obesity in a population sample or to evaluate possible changes in the distribution of BMI within the population can be misleading. An increase in mean BMI may be attributable either to a shift in the entire distribution or to an increase in the upper portion of the distribution only. It would be of interest to know, in the data reporting BMI increases, whether the entire population is becoming heavier or whether only heavy individuals are heavier than before, and lighter individuals show little change.

Comparisons of BMI in children from Lorraine in France (Rolland-Cachera et al., 1987), and an adjacent and comparable population from the Luxembourg region of Belgium showed no differences in mean BMI (Guillaume et al., 1995). However, when the distribution of BMI was analysed, the higher centiles of the Belgian population (above the 50th centile) showed considerably higher values than the same sections of the distribution curve for the French children. The pattern was similar in both sexes. The heaviest children in Belgium seemed to be heavier than those in France. However, the differences are probably attributable to

Table 2.4. Secular trends in prevalence (%) of obesity in children and adolescents

Region	Country and reference	Definition	Year	Prevalence by age and sex (%)			
Europe							
	Italy – Pavia (Salvatoni et al., unpublished data)			6–8 years (boys)		10–12 years (boys)	
		IBW > 120%	1977/78	3.5		11	
		Tanner reference	1991/92	18.8		20	
	Italy – Milan (Ceratti et al., 1990)			7–8 years		11–13 years	
		Weight-for-height > 120%	1986	6	16		
		Tanner reference	1990	10	17		
	France-Lorraine (Rolland-Cachera *et al.*, 1992)			4–17 years			
		BMI ≥ 90th centile	1980	12.5			
		French reference	1990	14.9			
	The Netherlands (Brugman et al., 1995, Spee van der Wekke et al., 1994)			4– ⩾ 13 years			
		BMI ⩾ 97th centile	1991/93	8			
		French reference	1993/94	10			
	Finland (Nuutinen et al., 1991)			9–18 years (boys)		9–18 years (girls)	
		BMI > 90th centile	1980	3.6		2.1	
		US reference	1986	4.3		2.6	
	Hungary			6–18 years			
		Triceps > 90th centile	1980	11.8			
		Tanner reference	1990	16.3			

				6–11 years (boys)	6–11 years (girls)	12–17 years (boys)	12–17 years (girls)
USA	NHANES I,II,III (Troiano & Flegal, 1998)	BMI > 85th centile	1971/74	3.8	3.7	5.5	5.8
		US reference	1976/80	6.5	4.9	4.6	4.2
			1988/94	11.2	9.1	12.2	9.4
				18 years (boys)			
South America	Argentina (Carmuega et al., 1996)	BMI 25– < 30	1969	11.8			
			1974	14.4			
			1975	15.4			
				6–14 years (boys)		6–14 years (girls)	
Asia	Japan (Shirai et al., 1990)	EBW > 120%	1979	6.4		7.7	
			1988	9.8		8.8	

Abbreviations: BMI, body mass index; EBW, expected body weight; IBW, ideal body weight.

Table 2.5. Secular trends in the prevalence (%) of obesity/overweight compared to super-obesity/obesity

Country	Definition	Year	Age range (years)	Prevalence (%)	
				Overweight/obesity	Superobesity/obesity
USA	BMI	From 1963/70 to	6–11	> 85th centile	> 95th centile
	US reference	1976/80	12–17	+54%[a]	+98%[a]
				+39%[a]	+64%[a]
France	BMI	1980	4–17	> 90th centile	> 97th centile
	French reference	1990		10.0	2.5
				11.7	3.2
Hungary	Skinfolds	1980	6–18	> 120%	> 140%
	Tanner reference	1990		11.8	3.4
				16.3	5.9
Japan	EBW	1974	6–14	> 120%	> 140%
		1993		5	1
				10	2

Abbreviations: BMI, body mass index; EBW, expected body weight.

[a]USA data indicate changes in prevalance, not actual values.

the secular trends reported everywhere, since the French study was performed 10 years earlier than the Belgian one.

The BMI distribution has also been compared across US national studies. No differences were observed between surveys at the lower BMI centiles but increasing differences were observed at the higher centiles in both sexes (Troiano & Flegal, 1998). These findings suggest that the increased obesity relates mainly to already overweight children and adolescents who are becoming heavier with time. Other comparisons of secular trends in the prevalence of obesity and super-obesity support this finding. Table 2.5 shows that in France, USA, Japan and Hungary, prevalences of super-obesity have increased dramatically. For example, French children born 1980–85 show a five-fold increase in massive obesity, compared with only a two-fold increase for moderate obesity.

2.3.4 Risk factors

Several factors have been highlighted as affecting the chance of a child becoming obese.

Heritability

Both genes and environment have an impact on obesity (Sørensen & Lissau, 1991). However, the relative contributions of genes and inherited lifestyle factors to the parent–child fatness association remain largely unknown. A recent systematic review concluded that the offspring of obese parents are consistently at increased risk of fatness, although few studies have followed this relationship from childhood into adult life (Parsons et al., 1999). Parental obesity increases the risk of obesity in the offspring (Garn & Clark, 1976; Poskitt & Cole, 1978; Garn & La Velle, 1985; Maffeis et al., 1994; Whitaker et al., 1997; Sørensen et al., 1998). The heritability of fatness has been studied in family, twin and adoption studies. Adoption studies show that the genetic effect on BMI is fully expressed in childhood (Sørensen et al., 1992) and that children have BMIs closer to those of their biological parents than to those of the parents who raised them (Stunkard et al., 1986). Twin studies suggest a heritability in fat mass and in disorders of energy balance arising from genetic defects. In the last 3 years, five single (and very rare) gene disorders resulting in early onset obesity have been characterized (Farooqi and O'Rahilly, 2000).

In a review, Maes et al. (1997) concluded that genetic factors explain 50–90% of the variation in BMI. Family studies generally report estimates of parent–offspring and sibling–sibling correlations in agreement with heritability of 20–80%. Data from adoption studies suggest genetic factors account for 20–60% of the variation in BMI. Reviewing family studies, Perusse & Bouchard (1999) concluded that the maximal heritability of obesity phenotypes ranges from about 30–50% and that the majority of effects on body fat content, energy intake and energy expenditure are also strongly affected by genetic influences. In addition to all this, there is increasing evidence that the response of the obese to dietary intervention is genetically determined. The genetic environment is undoubtedly important and worthy of considerable interest in the epidemiology of obesity. However, the genetic background to obesity, which is largely outside the scope of interventions, should not overshadow the fact that the epidemic increase in the prevalence of obesity world-wide must relate more to changes in the environment than to changes in human genes.

Socioeconomic status

The prevalence of obesity shows an interesting relationship with social development. In developing societies, where life has been little better than subsistence living until very recently, overweight and obesity in childhood are virtually confined to children from affluent urban families. In westernized societies and societies in transition, obesity – in both adults and children – is usually most prevalent in areas of social deprivation and poverty. Yet it is also children in such situations who are most prone to failure to thrive, stunting and evidence of undernutrition. This conundrum probably indicates the complexity of the social issues contributing to the epidemiology of obesity. In practical terms, it also means that efforts to treat and prevent obesity in these environments must concentrate on programmes for healthy lifestyles which will accommodate problems of both under- and overnutrition, rather than directing attention solely at reducing energy intake.

The reasons for the prevalence of obesity in deprived populations in western society are not clear. Indeed, research does not consistently find this relationship. Thus, whilst an inverse relationship between socioeconomic status and overweight or obesity is frequent for adult women and sometimes adult men, studies in children show weaker and less consistent relationships or even no difference between the sexes (Sobal & Stunkard, 1989). In the USA (Troiano & Flegal, 1998) and in Belgium (Guillaume et al., 1999), there was little evidence for any significant relationship between overweight and the education level of the family reference person. Ethnic origin may alter these associations. Thus, there was a significant influence of family income on overweight white non-Hispanic girls in the USA (Troiano & Flegal, 1998). In a study of 2607 Belgian schoolchildren, obesity increased in prevalence and severity with lower social class in girls but not in boys. Boys and immigrant children of both sexes showed no social-class-related differences in prevalence of obesity (De Spiegelaere et al., 1998a). Reviewing Belgian schoolchildren by 2-yearly school medical examinations between ages 12 and 15 years, De Spiegelaere et al. (1998b) concluded that the association of low social class with obesity was accentuated in early adolescence in girls as a result of both the development of new cases and lower rates of improvement in obesity amongst the more disadvantaged girls.

If it was better understood why obesity was so strongly associated with social deprivation under certain circumstances, it might be easier to design prevention and treatment programmes that could tackle the causes of obesity successfully. Studies from Denmark suggest that it is the physical environment, both at family (Lissau & Sørensen, 1993) and at community level (Lissau & Sørensen, 1992), rather than the level of education or the buying power of the family, which is the determining factor for the development of obesity in young adults (Chapter 6).

School performance

Studies have shown that low school performance and obesity are associated. A prospective study showed that differences in the percentage of overweight among children with average and below average scholastic proficiency, persisted into young adulthood. The odds ratio of being obese (above the 95th BMI centile) was more than two-fold and highly significant at ages 10–11 years when controlling for parental BMI and social background. Children who had received special education at school had a higher prevalence of overweight in childhood and an increased risk of obesity in young adulthood (Lissau & Sørensen, 1993).

A cross-sectional study of black inner-city schoolchildren found that the proportion of obese children receiving special education or in remedial classes was twice that for nonobese children (Tershakovec et al., 1994). Similarly, being overweight or becoming overweight during adolescence (grades 7–9) in Thailand was associated with poor school performance, although there was no such association for younger children in grades 3–6 (Mo-Suwan et al., 1999).

In a study of 26 274 young Danish men, intelligence test scores and educational levels were highest in those with below median BMI and declined steadily with increasing BMI so that at BMI above 32 kg/m^2 both intelligence-test score and educational level were approximately half a standard deviation below average (Teasdale et al., 1992).

Ethnicity

The effect of immigration on obesity has been most extensively studied in North America. These studies indicate that some races are more prone to become obese than others in societies where there is superfluous food. For example, obesity is more common in blacks and Hispanics compared with whites. Asian immigrant groups usually show lower prevalence of fatness. The National Longitudinal Study of Adolescent Health shows significant increases in obesity amongst second and third generation US immigrants. Obesity rates were 24.2% amongst White non-Hispanics; 30.9% amongst black non-Hispanics; and 20.6% amongst Asian-Americans. Chinese (15.3%) and Filipino (18.5%) showed substantially lower percentage prevalence of obesity than non-Hispanic whites. Asian-American and Hispanic adolescents born in the US are more than twice as likely to be obese than first generation residents of the 50 states (Popkin & Udry, 1998). In a study of more than 65 000 US children aged 5–17 years, age-specific mean BMI was noticeably higher in black and Hispanic girls than in white girls. The proportion of children diagnosed as obese using the NHANES I reference was highest for Hispanic boys, and black and Hispanic girls.

Mean BMIs are higher in black and Hispanic children when compared with white children of the same age (Rosner et al., 1998).

First-generation Asian immigrants to Canada also show lower prevalences of obesity compared with children born to Asian immigrant families already in Canada (Pomerleau & Ostbye, 1997).

Prevalence of overweight in adult females is 46% in traditional Western Samoans and 80% in migrants to Hawaii. Five-year longitudinal data show striking gains in weight and fat, especially amongst younger adults and amongst females (McGarvey, 1991).

In France a higher proportion of North African (Maghrebian) immigrant children aged 0–4 years had BMIs above the 97th centile than nonimmigrant children of the same age. Forty six per cent of immigrants born in the 1970s had their adiposity rebound at or before 48 months, whereas 66% of Maghrebian children born in the 1990s had their adiposity rebound at or before this age (Roville-Sausse, 1999).

Amongst children and adolescents attending the outpatient obesity clinic at the University Hospital for Children, Brussels, non-European origin was a major risk factor for obesity (Guillaume & Burniat, 1999). Another Belgian study of 12-year-old children living in Brussels showed that obesity and severe obesity were more prevalent amongst immigrant children than Belgian born children (De Spiegelaere et al., 1998a) (Table 2.6).

These gender and ethnic differences may ultimately guide us to understanding the causes, and thus consequently strategies for the prevention of obesity (Rosner et al., 1998).

Critical periods of growth

Rolland-Cachera (1990) reported that children who have an early adiposity rebound are at higher risk for obesity and persistent obesity. In physiological conditions, fat mass at birth represents 12–15% of the total mass. It increases up to 4–6 months and remains around 21–23% until 1 year of age. Fat mass declines until 5–6 years of age then increases again to reach 11–17% in boys and 23–26% in

Table 2.6. Prevalence (%) of obesity by ethnicity

Country and reference	Year	Definition	Race of Origin		Prevalence (%)
					Both sexes
The Netherlands					
(Brugman et al., 1995)	1993/94	BMI > 97th centile	Netherlands		10
		(French reference)	Turkey/Morocco		19
			Surinam/Antilles		11
			Others		13
				Boys	Girls
Belgium-Brussels					
(De Spiegelaere et al., 1998a)	1990	BMI > 120% median	Belgian immigrants from		
		(French reference)	North Africa/Turkey (74%),	20	19
			Mediterranean region (18%),	24	20
			Others (8%)		

girls by the end of the adolescent growth spurt. Thus the adiposity rebound which starts normally around 6 years of age corresponds to the second phase of increase in fat mass (following the increase in immediate postnatal life). In the obesity clinic at the University Hospital for Children in Brussels, more than 70% of the obese children and adolescents had had an early adiposity rebound (Guillaume & Burniat, 1999).

This period of adiposity rebound is important, but Dietz (1994) has underlined that it is not the only important period for the development of obesity. Macrosomic babies, whether or not they were born to mothers with gestational diabetes, are at four times greater risk of becoming obese than normal-sized new-borns.

Adolescence is another critical period for the development of obesity or of behaviours predisposing to obesity, perhaps because of the significant psychosocial and behavioural changes which take place at this time (Dietz, 1994).

We referred above to studies from Denmark which showed the importance of the rearing environment on obesity in children (Lissau & Sørensen, 1992). Later obesity was much more strongly associated with parental 'neglect' than with parental education or occupation (Lissau & Sørensen, 1994). Preventive programmes need directing towards children from deprived home environments. Further studies are needed to determine the role of psychosocial risk factors in the later development of obesity.

2.4 Conclusions

Studies of the epidemiology of childhood obesity have been hampered in the past by lack of consensus in definition of obesity or overweight.

In adults, the comorbidities of obesity can be used to establish cut-off points. Making a distinction between central and peripheral obesity is useful because of the higher risk with the former (WHO, 1998). However, morbidity occurs less frequently in children than in adults, and the role of body fat distribution has not been thoroughly studied (Fox et al., 1993; Brambilla et al., 1994; Guillaume et al., 1996). One important problem in childhood obesity is the psychological distress, which can result from frequent exclusion of the obese from group activities. Because exclusion (Dietz, 1992; Hill & Silver, 1995; WHO, 1998) as well as metabolic comorbidity (WHO, 1998) follow BMI closely, use of the BMI may be justified when screening a population. However, how well BMI measures body fat mass in children may become a greater problem when different populations are screened and compared.

So far, concerns for childhood obesity have led to numerous studies of the prevalence of childhood obesity in different communities – studies which are not directly comparable. The prevalence of overweight and obesity is increasing rapidly. The most concerning increase is at the upper extreme of the BMI distribution. The risk of obesity persisting into adult life is higher with more severe overweight and obesity (Guo et al., 1994). This risk also seems increased with early adiposity rebound (Rolland-Cachera, 1990), although what early adiposity rebound really signifies has recently been questioned (Dietz, 2000).

In addition to evidence of increasing childhood obesity with increasing prevalence of very severe obesity, there is consistent evidence that childhood obesity is common when there is a history of obesity in the family. The prevalence of obesity varies with age, to some extent with the sex of the child, and with socioeconomic circumstances. Only through consensus over the definition for obesity will it be possible to provide real comparisons between studies of different ethnic groups, ages and environments, and thus hone in on more precise epidemiology.

2.5 REFERENCES

Al-Nuaim, A.R., Bamgboye, E.A. & Al-Herbish, A. (1996). The pattern of growth and obesity in Saudi Arabian male school children. *International Journal of Obesity*, **20**, 1000–5.

Blaha, P. (1991). Body mass index of the current Czechoslovak population between the ages of 3 and 70. Males and Females. Prague: Ed Institute of Sports Medicine.

Brambilla, P., Manzoni, P., Sironi, S., Simone, P., Del Maschio, A., di Natale, B. & Chiumello, G. (1994). Peripheral and abdominal adiposity in childhood obesity. *International Journal of Obesity and Related Metabolic Disorders*, **18**, 795–800.

Brugman, E., Meulmeester, J.F., van der Wekke, J., Beuker, R.J. & Radder, J.J. (1995). Peilingen in jeugdgezondheidszorg: PGO-peiling 1993/1994. (Findings from preventive health studies on children between 1993–1994). *TNO Preventie en Gezondheid*, The Netherlands, report nr 95.061 (in Dutch).

Carmuega, E., O'Donnel, A.M. & Duran, P. (1996). *Project Tierra del Fuego: baseline health and nutrition survey*. Ediciones Fundacion Jorge Macri/CESNI.

Ceratti, F., Garavaglia, M., Piatti, L., Brambilla, P., Rondanini, G.F., Bolla, P., Ghisalberti, C. & Chiumello, G. (1990). Screening dell'obesit nella populazione scolastica della zona 20 di Milano ed intervento di educazione alimentare. *Epidemiologia Preventiva*, **12**, 1–6.

Cole, T.J., Freeman, J.V. & Preece M.A. (1995). Body mass index reference curves for the UK, 1990. *Archives of Disease in Childhood*, **73**, 25–9.

Cole, T.J., Bellizzi, M.C., Flegal, K.M. & Dietz, W.H. (2000). Establishing a standard definition for child overweight and obesity worldwide: international survey. *British Medical Journal*, **320**, 1240–3.

Dahlstrom, S., Viikari, J., Akerblom, H.K., Solakivi-Jaakkola, T., Uhari, M., Dahl, M., Lahde, P.L., Pesonen, E., Pietikainen, M., Suoninen, P. & Louhivuori, K. (1985). Atherosclerosis precursors in Finnish children and adolescents. II. Height, weight, body mass index, and skinfolds, and their correlation to metabolic variables. *Acta Paediatrica Scandinavica*, **Suppl. 318**, 65–78.

De Spiegelaere, M., Dramaix, M. & Hennart, P. (1998a). Social class and obesity in 12-year-old children in Brussels: influence of gender and ethnic origin. *European Journal of Pediatrics*, **157**, 432–5.

De Spiegelaere, M., Dramaix, M. & Hennart, P. (1998b). The influence of socioeconomic status on the incidence and evaluation of obesity during early adolescence. *International Journal of Obesity*, **22**, 268–74.

Dietz, W.H. (1992). Childhood obesity. In *Obesity*, eds. P. Björntorp & B.N. Bodoff, pp. 606–8. Philadelphia: JB Lippincott Co.

Dietz, W.H. (1994). Critical periods in childhood for the development of obesity. *American Journal of Clinical Nutrition*, **59**, 955–9.

Dietz, W.H. (2000). 'Adiposity rebound': reality or epiphenomenon? *Lancet*, **356**, 2027–8.

Farooqi, I.S. & O'Rahilly, S. (2000). Recent advances in the genetics of severe childhood obesity. *Archives of Disease in Childhood*, **83**, 31–4.

Fox, K., Peters, D., Armstrong, N., Sharpe, P. & Bell, M. (1993). Abdominal fat deposition in 11-year-old-children. *International Journal of Obesity*, **17**, 11–16.

Freedman, D.S., Srinavasan, S.R., Valdez, R.A., Williamson, D.F. & Berenson, G.S. (1997). Secular increases in relative weight and adiposity among children over two decades: the Bogalusa Heart Study. *Pediatrics*, **99**, 420–6.

Frelut, M.-L., Cathelineau, L., Bihain, B.-E. & Navarro, J. (1995). Prévalence de l'obésité infantile dans le monde. Quelle évolution? *Médecine et Nutrition*, **31**, 293–7.

Fung, K.P., Lee, J., Lau, S.P., Chow, O.K.W., Wong, T.W. & Davies, D.P. (1990). Properties and clinical implications of body mass indices. *Archives of Disease in Childhood*, **65**, 516–19.

Garn, S.M. & Clark, D.C. (1976). Trends in fatness and the origins of obesity: Ad Hoc Committee to review the Ten-State Nutrition Survey. *Pediatrics*, **57**, 443–56.

Garn, S.M. & La Velle, M. (1985). Two-decade follow-up of fatness in early childhood. *Archives of Disease in Childhood*, **139**, 181–5.

Guillaume, M. (1999). Defining obesity in childhood: current practice. *American Journal of Clinical Nutrition*, **70**, 126S–30S.

Guillaume, M.L. & Burniat, W. (1999). L'excès pondéral et l'obésité chez l'enfant: un réel problème de santé publique. *Revue de la Médecine Générale*, **163**, 213–17.

Guillaume, M.L., Lapidus, L., Beckers, F., Lambert, A.E. & Björntorp, P.A. (1995). Familial trends of obesity through three generations: The Belgian Luxembourg Child Study. *International Journal of Obesity*, **Suppl. 19**, 5–9.

Guillaume, M.L., Lapidus, L., Beckers, F., Lambert, A.E. & Björntorp, P.A. (1996). Cardiovascular risk factors in children from the Belgian Province of Luxembourg. The Belgian Luxembourg child study. *American Journal of Epidemiology*, **144**, 867–80.

Guillaume, M., Lapidus, L., Lambert, A. & Björntorp, P. (1999). Socioeconomic and psychosocial conditions of parents and cardiovascular risk factors in their children: the Belgian Luxembourg Child Study III. *Acta Paediatrica*, **88**, 866–73.

Guo, S., Roche, A., Chumlea, W., Gardner, J. & Siervogel, R. (1994). The predictive value of childhood body mass index values for overweight at age 35 years. *American Journal of Clinical Nutrition*, **59**, 810–19.

Hill, A.J. & Silver, E.K. (1995). Fat, friendless and unhealthy: 9 year old children's perception of body shape stereotypes. *International Journal of Obesity*, **19**, 423–30.

Kotani, K. (1997). Two decades of annual medical examinations in Japanese obese children: do obese children grow into obese adults? *International Journal of Obesity*, **21**, 912–21.

Lazarus, R., Baur, L., Webb, K., Blyth, F. & Gliksman, M. (1995). Recommended body mass index cut off values for overweight screening programmes in Australian children and adolescents: comparisons with North American values. *Journal of Paediatrics and Child Health*, **31**, 143–7.

Lissau, I. (1997). Prevalence of childhood obesity. The need for new data. *International Journal of Obesity*, **21** (**Suppl. 1**), S48.

Lissau, I. & Sørensen, T.I. (1992). Prospective study of the influence of social factors in childhood on risk of overweight in young adulthood. *International Journal of Obesity*, **16**, 169–75.

Lissau, I. & Sørensen, T.I. (1993). School difficulties in childhood and risk of overweight and obesity in young adulthood: a ten year prospective population study. *International Journal of Obesity*, **17**, 169–75.

Lissau, I. & Sørensen, T.I.A. (1994). Parental neglect during childhood and increased risk of obesity in young adulthood. *Lancet*, **343**, 324–7.

Maes, H.H., Neale, M.C. & Eaves, L.J. (1997). Genetic and environmental factors in relative body weight and human adiposity. *Behavioral Genetics*, **27**, 325–51.

Maffeis, C., Schutz, Y., Piccoli, R., Gonfiantini, E. & Pinelli, L. (1993). Prevalence of obesity in children in North-East Italy. *International Journal of Obesity*, **17**, 287–94.

Maffeis, C., Micciolo, R., Must, A., Zaffanello, M. & Pinelli, L. (1994). Parental and perinatal factors associated with childhood obesity in north-east Italy. *International Journal of Obesity*, **18**, 301–5.

Mamalakis, G. & Kafatos, A. (1996). Prevalence of obesity in Greece. *International Journal of Obesity*, **20**, 488–92.

McGarvey, S.T. (1991). Obesity in Samoans and a perspective on its etiology in Polynesians. *American Journal of Clinical Nutrition*, **53** (Suppl.), 1586S–94S.

Mo-Suwan, L. & Geater, A.F. (1996). Risk factors for childhood obesity in a transitional society in Thailand. *International Journal of Obesity*, **20**, 697–703.

Mo-Suwan, L., Lebel, L., Puetpaiboon, A. & Junjana, C. (1999). School performance and weight status of children and young adolescents in a transitional society in Thailand. *International Journal of Obesity*, **23**, 272–7.

Must, A., Dallal, G.E. & Dietz, W.H. (1991). Reference data for obesity: 85th and 95th percentiles of body mass index (wt/ht^2) and triceps skinfold thickness. *American Journal of Clinical Nutrition*, **53**, 839–46.

Nuutinen, E.M., Turtinen, J. & Pokka, T. (1991). Obesity in children, adolescents and young adults. *Annals of Medicine*, **23**, 41–6.

Parsons, T.J., Power, C., Logan, S. & Summerbell, C.D. (1999). Childhood predictors of adult obesity: a systematic review. *International Journal of Obesity*, **23** (Suppl. 8), S1–S107.

Perusse, L. & Bouchard, C. (1999). Role of genetic factors in childhood obesity and in susceptibility to dietary variations. *Annals of Medicine*, **31** (Suppl. 1), 19–25.

Pinelli, P., Cirillo, D., Golinelli, M., Gonfiantini, E., Leveghi, R., Maffeis, C., Olivieri, A., Piccoli,

R. & Gaburro, D. (1987). Anthropometric data and dietary habits of 1177 children in Verona. *Rivista Italia Pediatrica*, **13**, 6648–73.

Pomerleau, J. & Ostbye, T. (1997). [The relationship between place of birth and certain health characteristics in Ontario]. *Canadian Journal of Public Health*, **88**, 337–45.

Popkin, B.M. & Udry, J.R. (1998). Adolescent obesity increases significantly in second and third generation U.S. immigrants: the National Longitudinal Study of Adolescent Health. *Journal of Nutrition*, **128**, 701–6.

Poskitt, E.M.E. (1995). Committee report, Defining childhood obesity: The relative body mass index. *Acta Paediatrica*, **84**, 961–3.

Poskitt, E.M.E. & Cole, T.J. (1978). Nature, nurture, and childhood overweight. *British Medical Journal*, **1**, 603–5.

Rajan, U. (1994). Obesity among Singapore students. *International Journal of Obesity*, **Suppl. 18**, 27.

Rolland-Cachera, M.F. (1990). Timing weight-control measures in obese children. *Lancet*, 918.

Rolland-Cachera, M.-F., Deheeger, M., Guilloud-Bataille, M., Avons, P., Patois, E. & Sempé, M. (1987). Tracking the development of adiposity from one month of age to adulthood. *Annals of Human Biology*, **14**, 219–29.

Rolland-Cachera, M.F., Spyckerelle, Y. & Deschamps, J.P. (1992). Evaluation of pediatric obesity in France. *International Journal of Obesity*, **Suppl. 1**, 5.

Rosner, B., Prineas, R., Loggie, J. & Daniels, S.R. (1998). Percentiles for body mass index in U.S. children 5 to 17 years of age. *Journal of Pediatrics*, **132**, 211–22.

Roville-Sausse. F. (1999). [Increase during the last 20 years of body mass of children 0 to 4 years of age born to Maghrebian immigrants]. *Revues Epidemiologique Sante Publique*, **47**, 37–44.

Salvatoni, A., Livieri, C., Riganti, G., Chiesa, L., Bisio, P., Federico, M., Albertini, A. & Lorini, R. (1992). Obesity prevalence in schoolchildren of Pavia in the last 14 years: a rising problem? *Proceedings 3rd European Childhood Obesity Group*, Napoli.

Shirai, K., Shinomiya, M. & Umezono, T. (1990). Incidence of childhood obesity over the last ten years in Japan. *Diabetes Research Clinical Practice*, **Suppl. 10**, 65–70.

Sobal, J. & Stunkard, A.J. (1989). Socioeconomic status and obesity: a review of the literature. *Psychological Bulletin*, **105**, 260–75.

Sørensen, T.I. & Lissau-Lund-Sørensen, I. (1991). [Genetic–epidemiological studies of causes of obesity]. *Nordic Medicine*, **106**, 182–3, 204.

Sørensen, T.I., Holst, C. & Stunkard, A.J. (1992). Childhood body mass index – genetic and familial environmental influences assessed in a longitudinal adoption study. *International Journal of Obesity*, **16**, 705–14.

Sørensen, T.I., Holst, C. & Stunkard, A.J. (1998). Adoption study of environmental modifications of the genetic influences on obesity. *International Journal of Obesity*, **22**, 73–81.

Spee van der Wekke, J., Meulmeester, J.F., Radder, J.J., Verloove-Vanhorick, S.P. & Schalk van der Weide, Y. (1994). Peilingen in de jeugdgezondheidszorg: PGO-peiling 1992/1993. (Findings from preventive health studies on children between 1992–1993). *TNO Preventie en Gezondheid*, The Netherlands, report nr 94.091.

Stunkard, A.J., Sørensen, T.I., Hanis, C., Teasdale, T.W., Chakraborty, R., Schull, W.J. & Schulsinger, F. (1986). An adoption study of human obesity. *New England Journal of*

Medicine, **314**, 193–8.

Tanner, J.M., Whitehouse, R.H. & Takaishi, M. (1966a). Standards from birth to maturity for height, weight, height velocity, weight velocity in British children 1965 Part I. *Archives of Disease in Childhood*, **41**, 454–71.

Tanner, J.M., Whitehouse, R.H. & Takaishi, M. (1966b). Standards from birth to maturity for height, weight, height velocity, weight velocity in British children 1965 Part II. *Archives of Disease in Childhood*, **41**, 613–35.

Teasdale, T.W., Sørensen, T.I. & Stunkard, A.J. (1992). Intelligence and educational level in relation to body mass index of adult males. *Human Biology*, **64**, 99–106.

Tershakovec, A.M., Weller, S.C. & Gallagher, P.R. (1994). Obesity, school performance and behaviour of black, urban elementary school children. *International Journal of Obesity*, **18**, 323–7.

Troiano, R.P. & Flegal, K.M. (1998). Overweight children and adolescents: description, epidemiology, and demographics. *Pediatrics*, **Suppl. 101**, 497–504.

Van Meerbeeck, R. (1988). La condition physique des miliciens à l'armée belge en 1987. *Olympics*, Juin, 11–13.

Whitaker, R.C., Wright, J.A., Pepe, M.S., Seidel, K.D. & Dietz, W.H. (1997). Predicting obesity in young adulthood from childhood and parental obesity. *New England Journal of Medicine*, **337**, 869–73.

WHO (1998). Obesity: preventing and managing the global epidemic. *Report of a WHO consultation on obesity*, Geneva, 3–5 June 1997. WHO/NUT/NCD/98.1.

Molecular and biological factors with emphasis on adipose tissue development[1]

Martin Wabitsch

Department of Paediatrics, University of Ulm

3.1 Introduction

The energy content of the human body is under the control of several regulatory systems (Rosenbaum & Leibel, 1998). Changes in body energy content and changes in the size of adipose tissue – the major energy store of the body – result from alterations in the balance between energy intake and energy expenditure. The various regulatory systems produce different signals of which the main messages are integrated in the hypothalamus, where appetite and satiety, as well as the sympathetic and parasympathetic nervous systems, the hypothalamo-hypophysio-thyroid axis, and other endocrine systems are controlled.

Recent scientific data have clearly discarded the once widespread idea that obesity, which is an increase in body energy stores, just reflects a lack of willpower. It is evident that obesity results from changes in the above-mentioned regulatory systems with a lack of adequate counter-regulation, thus leading to positive energy balance. Recently, a few monogenetic defects, which occur rarely, have been shown to be associated with severe and early-onset obesity in humans. However, it is evident that the development of obesity, in the vast majority of cases, is a multifactorial event with a genetic predisposition affected by environmental factors which, so far, are not fully understood.

The storage of energy in white adipose tissue is physiologically important for survival during times of starvation, for fertility, for adequate function of the immune system and thus for overall well-being and health.

Interestingly, recent investigations of the regulation of energy balance in rodents and men have not only revealed the complex systems stabilizing energy balance but have also shown that the amount of energy stored in adipose tissue is related to various biological functions, including regulation of growth, puberty,

---

[1] Note added in proof. Since knowledge in this field has increased rapidly after 1998 the reader is also referred to recent reviews (Barsh et al. 2000, Lowell et al. 2000, Rosen and Spiegelman, 2000).

reproduction and the immune system. In the context of obesity, the advantages of a pathological enlargement of energy stores are not apparent, rather, a variety of comorbidities resulting from increased body fat are known to occur.

Since the regulation of energy stores in the human body is a crucial part of the complex regulatory system of energy balance and since in the author's laboratory much effort has been put into elucidating the regulation of adipose tissue growth, differentiation and metabolism, the main part of this chapter will focus on molecular and biological factors involved in the function of adipose tissue as the main energy stores of humans.

3.2 Regulation of body weight

The studies of Lavoisier in the 18th century were the foundation for the so-called 'New Chemical Sciences' and thus sowed the seed for the later development of the principles of thermodynamics. In relation to body-weight regulation these fundamental physical principles became significant when their applicability to biological systems was recognized. The first signals postulated in this system involved nutritional metabolites such as glucose and the amino acids. The historical 'gluco-stat' hypothesis postulated that the central nervous system senses glucose concentrations in the circulation (Mayer, 1953, 1955; Rosenbaum & Leibel, 1998). This hypothesis was first suggested by Mayer in the 1950s (Mayer, 1953, 1955; Rosenbaum & Leibel, 1998). Later, Mayer showed that disruption of the ventro-medial nuclei of the hypothalamus in rats led to a lack of satiety, whereas a disruption of the lateral areas of the hypothalamus led to a lack of hunger and death due to starvation. These early experiments localized the neuroanatomical systems which integrate the signals controlling hunger and satiety.

Parabiotic experiments with ob/ob mice and normal lean mice, appear to support the 'lipo-stat' hypothesis. Ob/ob mice, when put into parabiosis with lean mice, lose their excess weight and show reduction and/or normalization of their increased body fat stores, indicating the probable lack of some factor which reflects energy stores in the body and is produced in the white adipose tissue of ob/ob mice and sensed by the central nervous system.

Today, scientific work has begun characterizing short- and long-term systems regulating energy homeostasis. In the short term, regulatory signals from the gastrointestinal tract (e.g. quantity and quality of nutrients in the stomach) and signals generated during the metabolism of food, inform the central nervous system about food intake and thus regulate actual hunger and satiety. However, there is evidence for long-term systems which also regulate bodily energy stores. If this were not so, then one glass of milk of about 150 calories as an additional caloric intake above weight maintenance per day would result in an annual caloric excess of about 55 000 kcal or a weight gain of more than 10 kg (Rosenbaum & Leibel, 1998). One recently recognized example of a signal involved in the long-term regulation of body weight could be leptin which might also have short-term regulatory functions in humans.

Energy homeostasis of the body is equally dependent on systems regulating energy expenditure. Total energy expenditure is the sum of the energy expended for basal metabolic rate, for thermogenesis, for growth, for immune function and for physical activity. (Chapter 5 discusses this more extensively.)

It is evident from animal studies, including those with genetically obese rodents, and from studies in humans, including twin, adoption and family studies, that body weight is regulated and that a substantial part of this regulation is genetically determined. The body mass index (BMI) of children reflects body fat content and is strongly dependent on the BMI of children's biological parents (Rosenbaum & Leibel, 1998). Such genetic determinants have been recognized for many years with other biological characteristics such as height.

Human studies also indicate a genetic basis for obesity and subsequent studies have suggested that one part of the body's energy balance, namely the resting metabolic rate, is a major determinant of body weight development and itself might be mainly genetically determined (Levine et al., 1999). This possibility has strengthened the hypothesis that daily energy expenditure is at least partly regulated by genetic factors. Levine et al. (1999) demonstrated that the physiological basis for the considerable interindividual variation in susceptibility to weight gain in response to overeating might be a genetically determined difference in individuals' nonexercise activity thermogenesis.

Most recently, monogenetic defects causing obesity in humans have been reported, all but one of them showing a disturbed appetite regulation as the main cause for increased body fat stores (see below).

Principally, all regulatory systems involved in the control of energy balance involve several crucial steps where candidate genes, which could be important for body weight regulation, can be found. An updated overview on some of the regulatory systems involved in body weight regulation has been published recently (Rosenbaum & Leibel, 1998).

3.3 Single gene defects

At the time of writing, there are only six monogenetic forms of human obesity, all of which seem very rare. All newly described *endocrine disorders* resulting in early-onset obesity and associated symptoms are outlined below.

3.3.1 Congenital leptin deficiency

Montague et al. (1997) were the first to describe two patients with congenital leptin deficiency. Further individuals with leptin deficiency in a Turkish family have been described (Strobel et al., 1998). The two children described by Montague et al. (1997) are cousins within a highly consanguineous family of Pakistani origin. The children had normal birth weights but developed severe obesity within the first months of life. Patient 1 had a weight of 86 kg at the age of 8 years and patient 2 had a weight of 29 kg at the age of 2 years. Both children had normal heights when leptin deficiency was diagnosed. They were characterized by hyperphagia due to impaired satiety. The genetic defect consisted of a deletion of a single guanine nucleotide of the leptin gene. The children are currently treated with recombinant human leptin and are losing significant weight and adipose tissue mass thus providing the first evidence that leptin is an important regulator of energy balance in man.

3.3.2 Leptin receptor defect

Clement and coworkers (1998) described obese subjects in one family with a mutation in the human leptin receptor gene associated with obesity and pituitary dysfunction. The mutation resulted in a truncated leptin receptor lacking both the transmembrane and the intracellular domains. Affected individuals were characterized by early-onset morbid obesity although they had normal birth weight. By contrast to the two girls with leptin deficiency, these sisters affected by a leptin receptor defect were diagnosed after the normal age of puberty but showed no detectable mammary glands, no axillary hair, sparse pubic hair and amenorrhoea due to hypogonadotropic hypogonadism. Although obese, they showed no advance in bone age nor accelerated growth, but mild growth delay during early childhood associated with decreased serum concentrations of insulin-like growth factor (IGF)-1 and IGF binding protein (IGFBP)-3. In addition, there was evidence of hypothalamic hypothyroidism. Like the children with leptin deficiency, these girls were characterized by hyperphagia and abnormal eating behaviour. A functional leptin receptor would seem to be required not only for regulation of body weight, but also for sexual maturation and for the secretion of growth and thyrotropic hormones. Leptin is thus a potentially critical link between energy stores and hypothalamic pituitary functions in humans.

3.3.3 Prohormone convertase 1 (*PC 1*) defect

Jackson and coworkers (1997) described a woman who was heterozygotic for mutations in the prohormone convertase 1 gene (*PC 1*). Before the genetic defect was detected, this woman already had extreme childhood-onset obesity. Unusual associated features were abnormal glucose homeostasis despite low insulin levels and postprandial hypoglycaemia, both due to increased serum concentrations of proinsulin. In addition, the woman showed hypogonadotropic hypogonadism and hypocortisolism. These findings could be explained by defective functioning of PC 1. PC 1 acts proximally to CPE (carboxypeptidase E), the enzyme mutated in the fat/fat mouse. PC 1 is active in the post-translational processing and sorting of prohormones and neuropeptides. Products of PC 1 (and CPE) action have been implicated in the neuroendocrine control of energy balance and include α-MSH (melanocyte-stimulating hormone) and glucagon-like peptide (GLP)-1 derived from POMC (pro-opiomelanocortin) and proglucagon, respectively.

3.3.4 POMC deficiency

Krude et al. (1998) studied two patients with severe early-onset obesity, adrenal insufficiency and red hair. Stimulated by studies in the yellow obese mouse, in which α-MSH has a central role in the regulation of food-intake, this group was prompted to search for mutations within the POMC genes of these patients. In patient 1 they found two mutations interfering with synthesis of adrenocortico-trophic hormone (ACTH) and α-MSH. In patient 2 they found a mutation which abolishes POMC translation. These two patients provide evidence that defects in POMC synthesis can result in early-onset obesity and further endocrine disorders resulting from the defect in this precursor protein which normally generates the melanocortin peptides adrenocorticotrophin (ACTH), the melanocyte-stimulat-ing hormones (MSH) α, β, γ as well as the opioid-receptor ligand β-endorphin. Since α-MSH is a ligand for the melanocortin-4-receptor which leads to decreased food intake (satiety) when activated, the hyperphagia observed in patients with POMC deficiency is at least partly due to a deficiency in α-MSH, itself essential for body weight regulation.

3.3.5 Melanocortin-4-receptor defect

Two groups have described mutations in the human melanocortin-4-receptor associated with human obesity (Vaisse et al., 1998; Yeo et al., 1998). A defect in melanocortin-4-receptor function leads to lack of satiety and uncontrolled overeating. Animal studies have previously shown that dysfunction in the α-MSH/ melanocortin-4-receptor system can cause obesity through hyperphagia.

3.3.6 Peroxisome-proliferator-activated receptor γ-2 (PPARγ-2) defect

Ristow et al. (1998) found four out of 121 grossly obese subjects had a missense mutation in the gene for PPARγ-2. Overexpression of the mutant gene in preadipocytes was associated with accelerated adipose differentiation. The authors suggested that the mutant gene in their subjects might cause increased adipocyte differentiation in adipose tissue. If so, this would be, so far, the only monogenetic form of human obesity in which the genetic defect was not associated with central regulation of energy homeostasis. The findings of Ristow et al., however, demonstrated a high prevalence of this mutation, a finding which needs confirming in other cohorts of obese patients.

3.4 Regulation of body energy stores at adipose tissue level

Adipocytes in white adipose tissue are the body's major energy stores. A lean child with a weight of 30 kg has approximately 4.5 kg of triglycerides stored in adipose tissue equivalent to 1.3 million kJ stored. In the same child, energy stored as protein (mainly in the muscles), is approximately 1.5 kg or 26 000 kJ and energy stored as glycogen (mainly in liver and muscle) only around 130 g or 2100 kJ. Chemically, the main energy store of the body therefore is triglycerides. One adipocyte has a mean content of 1 µg lipid or approximately 17 mJ.

The energy stored as triglycerides in adipose tissue is the result of the balance between energy intake and energy expenditure. Changes in the size of adipose tissue mass occur when changes in this balance are present. In the next section, the biological and molecular basis for changes in adipose tissue size in man is summarized (Ailhaud 1996; Ailhaud & Hauner, 1998).

3.5 Changes of body fat stores during development

The first adipose tissue is visible in the human fetus between the 14th and 24th weeks of gestation. First, a local agglomeration of mesenchymal cells occurs, resembling small tissue globules. Capillaries grow into these agglomerations and the first fat globules are present in cells with a high triglyceride content. During further development these cells acquire a single larger lipid droplet. Morphologically, the typical fat globule, found in the subcutaneous fat of the new-born has developed. The observation that the first structure to be identified in developing fat tissue is a capillary, demonstrates the direct association between the development of fat cells and angiogenesis. In the last third of gestation the subcutaneous tissue of the fetus contains differentiated adipose tissue at almost all locations.

Body fat content is around 13% at birth, and rises to 28% by the end of the first year in a normal-weight infant (Fig. 3.1 according to McLaren, 1987). Normally, infants possess a considerable panniculus adiposus. At the beginning of the 20th century, Stratz (1902) described the different periods during infancy, childhood and adolescence in which anthropometric changes related to percentage adipose tissue occur. The first increase of percentage body fat, lasting until the end of the first year of life, was called by Stratz the 'first filling period'. This is followed by the

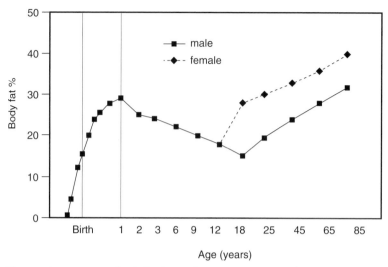

Figure 3.1   Changes in percentage body fat (according to McLaren 1987).

'first stretching period', during which subcutaneous adipose tissue mass decreases along with the percentage of body fat due to relative higher increases in lean body mass during growth. Interestingly, during this period longitudinal growth is not accelerated. Later, these cyclical changes are repeated, with percentage body fat increasing between the eighth and tenth years of life, in early puberty ('second filling period'). In boys, a second 'stretching period' occurs during the pubertal growth spurt. This second stretching period, during which the amount of subcutaneous fat remains constant over several months, can be observed, although it is not detectable in changes in the body mass index probably because of the concurrent significant increase in lean mass, especially muscle mass, during this period. In girls, the 'second filling period' continues after menarche with further increase in body fat mass until adulthood. The increase of body mass per se during growth and development can be divided into increases in fat-free and fat mass. The relation between these two increases is dependent on the biological age and shows sine wave-like changes over time. From this, critical periods of adipose tissue development can be assumed. Rolland-Cachera and coworkers (1984) showed that the time point when the second filling period begins (called by these authors 'adiposity rebound' and defined as the second increase in BMI values during childhood) is critical for the later development of obesity. The earlier this time point occurs the more likely obesity will develop. Normally, the second filling period does not begin before 5.5 years of age.

Generally, the BMI is a good measure of body fat content throughout childhood. The changes in body fat during childhood and adolescence are obviously also represented by the age-dependent curves for the body mass index.

Table 3.1. Distinguishable periods of increases in fat mass and lean mass during infancy, childhood and adolescence

0–1 years	1st filling period
3–7 years	1st stretching period
8–10 years	2nd filling period (pubertal filling period)
11–15 years	2nd stretching period (pubertal growth spurt)
16–20 years	3rd filling period (maturation)

After Stratz, 1902.

On the basis of results from studies on adipose tissue cellularity during these developmental periods, it was originally suggested that the total number of adipocytes of an adult is fixed during sensitive periods of adipogenesis in childhood and that there are no changes in the number of adipocytes during adulthood. This no longer seems the case (see below).

These periods of 'filling' and 'stretching' can also be demonstrated by following the development of the sum of triceps and subscapular skinfold thicknesses through infancy, childhood and adolescence (Brook, 1978). The growth periods during childhood and adolescence originally described by Stratz in 1902 are summarized in Table 3.1.

Early biological maturation brings together the cut-off points between the two filling periods described above. The second filling period occurs just before the pubertal growth spurt. It has long been hypothesized that the body needs a critical mass of energy stores and therefore of adipose tissue in order to induce puberty followed by fertility and reproduction. In this respect, it was recently suggested, on the basis of clinical observations, that critical concentrations of leptin are necessary for pubertal development and for successful reproduction (Hebebrand et al., 1997; Clement et al., 1998; Yeo et al., 1998).

Major changes in fat distribution take place through childhood into maturity. The gender-specific adipose tissue distribution pattern is genetically determined, with a predominance of body fat in the gluteo-femoral region in females and in the abdominal region in males, evident during puberty. These gender differences exist in minor forms even in infancy (Forbes, 1978).

3.6 Changes at cellular level related to changes in body fat

Hauner et al. (1989a), reviewing studies on adipose cellularity, identified two sensitive periods of development during childhood: one during the first year of life and the other just before puberty, coinciding with the two filling periods described by Stratz. During the first year of life the increase in body fat content is largely through increased adipocyte volume. Further growth in adipose tissue, especially

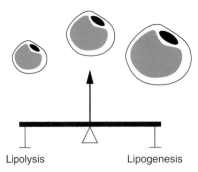

Lipolysis   Lipogenesis

Figure 3.2   Balance between lipolysis and lipogenesis determines adipocyte volume.

in the second filling period, is largely attributed to increased fat cell number without significant further change in fat cell volume. Mean fat cell volume remains relatively unchanged between the second year of life and adulthood. Whilst determining the activity of thymidine kinase in the stromal–vascular fraction of adipose tissue, two periods of high thymidine activity are found in the first year of life and in the period just before puberty. The activity of this enzyme is a marker for proliferative activity in the cell fraction containing preadipocytes. Again two sensitive periods become evident during which the numbers of undifferentiated adipocytes increase.

Thus, at the cellular level, changes in adipose tissue size result from changes in both adipocyte volume and adipocyte number. The volume of an adipocyte represents the balance between lipolysis and lipogenesis at the cellular level (Fig. 3.2). Changes in adipocyte number (increase or decrease) are the result of either a multiplication of preadipocytes and their subsequent differentiation into adipocytes resulting in an increase in fat mass or of dedifferentiation or apoptosis of existing adipocytes leading to a loss of adipose tissue mass. Although changes also leading to decreased numbers of adipocytes are theoretically possible, there are insufficient in vivo or in vitro data to know whether this ever happens.

Increased adipocyte volume leads to adipose tissue hypertrophy, whereas increased adipocyte number leads to adipose tissue hyperplasia. Recent reviews on the regulation of adipocyte volume and number in man are summarized in the paragraphs below (Hauner, 1992; Wabitsch et al., 1994b; Ailhaud, 1996; Ailhaud & Hauner, 1998).

3.7 Lipid storage in adipose tissue (lipogenesis)

The quantitatively most important method of lipid synthesis in the body is by uptake of fatty acids from the circulation. Triglycerides are present in the circulation as very-low-density lipoproteins (VLDL) or chylomicrons. They are hydrolysed by lipoprotein lipase. This enzyme is expressed and synthesized by fat cells and is localized after its secretion on the luminal side of the endothelial wall. Insulin is able to stimulate the activity of lipoprotein lipase. Circulating albumin-bound free fatty acids are another source of lipid for the adipocyte. Adipocytes are able to synthesize fatty acids from glucose acetate and pyruvate (de novo lipogenesis). The vast majority of fatty acids taken up by adipocytes or synthesized within adipocytes, are esterified and stored as triglycerides. The synthesis and the storage of other lipids are also possible in adipose tissue. For example, adipose tissue is a major store of cholesterol in the body.

Glucose enters fat cells by diffusion, facilitated by specific glucose transport proteins of which glucose transport protein 4 (GLUT 4) is the most important. Insulin is the main regulator of GLUT 4. Glucose is then phosphorylated and enters the metabolic pathways leading to the synthesis of α-glycerophosphate, fatty acids and glycogen. Some of the glucose incorporated into the cells is directly oxidized. Lactate seems to be the main metabolite of glucose breakdown in adipose tissue.

Insulin is the most important anabolic factor in adipose tissue. Besides its hormonal capacity to stimulate lipoprotein lipase, insulin stimulates the uptake of glucose and other metabolites into adipocytes. Insulin also stimulates triglyceride synthesis and inhibits lipolysis. Glucocorticoids, other steroid hormones, as well as other factors also modulate adipocyte lipid storage. By contrast, growth hormone (GH) stimulates lipogenesis and inhibits lipolysis (insulin-like effect) within its first minutes of action. This acute effect can be demonstrated in vivo as well as in vitro soon after starting GH treatment for GH-deficient children.

3.8 Lipid mobilization (lipolysis)

Fatty acids released from adipocytes are of major importance during periods of negative energy balance when fatty acids are essential for the supply of energy. There is a complex interaction between various hormones and other factors, which regulate the mobilization of lipids in adipose tissue. One important intracellular step is activation of hormone sensitive lipase (HSL) through stimulation of the adenylate-cyclase system and the subsequent protein phosphorylations. The result of the triglyceride breakdown in the adipocyte is the formation of free fatty acids and diacylglycerol, which itself is hydrolysed to free fatty acids and glycerol.

Lipid storage and lipogenesis, as well as lipid mobilization and lipolysis, can occur at the same time. The balance between these two metabolic processes at adipocyte level determines the changes in adipocyte volume.

Catecholamines are the major stimulators of lipolysis. In addition, GH has a direct lipolytic effect at the level of the adipocyte, which can be demonstrated through in vitro experiments. Small fat cells from new-borns seem to have a different capacity to respond to other lipolytic agents such as thyroid-stimulating hormone (TSH). This special characteristic of fat cells from neonates seems to be of physiological importance during the first hours of life (Marcus et al., 1988).

Currently, a paracrine/autocrine role for leptin in adipose tissue is debated (Friedman & Halaas, 1998). Recent data show a lipolytic effect of the hormone in rat adipocytes but these findings need confirming in human adipocytes.

3.9 Preadipocytes in human adipose tissue

The presence of preadipocytes in adipose tissue in postnatal life was originally suggested after demonstrating that cells of the stromal-vascular fraction of adipose tissue are able to incorporate [^{3}H]-thymidine and that this radioactive labelled thymidine can be found later in mature adipocytes. The stromal–vascular fraction of adipose tissue is a mixture of endothelial, blood and nerve cells together with macrophages and preadipocytes.

Today, it is possible to isolate preadipocytes from the adipose tissue of rodents to study cellular proliferation and differentiation in vitro. Earlier studies that tried to characterize preadipocytes in human adipose tissue were not very successful since only a small part of the stromal–vascular fraction of human adipose tissue developed into mature adipocytes in vitro. However, since Gerhard Ailhaud and coworkers (Hauner et al., 1989b), developed a serum-free chemically defined culture system for human preadipocytes it has become possible to follow in more detail the regulation of preadipocyte proliferation and adipose tissue differentiation in vitro. Almost all cells in the stromal–vascular fraction of human adipocyte tissue, when seeded in culture dishes according to established methods, were preadipocytes, capable of differentiating into adipocytes after adequate stimulation. These newly differentiated human adipocytes can then be cultured in monolayers for several days and further investigated.

At the undifferentiated stage, these preadipocytes possess multiple cytoplasmic arms and are macroscopically indistinguishable from fibroblasts. During adipose tissue differentiation the cells change. They become rounder and their cytoplasm gradually fills with multiple lipid droplets, which increase in size. These morphological changes result from various biochemical processes during differentiation. At the end of development, the preadipocytes not only have the phenotype of adipocytes with a univacuolar lipid droplet but also possess all the biochemical characteristics of mature fat cells.

The capacity of preadipocytes to differentiate depends on their anatomical origin and on the age of the donor. When preadipocytes from subcutaneous adipose tissue in the abdominal wall of young adults are cultured in an adipogenic medium containing physiological concentrations of insulin, cortisol and triiodothyronine, up to 80% of the preadipocytes are able to differentiate in vitro. By contrast, with cells from 80-year-old donors only around 20% cells seemed capable of differentiation. Nevertheless, these data show that even the adipose tissue of the elderly contains preadipocytes, which are able to differentiate with appropriate physiological stimulation.

3.10 Proliferation and differentiation of preadipocytes

Only one study which has investigated the proliferation and differentiation of preadipocytes in adipose tissue from children at different ages (Hauner et al., 1989a) is known to the author. Preadipocytes were isolated from adipose tissue according to established protocols. The results showed age-dependent differences in proliferative activity and in the capacity of cells to differentiate when cultured under serum-containing conditions. In parallel with the cyclic development of fat-free and fat mass during growth, the cells showed maximum proliferative ability and differentiation capacity in the first year of life and in the period just before puberty. These data support the view that the development of adipose tissue during childhood occurs mainly through the formation of new fat cells during sensitive periods – periods which might also be sensitive periods for the development of obesity. Another interesting finding in this study is the observation that the adipose tissue of children contains a much higher percentage of small fat cells with a diameter below 25 μm than that of adults. This seems to indicate higher rates of formation of new (small) fat cells during childhood and it is these cells which ultimately store more fat and increase their volume. These and other recent studies using serum-free culture conditions show that new fat cell formation is age-dependent and occurring extensively in childhood.

3.11 Adipogenic activity of human serum

The adipogenic activity of serum is defined as the capacity of the serum to stimulate differentiation of preadipocytes into adipocytes (Hauner et al., 1989c; Wabitsch et al., 1995). That human serum has significant adipogenic activity has been known since the time when clonal preadipocyte cell lines were established. When such cells were cultured in a serum containing medium, the number of cells differentiating into adipocytes depended on the origin of the serum. Although some of the factors responsible for the adipogenic activity of serum have been identified, some are still unknown. The adipogenic activity of serum from newborn human infants was almost twice as high as that of other sera. In adults, no differences have been found between the adipogenic activity of adipocytes from obese and normal weight persons. Likewise, no differences have been found between the adipogenic and the mitogenic activity of sera from obese and normal-weight children. However, there was a marked decrease in the adipogenic and also the mitogenic activity in the sera from obese children after they had lost around 10% of their body weight (Hauner et al., 1989c). This suggests that human serum contains factors which are affected by the nutritional state and which are able to influence the formation of new fat cells. Other studies show that the adipogenic activity of children's serum correlates significantly with the concentrations of IGF-1 and IGFBP-3. Furthermore, the decrease in adipogenic activity during weight loss is related to the decrease in serum free IGF-1 levels. Since the serum concentration of IGF-1 can be influenced by dietary changes, it is very likely that IGF-1 as its binding protein is one of the factors active in the cross-talk between nutritional intake on the one hand and fat cell formation on the other. In this context, it is also interesting that diets with high protein content lead to increased serum IGF-1 and thus the protein content of the diet might influence adipose tissue growth early in life (Wabitsch et al., 1994a, 1995).

The differentiation of adipocytes is strongly dependent on the presence of glucocorticoids. Clinical observation has shown that abdominal obesity is associated with increased hypothalamo-hypophysio-adrenal axis activity. Serum taken from individuals after ACTH-stimulation and added to cultures of primary human preadipocytes shows a significantly higher adipogenic activity than at baseline. This supports the idea that increased formation of new fat cells can occur, at least in defined anatomical locations, after adrenal stimulation with ACTH. Increased serum adipogenic activity in serum after ACTH-stimulation is directly related to glucocorticoid concentrations.

3.12 Hormonal and nutritional factors regulating adipose differentiation

There are different ways to identify and investigate hormonal and nutritional factors involved in the control of adipocyte differentiation. As mentioned above, studies on adipogenic activity in human serum show that glucocorticoids and IGF-1 are major determinants of the effect of human serum on adipocyte differentiation. Another approach is through study of the regulation of proliferation and differentiation of preadipocytes directly after stimulation with specific factors.

Several models have been described in the literature to study adipose tissue growth and metabolism: in vivo experiments using radioactive-labelled thymidine have successfully shown that differentiation of adipocytes can occur from cells of the stromal–vascular fraction of adipose tissue. A model using freshly isolated adipose tissue samples from rodents has been used mainly for incubation experiments to study the metabolic response of adipose tissue to various factors. Adipocyte differentiation cannot be studied with this model but a commonly used model to study adipocyte differentiation is the preadipocyte cell line which consists of clonal, immortalized cells. These primarily fibroblast-like cells are able to differentiate into adipocytes under certain culture conditions. Well-known cell lines are subclones of 3T3-cells, which have been derived from the mesenchymal tissue of the embryonic Swiss mouse, and ob-17-cells, which have been derived from the epidydimal fat pads of the ob/ob mouse. As well as being used to characterize different adipogenic and antiadipogenic factors involved in the control of adipocyte differentiation, these models have been used to investigate molecular mechanisms in adipose cell differentiation (see below). The physiological significance of the findings in studies using clonal cell lines derived from adipose tissue of rodents is not clear, since some results could not be confirmed when using human preadipocytes.

An adequate in vitro model for studying human adipocyte differentiation and metabolism has been described (Hauner et al., 1989a). This model has become an established method which is now also used for the study of hormonal regulation of leptin expression and secretion in human fat cells (Wabitsch et al., 1997).

The phenotypic and functional changes which occur during the differentiation of a preadipocyte into an adipocyte, are the results of molecular changes related to changes in the gene expression pattern. The differentiation process is characterized by an increase in the expression of adipocyte-specific genes (e.g. *LPL*, *GPDH*, *GLUT 4*, *Leptin* etc.) and the decrease in the expression of genes being predominant in preadipocytes (e.g. preadipocyte factor-1). Changes in gene expression are regulated by transcription factors. In the last few years, such 'key regulators' of adipocyte gene transcription have been described. It is known today that a combination of factors from the C/EBP-family and the PPAR-family will positively activate adipocyte gene transcription. PPAR isoforms have natural ligands, such as fatty acids, prostaglandins or leukotrienes or related metabolites. Further knowledge of the role of such natural ligands in activating PPARs and thus the transcription of adipogenic genes will help to understand better the link existing between the fatty acid composition of food and the formation of new fat cells (Ailhaud, 1996; Ailhaud & Hauner, 1998).

Clinical observations can be related to in vitro findings using the above mentioned models. These demonstrate important roles for glucocorticoids, GH, insulin and thyroid hormones in the control of adipose tissue cellularity (Ailhaud & Hauner, 1998). In vitro data also show that these hormones are important regulators of human adipocyte differentiation. Figure 3.3 presents a synopsis of these findings.

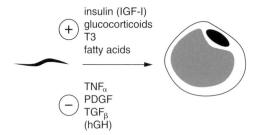

insulin (IGF-I)
glucocorticoids
T3
fatty acids

TNF_α
PDGF
TGF_β
(hGH)

Figure 3.3   Stimulation and inhibition of differentiation of human adipocytes.

Hypothyroidism is associated with a decreased number of fat cells with or without associated increased adipose tissue mass. Proliferation of cultured human preadipocytes is dependent on triiodothyronine (T3) concentration in the culture medium. Physiological concentrations of T3 decrease proliferation and stimulate differentiation in the presence of other adipogenic hormones.

GH-deficient children have slightly increased body fat stores. Their adipose tissue consists of enlarged fat cells which are decreased in number when compared with adipose tissue from healthy children of the same age. In cultures of human preadipocytes, GH will stimulate the proliferation of preadipocytes by inducing IGF-1 expression and secretion. The cells are then ready to differentiate in the presence of adipogenic factors. In addition, GH also has a significant diabetogenic effect inhibiting glucose uptake and lipogenesis, and a direct lipolytic effect in mature human adipocytes, leading to reduced adipocyte volume.

Clinically, glucocorticoid excess leads to individuals with the phenotypic characteristics of Cushing's syndrome, particularly increased adipose tissue mass, especially in the abdominal region. At the cellular level, glucocorticoids are potent stimulators of adipocyte differentiation in cultured human preadipocytes. This effect could be partly explained by increased availability of arachidonic acid for prostacyclin production.

Insulin and IGF-1 receptors are expressed in undifferentiated human preadipocytes and in human adipocytes. Due to the structural similarity of the ligands, insulin and IGF-1 are both able to stimulate both receptors although at different concentrations. In physiological concentrations, IGF-1 is able to stimulate the proliferation of human preadipocytes but insulin can only produce the same effect at supra-physiological concentrations, possibly via the IGF-1 receptor. In mature adipocytes, insulin at physiological concentrations and IGF-1 at supra-physiological concentrations are both able to stimulate glucose uptake and lipogenesis as well as to inhibit lipolysis, probably through the insulin receptor. The IGF-1 receptor is present in mature adipocytes but does not seem to induce any detectable biological effect.

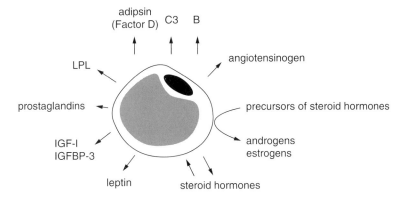

Figure 3.4   Human adipocyte as a secretory cell.

Insulin is necessary in physiological concentrations for differentiation of preadipocytes into adipocytes, although at supra-physiological concentrations IGF-1 can substitute for insulin.

The role of retinoids and fatty acids in the control of differentiation of human preadipocytes needs clarifying. Both groups of substances have been shown to stimulate adipose conversion in clonal cell lines.

Besides these examples of adipocyte stimulating factors there are also several antiadipogenic factors which inhibit the differentiation of human preadipocytes. Examples are TGFβ (transforming growth factor), TNFα (tumour necrosis factor), EGF (epidermal growth factor) and PDGF (platelet derived growth factor). In one sense, GH also belongs to these factors since its metabolic anti-insulin-like activity inhibits the phenotypic appearance of mature fat cells in vitro. There are certainly other as yet unknown factors in human serum which are able to inhibit and therefore control adipose cell differentiation in man.

3.13 Human adipocytes are secretory cells

Figure 3.4 summarizes how adipocytes might be able to interact in the control of various endocrine and metabolic systems, including the control of blood pressure through the expression and secretion of angiotensinogen which is then metabolized to angiotensin II.

One special function of adipocytes is the secretion of leptin. In human adipocytes, leptin production has been demonstrated as under glucocorticoid, insulin and IGF-1 (all stimulatory) control as well as that of androgens, GH, adrenergic agonists and fatty acids (all inhibitory). The rate of leptin production in adipocytes depends also on the anatomical origin of the cultured cells and on their size. It can be clearly shown that there is a direct connection between adipocyte volume and leptin secretion. Current knowledge about the regulation of leptin secretion in adipocytes suggests two forms of regulation. One regulating factor has a relatively long-term influence on the lipid content of adipocytes and affects the volume of the adipocyte and thus its lipid content. This effect may explain the observation that, in man, an increase in adipose tissue mass (from both cellular hyperplasia and hypertrophy) is paralleled by an increase in serum leptin levels. In addition to this 'long-term' regulation of leptin secretion, there is another determinant of leptin secretion responsible for short-term changes. It is suggested that the balance between lipogenic and lipolytic factors acting on the adipocyte represents this second determinant. This suggestion is based on the observation that almost all stimulatory factors for leptin secretion are also lipogenic factors (e.g. insulin) and all inhibitory factors show a lipolytic effect (e.g. GH). These short-term regulators might also account for the daytime variations in human serum leptin concentrations which are partly associated with times of eating and fasting.

3.14 Conclusions

Currently we understand only a minor part of the complex regulatory system of energy homeostasis in man. The acquisition of increased adipose tissue mass occurs during prolonged periods of positive energy balance. Energy homeostasis in most children and adults is strictly regulated and energy stores are kept within the defined age-dependent physiological range. The susceptibility to definitive increases in the level of energy balance during periods of reduced energy consumption and increased energy intake seem genetically determined. Studies in patients with rare monogenetic forms of obesity have elucidated some relevant genes and physiological relationships in this system. There is currently intense scientific interest in the central regulation of energy homeostasis. However it is clear that the acquisition of increased adipose tissue mass is also dependent on the susceptibility of preadipocytes to proliferate, to differentiate, and to enter into apoptosis.

Earlier studies have already revealed critical periods of adipogenesis during childhood. It seems that during these periods the systems regulating energy balance are sensitive to disequilibrating factors. These factors arise from an unfavourable environment supporting a sedentary lifestyle and high-energy high-fat diet. It is reasonable to assume that prevention of exposure to such factors will prevent the development of obesity. Very appropriately, the increasing prevalence of childhood obesity in European countries has led to calls for preventive action targeted at the ages critical for adipogenesis in childhood.

3.15 REFERENCES

Ailhaud, G. (1996). Molecular and cellular determinants of body weight regulation. In *Regulation of Body Weight: Biological and Behavioral Mechanisms*. Ed. C. Bouchard & G.A. Bray, pp. 211–22. Chichester: John Wiley & Sons.

Ailhaud, G. & Hauner, H. (1998). Development of white adipose tissue. In *Handbook of Obesity*, ed. G.A. Bray et al., pp. 359–78. New York: Marcel Dekker Inc.

Barsh, S.G., Farooqi S. I. & O'Rahilly, S. (2000). Genetics of body-weight regulation. *Nature*, **404**, 644.

Brook, C.G.D. (1978). Cellular growth: adipose tissue. In *Human Growth*, vol. II, eds. F. Falkner & J.M. Tanner, pp. 21–33. New York: Plenum Press.

Clement, K., Vaisse, C., Lahlou, N., Cabrol, S., Pelloux, V., Cassuto, D., Gourmelen, M., Dina, C., Chambaz, J., Lacorte, J.M., Basdevant, A., Bougneres, P., Lebouc, Y., Froguel, P. & Guy-Grand, B. (1998). A mutation in the human leptin receptor gene causes obesity and pituitary dysfunction. *Nature*, **392**, 398–401.

Friedman, J.M. & Halaas, J.L. (1998). Leptin and the regulation of body weight in mammals. *Nature*, **395**, 763–70.

Forbes, G.B. (1978). Growth of body fat. In *Human growth*, vol. II, eds. F. Falkner & J.M. Tanner, pp. 239–72. New York: Plenum Press.

Hauner, H. (1992). Physiology of the fat cell, with emphasis on the role of growth hormone. *Acta Paediatrica*, **383** (suppl.), 47–51.

Hauner, H., Wabitsch, M. & Pfeiffer, E.F. (1989a). Proliferation and differentiation of adipocyte precursor cells from children at different ages. In *Obesity in Europe 1988*, ed. P. Björntorp, pp. 195–200. London: John Libbey.

Hauner, H., Entenmann, G., Wabitsch, M., Gaillard, D., Ailhaud, G., Negrel, R. & Pfeiffer, E.F. (1989b). Promoting effect of glucocorticoids on the differentiation of human adipocyte precursor cells cultured in an chemically defined medium. *Journal of Clinical Investigation*, **84**, 1663–70.

Hauner, H., Widhalm, K. & Pfeiffer, E.F. (1989c). Adipogenic activity in sera from obese children before and after weight reduction. *American Journal of Clinical Nutrition*, **50**, 63–7.

Hebebrand, J., Blum, W.F., Barth, N., Coners, H., Englaro, P., Juul, A., Ziegler, A., Warnke, A., Rascher, W. & Remschmidt, H. (1997). Leptin levels in patients with anorexia nervosa are reduced in the acute stage and elevated upon short-term weight restoration. *Molecular Psychiatry*, **2**, 330–4.

Jackson, R.S., Creemers, J.W.M., Ohagi, S., Raffin-Sanson, M.L., Sanders, L., Montague, C.T., Hutton, J.C. & O'Rahilly, S. (1997). Obesity and impaired prohormone processing associated with mutations in the prohormone convertase 1 gene. *Nature Genetics*, **16**, 303–6.

Krude, H., Biebermann, H., Luck, W., Horn, R., Brabant, G. & Gruters, A. (1998). Severe early-onset obesity, adrenal insufficiency and red hair pigmentation caused by POMC mutations in human. *Nature Genetics*, **19**, 155–7.

Levine, J.A., Eberhardt, N.L. & Jensen, M.D. (1999). Role of nonexercise activity thermogenesis in resistance to fat gain in humans. *Science*, **283**, 212–14.

Lowell, B.B., Schwartz, M.W., Woods, S.C., Porte, D., Seeley, R.J. & Baskin, D.G. (2000). Central nervous system control and food intake. *Nature*, 404, 661.

Marcus, C., Ehren, H., Bolme, P. & Arner, P. (1988). Regulation of lipolysis during the neonatal period: importance of thyrotropin. *Journal of Clinical Investigation*, **82**, 1793–9.

Mayer, J. (1953). Glucostatic mechanisms of the regulation of food intake. *New England Journal of Medicine*, **249**, 13–43.

Mayer, J. (1955). Regulation of energy intake and the body weight. The glucostatic theory and the lipostatic hypothesis. *Annals of the New York Academy of Sciences*, **63**, 15–43.

McLaren, D.S. (1987). A fresh look at some perinatal growth and nutritional standards. *World Review of Nutrition and Dietetics* vol. 49, pp. 87–120, Basel: Karger.

Montague, C.T., Farooqi, S., Whitehead, J.P., Soos, M.A., Rau, H., Wareham, N.J., Sewter, C.P., Digby, J.E., Mohammed, S.N., Hurst, J.A., Cheetham, C.H., Earley, A.R., Barnett, A.H., Prins, J.B. & O'Rahilly, S. (1997). Congenital leptin deficiency is associated with severe early-onset obesity in humans. *Nature*, **387**, 903–8.

Ristow, M., Müller-Wieland, D., Pfeiffer, A., Krone, W. & Kahn, R. (1998). Obesity associated with a mutation in a genetic regulator of adipocyte differentiation. *New England Journal of Medicine*, **339**, 953–9.

Rolland-Cachera, M.F., Deheeger, M., Bellisle, F., Sempé, M., Guilloud-Bataille, M. & Patois, E. (1984). Adiposity rebound in children: a simple indicator for predicting obesity. *American Journal of Clinical Nutrition*, **39**, 129–35.

Rosen, E.D. & Spiegelman, B.M. (2000). Molecular regulation of adipogenesis. *Annual Review of Cellular and Developmental Biology*, **16**, 145.

Rosenbaum, M. & Leibel, R.L. (1998). The physiology of body weight regulation: relevance to the etiology of obesity in children. *Pediatrics*, **101**, 525–39.

Stratz, W. (1902). *Der Körper des Kindes*, vol. 1, Stuttgart.

Strobel, A., Camoin, T.I.L., Ozata, M. & Strossberg, A.D. (1998). A leptin missense mutation associated with hypogonadism and morbid obesity. *Nature Genetics*, **18**, 213–15.

Vaisse, C., Clement, K., Guy-Grand, B. & Froguel, P. (1998). A frameshift mutation in human MC4R is associated with a dominant form of obesity. *Nature Genetics*, **20**, 113–14.

Wabitsch, M., Blum, W.F., Heinze, E., Böckmann, A. & Teller, W. (1994a). Association of insulin-like growth factors and their binding proteins with anthropometric parameters in obese adolescent girls. In *Obesity in Europe* 1993, eds. H. Ditschuneit et al., pp. 155–60. London: John Libbey.

Wabitsch, M., Hauner, H., Heinze, E. & Teller, W. (1994b). In-vitro effects of growth hormone in adipose tissue. *Acta Paediatrica*, **406** (suppl.), 48–53.

Wabitsch, M., Hauner, H., Heinze, E. & Teller, W. (1995). The role of GH/IGF in adipocyte differentiation. *Metabolism*, **44** (suppl.), 45–49.

Wabitsch, M., Blum, W.F., Rascher, W. & Hauner, H. (1997). Studies on the regulation of leptin expression using in vitro differentiated human adipocytes. In *Leptin. The Voice of Adipose Tissue*, eds. W.F. Blum, W. Kiess & W. Rascher, pp. 102–9. Heidelberg: Johann Ambrosius Barth Verlag.

Yeo, G.S., Farooqi, I.S., Aminian, S., Halsall, D.J., Stanhope, R.G. & O'Rahilly, S. (1998). A frameshift mutation in MC4R associated with dominantly inherited human obesity. *Nature Genetics*, **20**, 111–12.

Nutrition

Marie Françoise Rolland-Cachera[1] and France Bellisle[2]

[1]ISTNA-CNAM, Paris. [2] Hotel Dieu-Unité Inserm 341, Paris

4.1 Introduction

Nutrition is a major determinant of body size (Forbes, 1962). In addition to the energy intake from food, other components, such as the balance of nutrients in the diet and the diurnal pattern of food consumption, have been related to body composition.

Some studies describe trends in nutritional intake and obesity over time. Others analyse associations between food intake and body weight status but the available information is not always easy to interpret. Most results derive from dietary surveys, which remain the main method for determining the intakes of large populations. The limitations of dietary surveys, particularly under-reporting by obese subjects, have been widely discussed. One reason, apart from the difficulties of data collection on diets, why the interpretation of nutritional data is often difficult in obesity, could be that the *present* nutritional intake of obese subjects is not the factor responsible for development of the obese constitution. Indeed, dietary restriction in obese adults is frequently reported (Ballard-Barbash et al., 1996). In children, however, dietary data should be more promising, because the current behaviour of obese children is closer than adult behaviour to the spontaneous obesity-promoting intake.

In the present chapter, we discuss the significance of data on food intake for obesity in children and try to identify the nutritional and/or behavioural factors, which promote obesity.

4.2 Secular trends of nutrition and obesity

Overweight and obesity affect an increasing proportion of children and adults in both industrialized (Gortmaker et al., 1987; Prentice & Jebb, 1995; Seidell, 1997; Oppert & Rolland-Cachera, 1998) and developing countries (Drewnowski & Popkin, 1997). In seeking potential causes for the increasing prevalence of

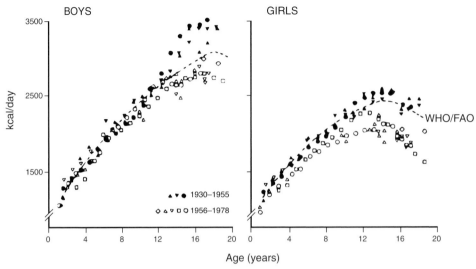

Figure 4.1   Energy intake (kcal/day) of boys and girls studied between 1930 and 1955 compared to more recent studies (1956–78), with reference to WHO/FAO (1973) recommendations (dashed lines) (Whitehead et al., 1982).

childhood obesity, several factors which influence body fatness should be considered. Increased body fatness in children is usually associated with other anthropometric features. Obese children display increased stature and muscle mass (Knittle et al., 1979). In many countries, children have been getting taller, heavier and maturing more rapidly (Eveleth & Tanner, 1990; Takaishi, 1994; Hughes et al., 1997). Both the increased prevalence of obesity and the changing patterns of growth may relate to changes in nutritional intake.

Table 4.1 lists details of some of the varied studies that have recorded food intakes over the last 70–80 years. Whitehead et al. (1982) examined time trends in energy intakes from studies made from the 1930s until 1978. Energy intakes of infants were higher before 1955 than later on, and these differences were maintained throughout childhood. A progressive reduction in energy intake was particularly apparent for girls (Fig. 4.1). The dietary intakes of 10-year-old children from the Bogalusa Heart Study (Nicklas et al., 1993) showed that total energy intakes had remained unchanged from 1973 to 1988. However, when expressed as energy/kilogram body weight, intakes were lower in 1988, because children's weights had increased. Negative linear trends over this time period were noted for fat intake (both as total intake and as percentage of total energy). There were also significant increases in percentage of energy from protein and carbohydrate (CHO). The trends in types of food consumed support these findings. For example, consumption of whole milk declined and consumption of 2% fat and skim milks increased. Despite stable energy intakes and decreased

Table 4.1. Trends in nutritional intake in various studies

Country	Period	Age (years)	Intake					Reference
			Energy	Nutrients (% energy)				
				Protein	Fat	CHO		
Children								
UK	1967–1993	1.5–2.5	↓	↑	↓	=		Gregory et al., 1995
USA	1977–1987	3–5	↓		↓			Schlicker et al., 1994
USA	1977–1987	6–11	↓		↓			Schlicker et al., 1994
Sweden	1967–1981	8				↓		Sunnegardh et al., 1986
France	1978–1995	10	↓	↑	↓	=		Rolland-Cachera et al., 1996a
USA	1973–1988	10	=	↑	↓	↑		Nicklas et al., 1993
Sweden	1967–1981	13	↓		↓	=		Sunnegardh et al., 1986
Finland	1970–1980	13–18	↓	↑	↓	=		Räsänen et al., 1985
USA, UK, Australia	1930–1978	0.5–18	↓					Whitehead et al., 1982
USA	1977–1987	12–19	↓		↓			Schlicker et al., 1994

Country	Period		Intake					Reference
			Energy	Nutrients (g)				
				Protein	Fat	CHO		
Whole population								
Britain	1970–1990		↓		↓			Prentice & Jebb, 1995
Japan	1950–1990		=	↑	↑	↓		Takaishi, 1994
Netherlands	1987–1993		↓	↑	↓	=		Seidell, 1997
USA	1976–1991		↓		↓			Heini & Weinsier, 1997

⇓ : decrease; = : no change; ⇑ : increase.

CHO: Carbohydrate.

dietary fat intakes, obesity increased and serum lipoprotein concentrations were unchanged over the same time period.

A study of the dietary intakes of 8- and 13-year-old Swedish children (Sunnegardh et al., 1986) showed that energy intakes had fallen in 8-year-old boys and girls, and in 13-year-old girls, but not in 13-year-old boys over the previous 10–15 years. Over the same time, body fatness increased.

Two studies conducted 17 years apart in 10-year-old French children (Rolland-Cachera et al., 1996a) showed mean daily energy intakes falling from 2326 kcal to 2108 kcal between 1978 and 1995. This trend was accounted for by a decrease in both fat and CHO intake (including sucrose). Total protein intakes remained constant, but the animal/vegetable protein ratio increased, mainly as a consequence of a decline in vegetable protein consumption. The percentage of energy provided by protein increased, the percentage of fat decreased and the percentage of CHO, including sucrose, remained constant. Over the same time period, children became taller, the percentage of obese children increased from 6.3% to 14.4%, and body fat showed a more android pattern of distribution.

Nutritional intakes recorded for a study of atherosclerosis precursors in Finnish children were compared with results of earlier surveys (Räsänen et al., 1985). Intakes of energy, fat and sucrose fell between 1970 and 1980. Over the same period the percentage of energy in the diet coming from protein rose, that from fat fell and the percentage of energy from CHO stayed the same.

As in western countries, secular trends to increased weight and height of Japanese children (Takaishi, 1994) are not matched by parallel increases in energy intake. Fat and animal protein intakes rose steeply between 1950 and 1990 whilst total CHO fell.

Similar trends are seen in young children. Data from the Nation-wide Food Consumption Survey (NFCS) show that 3- to 5-year-old American children consumed less fat and fewer calories in 1987 than in 1977 (Schlicker et al., 1994). Energy intakes in 1.5- to 2.5-year-old English children fell from 1264 kcal/day to 1045 kcal/day between 1967 and 1993 (Gregory et al., 1995). Over the same time period, the percentage of energy from protein rose, the percentage from fat fell and the percentage from CHO stayed the same. Similar changes in the balance of nutrients were recorded in 2-year-old French children between 1973 and 1986 (Deheeger et al., 1991).

Falls in energy intakes are likely to be associated with decreasing energy expenditures. However, this association seems less likely to account for falling energy intakes in very young, as opposed to older, children. Infant diets in industrialized countries are characterized by high protein and low fat content (Table 4.2). Reduced energy intakes may relate to changes in the composition of the diet. Low-fat foods reduce the energy density of diets and thus reduce total

Table 4.2. Nutritional intake in infants from different countries

Country	Age (months)	Intake (g/kg)	Protein (% energy)	Fat (% energy)	CHO (% energy)	Reference
Belgium	12–36	3.8	15.8	29.2	55	Mozin, unpublished data
Denmark	12	3.3	15	28	57	Michaelsen & Jorgensen, 1995
France	10	4.3	15.6	27.4	57	Deheeger et al., 1994
Israel	30	3.6	17.4	—	—	Palti et al., 1979
Italy	12	5.1	19.5	30.5	50	Bellù et al., 1991
Spain	9	4.4	15.7	26.4	57.9	Capdevilla et al., 1998

energy intake (Michaelsen & Jorgensen, 1995). In addition, low-fat, high-protein diets can reduce energy intakes as young children prefer flavours associated with high dietary fat (Johnson et al., 1991) and because of the high satiating power of protein (Blundell & Tremblay, 1995).

The prevalence of obesity is rising even in developing countries. This rise parallels changes in nutritional intake but, in contrast to industrialized countries, obesity is increasing in parallel with increases in fat intake (Drewnowski & Popkin, 1997).

In summary, today's children, in both developing and industrialized countries, are taller and heavier than in the past, in spite of relatively stable or falling energy intakes amongst children from industrialized countries. Their fat intakes are falling and the percentage of total energy derived from protein is rising. Lower energy intakes are apparent even amongst young children and seem to be more pronounced in girls than in boys.

The increase in stature suggests that some important factors may be operating in early life. Most of the secular increase in height happens during the first years of life (Bock & Sykes, 1989; Takaishi, 1994). Thus, trends to larger body size may be more strongly associated with early feeding practices than with nutritional intakes at older ages (Rolland-Cachera et al., 1999).

4.3 Relationship between nutrition and adiposity

Dietary records have been used to examine the relationship between nutrition and adiposity. The development of methods for measuring energy expenditure have led to abundant criticism of dietary methodology in recent years. In several studies, energy intake and expenditure data seemed incompatible. The usual conclusion was that subjects under-reported their intake in proportion to their excess body weight. This bias probably affected the results of many studies. In the present chapter, survey data will be reviewed as they were published, accepting some probable under-reporting in the child populations described. Even if there are some errors in reported intakes, consistent tendencies do emerge from diverse studies. The associations between adiposity and food intakes reported in many studies can inspire hypotheses about the various mechanisms leading to the development of obesity.

4.3.1 Relationship between nutrition and total adiposity
Cross-sectional studies

The simplest approach to investigating the dietary component of obesity is to analyse associations between food intake and fatness on the basis of cross-sectional studies.

Thirty-five years ago, Hampton et al. (1967), whilst studying teenagers, found no association between energy intake and body fat. Indeed, the association was a negative one if energy was expressed as energy/kilograms of body weight or energy for unit height. Similarly, no association was found between fatness level and energy intake of 1- to 3-year-old French children (Rolland-Cachera et al., 1988). Dietary intakes recorded in a subsample of 10-year-old American children from the Bogalusa Heart Study were examined for cardiovascular risk factors (Frank et al., 1978). No correlation was found between diet composition and risk factor levels. However, children with the highest indices of obesity ingested significantly more protein. Another study in 9- to 11-year-old children participating in the Muscatine Risk Factors Survey (Gazzaniga & Burns, 1993) found obese children consumed significantly more energy (kJ/day) than their nonobese peers but, again, the association became negative when energy was expressed as kiloJoules/ kilogram body weight. Fatness correlated positively with fat, negatively with CHO and showed no association with protein intakes. A similar analysis in 9- and 10-year-old children (Tucker et al., 1997) showed per cent body fat negatively associated with energy and with CHO intakes. When the nutrient content of the diet was expressed as a percentage of the total energy intake, body fatness was positively associated with fat, negatively with CHO and positively with protein, after controlling for gender and energy intake. In 11- to 16-year-old Tasmanian children, fatter girls were less likely to have high intakes of energy and CHO, while no association appeared between fatness and the nutritional intake of boys (Woodward, 1985).

A weight-control programme conducted in children aged 8–12 years (Valoski & Epstein, 1990) found, at baseline, no significant differences in the caloric and fat content of the diets eaten by obese and nonobese children, although the obese children consumed more protein. No differences were found between energy intakes of normal-weight and obese Spanish adolescents (Ortega et al., 1995), although obese adolescents derived a greater proportion of their energy from protein and fat and less from CHO.

A study of 7- to 12-year-old French children by Rolland-Cachera & Bellisle (1986) examined correlations between nutritional intakes and body fatness assessed by body mass index (BMI) or subscapular skinfolds. The only significant finding was that a high percentage of protein in the diet was positively associated with both high BMI and high subscapular skinfold thicknesses. In another study with French adolescents, the ponderal index was negatively associated with energy intake and positively associated with the percentage of energy derived from protein (Spyckerelle et al., 1992). Finally in a study of very young British children aged 1.5–4.5 years, no association at all was recorded between diet composition and body size (Davies, 1997).

Retrospective analysis and longitudinal studies

The relationship between adiposity and food intake has been widely investigated using cross-sectional studies. These studies fail to explain the development of obesity, probably because the determinants of obesity have their main effect at an early period of growth. In order to elucidate the relationships between nutritional intake and the development of obesity, longitudinal growth studies may be more appropriate. In addition, such studies should show less bias in reported nutritional intakes, since many children would be interviewed before the development of excessive adiposity.

While less informative than prospective studies, retrospective analyses can provide useful information. The relative importance of dietary factors in determining weight was studied in 5-year-old children (Poskitt & Cole, 1978). Neither the energy intakes recorded in infancy, nor the intakes from dietary recall at 5 years correlated significantly with relative body weight at age 5 years. Further, children of overweight mothers did not have higher energy intakes than children of underweight mothers. In another British study, infants initially either below the 10th centile or above the 90th centile weight-for-age were enrolled in an 18 months longitudinal study (Mumford & Morgan, 1982). All children were under 1 year of age on the first examination. Although the two groups of children remained different in terms of body size and skinfold measurements throughout the study, there were no differences in nutritional intakes at any time.

To examine whether or not obesity at 3 years of age was related to feeding practices in early infancy, daily nutrient intakes were studied from birth in Canadian infants (Vobecky et al., 1983). In overweight infants, energy (expressed as kilocalories/kilogram body weight), fat and CHO intakes were lower than in thinner infants There was no difference in protein intake according to relative weight, although intake was higher than recommended. The authors concluded that overfeeding in early infancy might not be a major cause of obesity in later life.

A longitudinal study of nutrition and growth investigated the early determinants of the age at adiposity rebound (Rolland-Cachera et al., 1995). The only significant association between nutritional intake at the age of 2 years and age at adiposity rebound was a high percentage of energy derived from protein in the diet, that is the higher the percentage of protein, the earlier the adiposity rebound. These results have underlined the inadequate nutrient balance of the infant diet in industrialized countries (Rolland-Cachera et al., 1999). By the age of 1 year, infant diets are characterized by high intakes of protein (~4 g/kg body weight or 16% of total energy) and low intakes of fat (~28% total energy) (Table 4.2). Protein intake represents three to four times as much as requirements (WHO, 1985). This imbalance in protein and fat intake is attributable to excessive consumption of animal products, particularly low-fat dairy products, and to low intakes of veg-

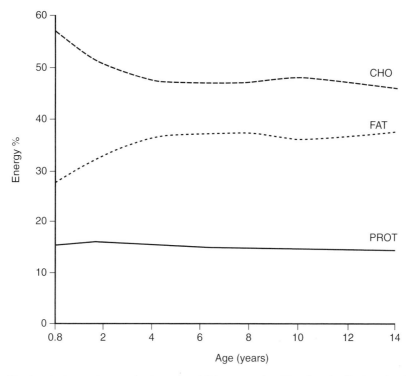

Figure 4.2   Nutrient balance changes in the same children examined in a longitudinal study of nutrition and growth (Deheeger et al., 1994). The proportion of fat in the diet is low in infancy and increases with age and the proportion of protein is high at all ages. The infant diet should be high in fat and low in protein, like human milk. Subsequently the proportion of fat in the diet should decrease while the proportion of protein should increase with age.

etable oil (Deheeger et al., 1994). High-protein, low-fat diets do not provide a nutrient balance in proportion to infants' needs. This imbalance is remarkable because the diet during the first months of life, when human milk is the only food, provides 7% of energy as protein and 50% as fat. Figure 4.2 presents changes in the nutrient balance in the children from the Rolland-Cachera et al. (1999) studies between the age of 10 months and 14 years. Fat intakes are too low in early life and too high later on. At all ages, the protein content of the diet is high, but particularly so in infancy.

Childhood obesity is characterized by increased stature and increased muscle mass (Knittle et al., 1979). Early high protein intakes could account for these anthropometric characteristics, perhaps as a result of changes in hormonal status since obesity is associated with alterations in hormonal status. High plasma insulin-like growth factor-1 (IGF-1) concentrations and reduced growth hormone (GH) secretion (spontaneous or in response to a wide variety of stimuli) are

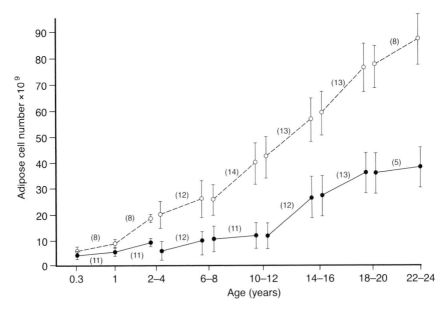

Figure 4.3   Longitudinal development of adipose cell number as a function of age (Knittle et al., 1979). (Dashed lines: obese; continuous line: controls.)

characteristic features of children with simple obesity (Van Vliet et al., 1986; Loche et al., 1987; Rosskamp et al., 1987).

Nutrition is one of the main regulators of IGF-1 and GH. Low IGF-1 and high GH are reported in malnourished children (Waterlow, 1992). Energy and protein intakes have independent effects on hormonal status (Thissen et al., 1994). We have previously proposed (Rolland-Cachera, 1995) that the altered hormonal status of obese children (high IGF-1 and low GH) could be the mirror image of protein deprivation, that is the consequence of excess protein intake, since high protein intakes are often recorded in the obese. High protein intakes could stimulate increased IGF-1 levels and in turn, high IGF-1 levels could stimulate protein synthesis and cell proliferation. As IGF-1 promotes the differentiation of preadipocytes into adipocytes (Ailhaud et al., 1992), high protein intakes might induce hyperplasia in adipose tissue. The early increase in adipocyte number reported in obese children (Knittle et al., 1979) (Fig. 4.3) might explain early adiposity rebound. In addition, high protein intakes, at all ages, might lead to lower GH levels, reduced lipolysis and the development and maintenance of fat stores (Table 4.3).

4.3.2 Relationship between macronutrient intake and body fat distribution

Protein excess seems particularly associated with fat located at the abdominal level rather than other sites (Rolland-Cachera et al., 1996b). This association has been

Table 4.3. Hypotheses on the various origins of obesity and associated disorders

Risk factors	Consequences
Early childhood	
Excess protein intake	$\Uparrow$ IGF-1 $\Rightarrow$ Cell proliferation in all tissues
	Accelerated growth
	Adipose tissue hyperplasia
All ages	
Excess protein intake	$\Downarrow$ Growth hormone $\Rightarrow$ $\Downarrow$ Lypolysis
	$\Uparrow$ Abdominal fat ('Syndrome X')
High energy intake and/or low energy expenditure	Positive energy balance $\Rightarrow$ $\Uparrow$ Body fat

shown in both cross-sectional (Rolland-Cachera et al., 1986; Buemann, 1995) and longitudinal studies (Rolland-Cachera et al., 1995). The hypothesis of an association between excessive protein intake and decreased GH is consistent with an association between high protein intake and android body fat distribution, as this fat pattern is also characteristic of GH deficiency (Zachmann et al., 1980). Such an association would suggest a role for excessive protein intake in the development of the metabolic complications of obesity such as insulin resistance, cardiovascular disease and some cancers (Vague, 1956; Björntorp, 1996).

In summary, it is often suggested that high energy or high fat intakes predispose to obesity. No clear evidence for this emerges from epidemiological studies conducted in children – although similar inconsistencies are reported in adults (Seidell, 1998; Willett, 1998). Thus, contrary to the usual views, protein excess, rather than fat excess, may well account for the various characteristics associated with obesity during growth.

4.4 Qualitative assessment of intake behaviour

Food intakes can be investigated qualitatively as well as quantitatively. The quantity of food ingested daily is obviously important, but meal patterns and the selection of particular foods are other important aspects of feeding behaviour which can have decisive influences on growth and development.

4.4.1 Circadian distribution of food intake and adiposity

In both adults and children, epidemiological data reveal wide differences in patterns of eating which seem to relate to fatness. Obese individuals eat less than nonobese controls in the morning and more in the evening. For example, in a group of 339 French 7- to 12-year-old children, breakfast represented 15.7% of daily energy intake in the obese ($n = 48$) whereas it accounted for 19.2% of daily energy intake in controls of average BMI ($n = 172$). By contrast, dinner accounted for 32.5% of total daily energy intake in the same group of obese children and only 28.7% in controls of average BMI (Bellisle et al., 1988).

In obese adults, Stunkard (1955) has described extreme cases characterized by morning anorexia and massive eating in the late hours of the day or even during the night. The 'night eating syndrome' may be present, perhaps in milder form, in many obese children.

In animal models of obesity, one significant behavioural characteristic is disappearance, or at least disturbance, of the normal day/night feeding cycle. In normal-weight animals, feeding is restricted to one phase of the daily illumination cycle (the light or the dark phase). During the alternate phase, the animal does not eat. A superimposed metabolic cycle facilitates lipogenesis in the active phase when the animal periodically eats and lipolysis in the inactive phase. Such alternation of lipogenesis and lipolysis appears essential for body weight regulation (Le Magnen, 1992). When an animal is made obese with surgical, chemical, or dietary manipulations, one of the first behavioural signs of the developing body adiposity is the loss of alternating day/night-feeding cycles.

In children, it is not clear whether some primary defect in diurnal metabolism induces peculiar feeding patterns or whether eating habits, perhaps reinforced by attempts to lose weight, alter diurnal rhythm with potential obesity-promoting metabolic effects. Cause and effect remain unclear. However, weight-reduction programmes often redistribute the energy ration over the waking hours, with a special emphasis on breakfast. The contribution of this aspect of behaviour modification on long-term treatment outcome is unknown.

4.4.2 Daily meal number

Following several observations of an inverse relationship between body adiposity and daily meal number, Fabry et al. (1966) performed an intervention study in which two schools for 6- to 16-year-olds were selected for comparison of three-meal-a-day versus seven-meal-a-day regimes. A third school remained on its normal five meals a day regimen ($n = 226$). Energy intakes were planned to be the same in all three groups. After one year, some anthropometric parameters suggested an increase in adiposity in 10- to 16-year-old subjects who ingested three daily meals as compared to five or seven. No such indication appeared in younger children.

The study has been replicated many times, mostly in adults, and the findings repeated (Bellisle et al., 1997). However, recent questions about the validity of estimated nutrient intakes, due to the high levels of under-reporting, have cast doubt on the existence of any relationship between meals per day and weight status. Even so, under-reporting has been demonstrated to affect energy intake records, but not recorded numbers of eating episodes.

The uneven eating patterns of many obese subjects, with low intakes in the morning, frequent breakfast skipping, and substantial eating starting in the afternoon, suggest that energy intakes are met by fewer, larger meals than with lean subjects. The direction of causality here is unknown. Does gorging (few, large meals) late in the day facilitate fat accumulation, or does obesity, with irrational efforts at dieting, induce peculiar meal patterns?

Current literature confirms, without reasonable doubt, that diets are no more successful when offered as several small meals a day or as a few larger ones (Bellisle et al., 1997). The amount of weight lost during dieting is critically dependent on the energy deficit, irrespective of the number of meals eaten.

Eating a few meals a day may facilitate weight gain, but eating several daily meals a day does not help weight loss.

4.4.3 Snacking

Large quantities of energy can be ingested outside mealtimes as snacks – a frequent part of the daily eating schedule in children – and as semi-automatic nibbling where the consumer is not fully aware of the amount of food ingested. Long hours in front of the television set are potentially free for semi-conscious stomach filling with 'junk' foods. Obviously, such intake is unlikely to be reported precisely in dietary surveys.

Extra-prandial eating is practised by both obese and nonobese (Basdevant et al., 1993). How much snacking and nibbling contribute to energy intakes is difficult to assess. The nature of foods selected for extra-prandial intake also deserves consideration. In obese women, the nutrient content of snack foods was closer to nutritional recommendations than the nutrient content of meals. Again, under-reporting or selective reporting is suspected.

4.4.4 Binge eating

Binge eating occurs not only in bulimia nervosa, but in the obese as well (American Psychiatric Association, 1990). Some obese individuals report binges, with rapid ingestion of large amounts of food, accompanied with feelings of loss of control. Whether this behaviour only follows periods of dieting or whether it is a primary feature of disordered eating is still debated. In obesity (in contrast to bulimia nervosa), no 'corrective' behaviours such as purging or self-induced vomiting take place. Thus excessive energy intakes during binges create a positive energy balance, which is unlikely to be counterbalanced by strict dieting or fasting. Frequent nonbulimic bingers are thus heading for obesity.

4.4.5 Other behavioural symptoms

Some obese subjects have a tendency to eat faster than their lean controls (Bellisle & Le Magnen, 1981). They fail to respond to sensations of satiety (Meyer & Pudel, 1972). In the clinical context, some obese patients claim that they never experience satiety (Stunkard, 1955). These characteristics could be secondary to chronic dieting but could reflect fundamental metabolic and/or behavioural problems. There is need for further investigation.

It should always be remembered that, whilst some obese subjects have obvious behavioural problems such as nibbling, gorging and bingeing, many never show this sort of behaviour. Human behaviour is extremely diverse and we must be very cautious when we make generalizations.

4.4.6 Food preferences

Contrary to popular belief, a sweet tooth is not characteristic of obese children and adults. Obese subjects usually have only a modest appetite for sweet foods and, by contrast, heavy consumers of sweet foods are rarely obese (Garn et al., 1980; Bolton-Smith, 1996). In a group of 6-year-old children, daily sucrose consumption ranged between 22 g and 88 g (Rolland-Cachera et al., 1993). However, the mean BMI of children in each of the quartiles of sucrose consumption were the same. Apparently, children with high intakes of sucrose, who also eat more of other nutrients, have higher energy needs than low-intake peers. They find rapidly available energy in sucrose and use it. Their dietary intake is also closer to recommended nutrient distributions than that of their lower-sucrose-intake peers.

Most dietary surveys suggest a preference for dietary fats in obese children and adults (Drewnowski & Schwartz, 1990). High-fat sweet foods are highly rated by both obese (Drewnowski, 1985; Drewnowski et al., 1985, 1992) and normal-weight individuals. In North America, foods preferred by most (obese and nonobese) children are rich in energy (Drewnowski, 1988). Epidemiological surveys, which show no correlations between energy intakes and body weight status, are inconsistent in finding positive correlations between fat intake and relative adiposity.

Progress in the understanding of dietary fat metabolism has shown how dietary lipids facilitate fat deposition (Flatt, 1987; Dreon et al., 1988; Datillo, 1992; Gazzaniga & Burns, 1993; Bolton-Smith & Woodward, 1994; Lissner & Heitmann, 1995; Nguyen et al., 1996; Tremblay & Saint-Pierre, 1996). Fat intake levels in children predict body adiposity (Gazzaniga & Burns, 1993; Nguyen et al., 1996). In North America, fat children of fat parents enjoy fatty foods and eat them in large quantities (Johnson & Birch, 1994; Fisher & Birch, 1995).

Fat children also consume more protein than their lean peers. Obese children on very-low-calorie diets (VLCD) are usually encouraged to perpetuate the high protein content of their usual diet, often beyond the level of their protein needs. The rationality of this strategy has been questioned recently (Rolland-Cachera et al., 1998). Dieting adolescents lose weight as successfully on low-calorie diets that meet protein needs, as on classical low-calorie, high-protein, highly unbalanced diets.

4.5 Lifestyle

Eating occurs within a particular environment. The food environment of obese children is different from that of nonobese children (Fisher & Birch, 1995). Socioeconomic factors for example influence the intakes acceptable to families, and thus children's reactions to foods and diets. Obesity is more prevalent in those social strata where typical nutrient intakes are relatively high (Rolland-Cachera & Bellisle, 1986). Fat parents create specific food environments for their children (Fisher & Birch, 1995) since, in addition to their genetically transmitted predisposition to overweight, fat parents often raise their children in environments where the selection of fatty food is easy and encouraged.

Work by Birch and collaborators (1980, 1982, 1984, 1985, 1986, 1990) has demonstrated the importance of learning mechanisms in the acquisition of food likes and dislikes. Children learn to accept and like a wide variety of foods during childhood and adolescence. As new substances are presented to growing children, a hierarchy of likes and dislikes is formed. Repeated exposure to foods with diverse appearance and diverse nutritional content shapes the development of taste for a variety of foods and facilitates the selection of a varied diet (Pliner, 1982). In the same way, repeated exposure to high-fat foods is likely to encourage a 'taste' for them (Johnson et al., 1991).

Parental strategies orientating the food choices of their children can be very influential, but not necessarily in the directions expected. For example, foods used as rewards for the performance of 'good' behaviour can lead to reinforcing their positive value with children. Sweets given as reward become more desirable. Foods whose consumption is seen as worthy of reward by other foods, become less attractive. Foods only consumed under duress become frankly aversive. Peer influences play a major role in the evolution of preferences in school-aged children. Children who accept few foods at home are often perfectly happy to eat much more varied diets in the school cafeteria, especially under a leading peer's influence. These learned attitudes contribute to the acquisition of particular food selections by a particular culture (Rozin, 1998) and specific social and family environments. It is not known whether obese subjects respond differently to these processes. Fussy though these children sometimes are, their problem is hardly one of getting to like foods but of learning how to limit intakes of very enjoyable foods so as to maintain energy balance.

Children are, reportedly, 'good regulators' of energy balance. Four- to five-year-olds adjust their spontaneous intakes at a meal to the energy density of earlier food consumption (Birch & Deysher, 1985, 1986). Children also show considerable ability to associate the sensory characteristics of foods with the level of satiety experienced following ingestion. This subconscious skill, dependent on both unconditioned and conditioned mechanisms, makes children very competent at adjusting intakes to needs. Perhaps some obese children are less competent than their normal-weight peers. Parental directives ('Eat your plate up') can lead to the loss or the weakening of these seemingly innate abilities in children. The effects of such parental orders are to focus on arbitrary cues (for example the size of a serving) as a guide to behaviour, rather than on internal signals of hunger or satiety. Such 'external' control of eating behaviour makes internal biological signals irrelevant and can leave children progressively less capable of responding to them. These mechanisms can exert adverse effects on body weight control but are obese children more easily affected by them than their lean peers? The chronic dieting often imposed on overweight children creates circumstances where internal signals of hunger are disregarded and where the 'diet' determines meal size and meal number. Intermittent hyperphagia or eating binges in some dieters show that internal signals do recover their influence sometimes. However, responses to subtle, changing biological cues are highly likely to be altered as a result of chronic dieting (Herman & Polivy, 1988; Wilson, 1995).

Energy expenditure in physical activity has been decreasing steadily over many years. Children and adults move less and less. Television and computer games have added to the energy-saving effects of private cars, elevators and central heating. The cumulative effect of these factors is difficult to quantify precisely. Television viewing alone plays an important role in the daily energy balance (see Chapter 12).

Physical activity can take place as part of a formal sporting occasion, or as an intimate part of everyday life. The latter, whilst perhaps unnoticed, is not unimportant. Minor, but repeated, behavioural choices (e.g. stairs preferred to lift) can add up to large energy expenditures and thus contribute significantly to energy balance. Recent data in French children (Deheeger et al., 1997) suggest that daily energy expenditure acts not only directly on energy balance but also indirectly, through affecting food choices. The most active children in a population ($n = 84$) of 10-year-olds had the same BMI as their less active peers. However, they ate

much more. The nutrient source that was significantly augmented in the most active children was CHO. These children had larger breakfasts and afternoon snacks. They ingested more cereal and dairy products. Since they consumed more CHO, the percentage of fat in the diet was lower and, consequently, their macronutrient distribution was closer to recommendations. Although it is not possible to claim any causal effects, it can be hypothesized that higher needs in the more active children led to different food choices, at different times during the day, and that rapid energy sources (CHO) were often preferred to high fat foods. More research is needed in this area in order to disclose exact cause and effect relationships.

4.6 Conclusions

There is abundant literature about the nutrition of obese individuals, particularly obese children. Some clear observations emerge from this analysis.

- In industrialized countries, the prevalence of obesity is rising, in spite of falling energy intakes. The diminished energy intake is largely due to decreased fat intake, with inconsistent changes in CHO intake and often increases in the percentage of energy provided by protein. The changes also reflect a decrease in foods of vegetable origin and an increase in animal products.

- Energy intakes in the obese are not higher than those of nonobese controls when assessed in epidemiological studies. The results could be explained by bias due to under-reporting in the obese. Protein intakes are always very high. Many studies show protein intakes are higher in obese than in lean children. CHO intakes are negatively correlated with adiposity. There is a ubiquitous nutritional imbalance in children's diets: too little fat in weanlings; too much fat a few years later; excessive protein intake at all ages once breast feeding ceases.

- Excess body fat is associated with alterations in lean body mass (LBM) and hormonal status (decreased IGF-1 and raised GH). These characteristics could be attributed to infants' early excessive protein intakes.

- Obese and nonobese children show different diurnal eating patterns. The obese children eat less in the morning and more later in the day.

- Some behavioural traits, present in certain individuals (snacking, bingeing, late-day or night eating, etc.) facilitate the development or persistence of obesity. These are not present in all obese individuals, whether children or adults.

- Obese children and adults do not exhibit excessive appetite for sweet foods. They enjoy high-fat foods. High-fat sweet foods (cakes, biscuits, pies, ice cream, etc.) are highly popular with obese and nonobese individuals alike. Conversely, most studies find high consumers of sweet foods are not fatter than low consumers of sweet foods.

- Physical activity reduces the risk of obesity, via its role in energy expenditure. In addition it is associated with high CHO intake, which brings daily nutrient intakes closer to recommended macronutrient distribution.
- Children appear to have an innate ability to adjust energy intakes to nutritional status. The amount of food taken at a meal is influenced by what has been ingested at recent meals. This precious competence seems to be lost during growth, perhaps due to parents' control over their children's behaviour. It is not known whether this regulatory competence is absent in obese children or whether it is disrupted by early attempts at dieting.

Despite existing knowledge, it is difficult to draw clear conclusions and develop potent nutritional strategies with which to treat or prevent obesity in children. Although hypotheses have been proposed regarding high fat and/or high sugar intakes, they are not supported by epidemiological data. Excessive protein intakes are proposed as a causal factor, more research is needed in this area.

We recommend:

- the nutrient balance of the diet should be adapted to meet specific needs at each period of growth;
- behaviours and lifestyles can be shaped to facilitate healthy eating practices such as daily breakfast, adequate distribution of eating over the waking hours and appropriate stimulus control so as to reduce overeating.

In other words, healthy lifestyles should be adopted by all, obese and nonobese alike, in order to counter our 'increasingly obesogenic environment' (Egger & Swinburn, 1997).

4.7 REFERENCES

Ailhaud, G., Grimaldi, P. & Négrel, R. (1992). A molecular view of adipose tissue. *International Journal of Obesity*, **16**, 17–21.

American Psychiatric Association (1990). *Diagnostic and Statistical Manual of Mental Disorders*, 4th edn. Washington DC: American Psychiatric Association.

Ballard-Barbash, R., Graubard, I., Krebs-Smith, S.M., Schatzkin, A. & Thompson, F.E. (1996). Contribution of dieting to the inverse association between energy intake and body mass index. *European Journal of Clinical Nutrition*, **50**, 98–106.

Basdevant, A., Craplet, C. & Guy-Grand, B. (1993). Snacking patterns in obese French women. *Appetite*, **21**, 17–23.

Bellisle, F. & Le Magnen, J. (1981). The structure of meals in humans: eating and drinking patterns in lean and obese subjects. *Physiology and Behaviour*, **27**, 649–58.

Bellisle, F., Rolland-Cachera, M.F., Deheeger, M. & Guilloud-Bataille, M. (1988). Obesity and food intake in children: Evidence for a role of metabolic and/or behavioral daily rhythms. *Appetite*, **11**, 111–18.

Bellisle, F., McDevitt, R. & Prentice, A.M. (1997). Meal frequency and energy balance. *British Journal of Nutrition*, **77**, Suppl. 1, S57–S70.

Bellù, R., Ortisi, M.T., Incerti, P., Mazzoleni, V., Martinoli, G., Agostini, C., Galluzzo, C., Riva, E. & Giovanini, M. (1991). Nutritional survey on a sample of one year old infants in Milan: intake of macronutrients. *Nutrition Research*, **11**, 1221–9.

Birch, L.L. & Deysher, M. (1985). Conditioned and unconditioned caloric compensation: Evidence for self regulation of food intake in young children. *Learning and Motivation*, **16**, 341–55.

Birch, L.L. & Deysher, M. (1986). Caloric compensation and sensory specific satiety: Evidence for self regulation of food intake by young children. *Appetite*, **7**, 323–31.

Birch, L.L., Zimmerman, S. & Hind, H. (1980). The influence of social-affective context on the formation of children's food preferences. *Child Development*, **51**, 856–61.

Birch, L.L., Birch, D., Marlin, D.W. & Kramer, L. (1982). Effects of instrumental consumption on children's food preference. *Appetite*, **3**, 125–34.

Birch, L.L., Marlin, D.W. & Rotter, J. (1984). Eating as the 'means' activity in a contingency: effects on young children's food preferences. *Child Development*, **55**, 431–9.

Birch, L.L., McPhee, L., Steinberg, L. & Sullivan, S. (1990). Conditioned flavor preferences in young children. *Physiology and Behaviour*, **47**, 501–5.

Björntorp, P. (1996). The regulation of adipose tissue distribution in humans. *International Journal of Obesity*, **20**, 291–302.

Blundell, J.E. & Tremblay, A. (1995). Appetite control and energy (fuel) balance. *Nutrition Research Reviews*, **8**, 225–42.

Bock, R.D. & Sykes, R.C. (1989). Evidence for continuing secular increase in height within families in the United States. *American Journal of Human Biology*, **1**, 143–6.

Bolton-Smith, C. (1996). Intake of sugars in relation to fatness and micronutrient adequacy. *International Journal of Obesity*, **20** suppl. 2, S31–S33.

Bolton-Smith, C. & Woodward, M. (1994). Dietary composition and fat to sugar ratios in relation to obesity. *International Journal of Obesity*, **18**, 820–8.

Buemann, B., Tremblay, A. & Bouchard, C. (1995). Social class interacts with the association between macronutrient intake and subcutaneous fat. *International Journal of Obesity and Related Metabolic Disorders*, **19**, 770–75.

Capdevilla, F., Vizmanos, B. & Marti-Henneberg, C. (1998). Implications of the weaning pattern on macronutrient intake, food volume and energy density in non-breast fed infants during the first year of life. *Journal of the American College of Nutrition*, **17**, 256–62.

Datillo, A.M (1992). Dietary fat and its relationship to body weight. *Nutrition Today*, **27**, 13–19.

Davies, P.S.W. (1997). Diet composition and body mass index in pre-school children. *European Journal of Clinical Nutrition*, **51**, 443–8.

Deheeger, M., Rolland-Cachera, M.F., Péquignot, F., Labadie, M. & Rossignol, C. (1991). Evolution de l'alimentation des enfants de 2 ans entre 1973 et 1986. *Annals of Nutrition and Metabolism*, **140**, 132–46.

Deheeger, M., Rolland-Cachera, M.F., Labadie. M.D. & Rossignol, C. (1994). Etude longitudinale de la croissance et de l'alimentation d'enfants examinés de l'âge de 10 mois à 8 ans. *Cahiers de Nutrition et de Diététique*, **1**, 16–23.

Deheeger, M., Rolland-Cachera, M.F. & Fontvieille, A.M. (1997). Physical activity and body composition in 10-year-old French children: linkages with nutritional intake? *International Journal of Obesity*, **21**, 372–9.

Dreon, D.M., Frey-Hewitt, B., Ellsworth, N., Williams, P.T., Terry, E.B. & Wood, P.D. (1988). Dietary fat: carbohydrate ratio and obesity in middle-aged men. *American Journal of Clinical Nutrition*, **47**, 995–1000.

Drewnowski, A. (1985). Food perceptions and preferences of obese adults: a multidimensional approach. *International Journal of Obesity*, **9**, 201–12.

Drewnowski, A. (1988). Sweet foods and sweeteners in the U.S. diet. In *Diet and Obesity*, ed. G.Bray, pp. 153–61. Basel: Karger.

Drewnowski, A. & Popkin, B.M. (1997). The nutrition transition: new trends in the global diet. *Nutrition Reviews*, **55**, 31–43.

Drewnowski, A. & Schwartz, M. (1990). Invisible fats: sensory assessment of sugar/fat mixtures. *Appetite*, **14**, 203–17.

Drewnowski, A., Brunzell, J.D., Sande, K., Iverius, P.H. & Greenwood, M.R.C. (1985). Sweet tooth reconsidered: taste responsiveness in human obesity. *Physiology and Behaviour*, **35**, 617–22.

Drewnowski, A., Krahn, D.D., Demitrack, M.A., Nairn, K. & Gosnell, B.A. (1992). Taste responses and preferences for sweet high-fat foods: evidence for opioid involvement. *Physiology and Behaviour*, **51**, 371–9.

Egger, G. & Swinburn, B. (1997). An 'ecological' approach to the obesity pandemic. *British Medical Journal*, **315**, 477–80.

Eveleth, P. & Tanner, J.M. (1990). *World-wide Variation in Human Growth*, 2nd edn. Cambridge: Cambridge University Press.

Fabry, P., Hejda, S., Cerna, K., Osoncova, K., Pechor, J. & Zvolankova, K. (1966). Effect of meal frequency in schoolchildren: changes in weight–height proportion and skinfold thickness. *American Journal of Clinical Nutrition*, **18**, 358–61.

Fisher, J.O. & Birch, L.L. (1995). Fat preference and fat consumption of 3- to 5-year-old children are related to parental adiposity. *Journal of the American Dietetic Association*, **95**, 759–64.

Flatt, J.P. (1987). Dietary fat, carbohydrate balance, and weight maintenance: effects of exercise. *American Journal of Clinical Nutrition*, **45**, 296–306.

Forbes, G.B. (1962). Methods for determining composition of the human body. *Pediatrics*, **29**, 477–94.

Frank, G.C., Berenson, G.S. & Webber, L.S. (1978). Dietary studies and the relationship of diet to cardiovascular disease risk factor variables in 10-years-old children: the Bogalusa Heart Study. *American Journal of Clinical Nutrition*, **31**, 328–40.

Garn, S.M., Solomon, M.A. & Cole, P.E. (1980). Sugar-food intake of obese and lean adolescents. *Ecology of Food and Nutrition*, **9**, 219–22.

Gazzaniga, J.M. & Burns, T.L. (1993). Relationship between diet composition and body fatness, with adjustment for resting expenditure and physical activity in preadolescent children. *American Journal of Clinical Nutrition*, **58**, 21–8.

Gortmaker, S.L., Dietz, W.H. Jr, Sobol, A.M. & Wehler, C.A. (1987). Increasing pediatric obesity in the United States. *American Journal of Diseases of Children*, **141**, 535–40.

Gregory, J.R., Collins, D.L., Davies, P.S.W., Hughes, J.M. & Clarke, P.C. (1995). *National Diet and Nutrition Survey: Children Aged 1.5 to 4.5 years.* London: HMSO.

Hampton, M.C., Hueneman, R.L., Shapiro, L.R. & Mitchell, B.W. (1967). Caloric and nutritional intake of teenagers. *Journal of the American Dietetic Association*, **50**, 385–96.

Heini, A.F. & Weinsier, R.L. (1997). Divergent trends in obesity and fat intake patterns: the American paradox. *American Journal of Medicine*, **102**, 259–64.

Herman, C.P. & Polivy, J. (1988). Studies of eating in normal dieters. In *Eating Behavior in Eating Disorders*, ed. B.T. Walsh, pp. 97–111. Washington DC: American Psychiatric Association.

Hughes, J.M., Chinn, L.L. & Rona R.J. (1997). Trends in growth in England and Scotland, 1972 to 1994. *Archives of Disease in Childhood*, **76**, 182–9.

Johnson, S.L. & Birch, L.L. (1994). Parents' and children's adiposity and eating style. *Pediatrics*, **94**, 653–61.

Johnson, S.L., McPhee, L. & Birch, L.L. (1991). Conditioned preferences: young children prefer flavors associated with high dietary fat. *Physiology and Behaviour*, **50**, 1245–51.

Knittle, J.L., Timmers, K., Ginsberg-Fellner, F., Brown, R.E. & Katz, D.P. (1979). The growth of adipose tissue in children and adolescents. Cross sectional and longitudinal studies of adipose cell number and size. *Journal of Clinical Investigation*, **63**, 239–46.

Le Magnen, J. (1992). *Neurobiology of Feeding and Nutrition.* San Diego: Academic Press.

Lissner, L. & Heitmann, B.L. (1995). Dietary fat and obesity: evidence from epidemiology. *European Journal of Clinical Nutrition*, **49**, 79–90.

Loche, S., Cappa, M., Borrelli, A., Faedda, A., Crino, A., Cella, S.G., Corda, R., Müller, E.E. & Pintor, C. (1987). Reduced growth hormone response to growth hormone-releasing hormone in children with simple obesity: evidence for somatomedin-C mediated inhibition. *Clinical Endocrinology*, **27**, 145–53.

Meyer, J.E. & Pudel, V. (1972). Experimental studies on food intake in obese and normal weight subjects. *Journal of Psychosomatic Research*, **16**, 305–8.

Michaelsen, K.F. & Jorgensen, M.H. (1995). Dietary fat content and energy density during infancy and childhood: the effect on energy intake and growth. *European Journal of Clinical Nutrition*, **49**, 467–83.

Mumford, P. & Morgan, J.B. (1982). A longitudinal study of nutrition and growth of infants initially on the upper and lower centiles for weight and age. *International Journal of Obesity*, **6**, 335–41.

Nguyen, V.T., Larson, D.E., Johnson, R.K. & Goran, M.I. (1996). Fat intake and adiposity in children of lean and obese parents. *American Journal of Clinical Nutrition*, **64**, 507–13.

Nicklas, T.A., Webber, L.S., Srinivasan, S.R. & Berenson, G. (1993). Secular trends in dietary intakes and cardiovascular risk factors of 10-y-old children: The Bogalusa Heart Study (1973–1988). *American Journal of Clinical Nutrition*, **57**, 930–7.

Oppert, J.M. & Rolland-Cachera, M.F. (1998). Prévalence, évolution dans le temps et conséquences économiques de l'obésité. *Médecine/Sciences*, **14**, 939–43.

Ortega, R.M., Requejo, A.M., Andres, P., Lopez-Sobaler, A.M., Redondo, R. & Gonzalez-

Fernandez, M. (1995). Relationship between diet composition and body mass index in a group of Spanish adolescents. *British Medical Journal*, **74**, 765–73.

Palti, H., Reshef, A. & Adler, B. (1979). Food intake and growth of children between 30 and 48 months of age in Jerusalem. *Pediatrics*, **63**, 713–18.

Pliner, P. (1982). The effects of mere exposure on liking for edible substances. *Appetite*, **3**, 283–290.

Poskitt, E.M.E. & Cole, T.J. (1978). Nature, nurture and childhood overweight. *British Medical Journal*, **1**, 603–5.

Prentice, A.M. & Jebb, S.A. (1995). Obesity in Britain: gluttony or sloth? *British Medical Journal*, **311**, 437–9.

Räsänen, L., Ahola, M., Kara, R. & Uhari, M. (1985). Atherosclerosis precursors in Finnish children and adolescents. VII. Food consumption and nutrient intakes. *Acta Paediatrica Scandinavica*, **135** (Suppl. 318), 135–53.

Rolland-Cachera, M.F. (1995). Prediction of adult body composition from childhood measurements. In *Body Composition Techniques in Health and Disease*, eds. P.S.W. Davies & T.J. Cole, pp. 100–45. Cambridge: Cambridge University Press.

Rolland-Cachera, M.F. & Bellisle, F. (1986). No correlation between adiposity and food intake: why are working class children fatter? *American Journal of Clinical Nutrition*, **44**, 779–87.

Rolland-Cachera, M.F., Bellisle, F., Péquignot, F., Guilloud-Bataille, M. & Vinit, F. (1988). Adiposity and food intake in young children: the environmental challenge to individual susceptibility. *British Medical Journal*, **276**, 1037–8.

Rolland-Cachera, M.F., Deheeger, M., Bellisle, F., Péquignot, F. & Rossignol, F. (1993). Consommation de glucides chez l'enfant. *Information Diététique*, **1**, 18–25.

Rolland-Cachera, M.F., Deheeger, M., Akrout, M. & Bellisle, F. (1995). Influence of macronutrients on adiposity development: a follow-up study of nutrition and growth from 10 months to 8 years of age. *International Journal of Obesity*, **19**, 573–8.

Rolland-Cachera, M.F. Deheeger, M. & Bellisle, F. (1996a). Nutritional changes between 1978 and 1995 in 10 years old French children. *International Journal of Obesity*, **20** (suppl. 4), Abstr. 105, 53.

Rolland-Cachera, M.F., Deheeger, M. & Bellisle, F. (1996b). Nutrient balance and android body fat distribution: why not a role for protein? *American Journal of Clinical Nutrition*, **64**, 663–4.

Rolland-Cachera, M.F., Thibault, H., Soulié, D., Carbonel, P., Roinsol, D., Deheeger, M., Pons, C., Longueville, E. & Serog, P. (1998). Weight loss in two groups of obese children consuming diets containing different amounts of protein. *International Journal of Obesity*, **22** (suppl. 4), S32.

Rolland-Cachera, M.F., Deheeger, M. & Bellisle, F. (1999). Increasing prevalence of obesity among 18-year-old males in Sweden: evidence for early determinants. *Acta Paediatrica*, **88**, 365–7.

Rosskamp, R., Becker, M. & Soetadji, S. (1987). Circulating somatomedin-C levels and the effect of growth releasing factor on plasma levels of growth hormone and somatomedin-like immunoreactivity in obese children. *European Journal of Pediatrics*, **146**, 48–50.

Rozin, P. (1998). *Towards a Psychology of Food Choice*. Danone Chair Monograph. Brussels: Institut Danone.

Schlicker, S.A., Borra, S.T. & Regan, C. (1994). The weight and fitness status of United States children. *Nutrition Reviews*, **52**, 11–17.

Seidell, J.C. (1997). Time trends in obesity: an epidemiological perspective. *Hormone and Metabolic Research*, **29**, 155–8.

Seidell, J.C. (1998). Dietary fat and obesity: an epidemiologic perspective. *American Journal of Clinical Nutrition*, **67** (suppl.), 546S–50S.

Spyckerelle, Y., Herbeth, B. & Deschamps, J.P. (1992). Dietary behaviour of an adolescent French male population. *Journal of Human Nutrition and Dietetics*, **5**, 161–8.

Stunkard, A.J. (1955). Untoward reactions to weight reduction among certain obese persons. *Annals of the New York Academy of Sciences*, **63**, 4–5.

Sunnegardh, J., Bratteby, L.E., Hagman, U., Samuelson, G. & Sjolin, S. (1986). Physical activity in relation to energy intake and body fat in 8- and 13-year-old children in Sweden. *Acta Paediatrica Scandinavica*, **75**, 955–63.

Takaishi, M. (1994). Secular changes in growth of Japanese children. *Journal of Pediatric Endocrinology and Metabolism*, **7**, 163–73.

Thissen, J.P., Ketelsleger, J.M. & Underwood. L.E. (1994). Nutritional regulation of the insulin-like growth factors. *Endocrine Reviews*, **15**, 80–101.

Tremblay, A. & Saint-Pierre, S. (1996). The hyperphagic effect of a high-fat diet and alcohol intake persists after control for energy density. *American Journal of Clinical Nutrition*, **63**, 479–82.

Tucker, L.A., Seljaas, G.T. & Hager, R.L. (1997). Body fat percentage of children varies according to their diet composition. *Journal of the American Dietetic Association*, **97**, 981–6.

Vague, J. (1956). The degree of masculine differentiation of obesities: a factor determining predisposition to diabetes, arteriosclerosis, gout, and uric calculous diseases. *American Journal of Clinical Nutrition*, **4**, 20–34.

Valoski, A. & Epstein, L.H. (1990). Nutrient intake of obese children in a family-based behavioral weight control program. *International Journal of Obesity*, **14**, 667–77.

Van Vliet, G., Bosson, D., Rummens, E., Robyn, C. & Wolter, R. (1986). Evidence against growth hormone releasing factor deficiency in children with idiopathic obesity. *Acta Endocrinologica*, **279** Suppl., 403–10.

Vobecky, J.S., Vobecky, J., Shapcott, D. & Demers, P.P. (1983). Nutrient intake patterns and nutritional status with regard to relative weight in early infancy. *American Journal of Clinical Nutrition*, **38**, 730–8.

Waterlow, J.C. (1992) *Protein-Energy Malnutrition*. 2nd edn. London: Edward Arnold.

Whitehead, R.G., Paul, A.A. & Cole, T.J. (1982). Trends in food energy intakes throughout childhood from one to 18 years. *Human Nutrition: Applied Nutrition*, **36**, 57–62.

WHO (1985). *Energy and Protein Requirements. Report of a Joint Expert Consultation*. Food and Agriculture Organization, World Health Organization, United Nation University (WHO technical report series, No 274). Geneva: World Health Organization.

Willett, W.C. (1998). Is dietary fat a major determinant of body fat? *American Journal of Clinical Nutrition*, **67** (suppl.), 556S–62S.

Wilson, T.G. (1995). The controversy over dieting. In *Eating Disorders and Obesity*, eds. K.D. Brownell & C.G. Fairburn, pp. 87–91. New York: Guilford Press.

Woodward, D.R. (1985). What sort of teenager has high intakes of energy and nutrients? *British Journal of Nutrition*, **54**, 325–33.

Zachmann, M., Fernandez, F., Tassinari, D., Thakker, R. & Prader, A. (1980). Anthropometric measurements in patients with growth hormone deficiency before treatment with human growth hormone. *European Journal of Pediatrics*, **133**, 277–82.

Physical activity

Yves Schutz[1] and Claudio Maffeis[2]

[1]Institute of Physiology, University of Lausanne. [2]Department of Paediatrics, University Hospital, Verona

5.1 Introduction

Normal growth in children involves large fluctuations in both daily energy intake and expenditure and, hence, acute daily fluctuations in energy balance. This indicates the complex interaction of different control mechanisms that must coexist to maintain adequate body weight and body composition during growth and maturation (Rosenbaum & Leibel, 1998). The exact mechanisms involved in body weight regulation remain largely unknown.

In many adults, stability of body weight and body composition over long periods of time indicates that energy and macronutrient intakes and expenditures are balanced. By contrast, in growing children, energy and substrate intakes must be chronically greater than energy expenditures and total substrate oxidation, though not necessarily on a daily basis, in order to accommodate normal growth. Thus, obesity in children can be viewed as 'overgrowth' of the adipose tissue normally synthesized to achieve normal body composition.

This chapter will review current knowledge relating to physical activity and inactivity in the development of obesity during childhood.

5.2 Energy expenditure assessment

A number of methods have been developed to assess total energy expenditure (TEE) in free-living conditions (Schutz & Deurenberg, 1996). The most recent method is the doubly labelled water technique based on the utilization of stable isotopes using heavy water (deuterium and oxygen 18). Detailed explanation of the method is given elsewhere (Schoeller et al., 1986). With the use of new stable-isotope techniques, researchers now have a (relatively expensive) tool with which to investigate the relationship between energy balance and body weight change in much greater detail than before, and to develop working hypotheses relating to the aetiology of obesity in children. Other more traditional methods of assessing physical activity in the free living environment include heart-rate monitoring (after assessing the individual relationship between heart rate and energy expenditure), and less objective methods of documenting activity using diaries, time and motion records, and interviews. More recently accelerometry has also been used (Schutz et al., 2002).

5.3 Energy intake vs. energy expenditure

Prospective studies of the development of obesity in children clearly identify dietary intake as a risk factor for body fat gain (Klesges et al., 1995). A positive relationship between relative fat intake (expressed as a percentage of total energy intake) and the level of adiposity (expressed as percentage body fat) (Maffeis et al., 1996a) has been observed in obese children. Yet, recent data from the USA suggest that, on average, children's diets have been getting progressively lower in total energy for decades. This is in contrast to the steady increase in the prevalence of childhood obesity (Troiano & Flegal, 1998). The explanation for this paradox of higher prevalence of obesity despite reduced total energy intake must be a progressive decline in the total energy requirements of North American children. A similar situation applies in Europe.

Most available information indicates that the *self-reported* energy intakes of obese children are not higher but comparable, or even lower, than those of their lean counterparts (Johnson et al., 1956; Wilkinson et al., 1977; Elliot et al., 1989). Since TEE is higher in the obese than in the lean, one can infer that, in order to maintain normal body growth, the total energy intake of the obese must be greater than that of their lean peers. If we accept these self-reported intakes as accurate, obese children appear to have greater metabolic 'efficiency' and/or reduced levels of physical activity, when compared with nonobese children. However, energy balance studies have demonstrated that obese children and adolescents consume *more* food energy than their lean counterparts (Bandini et al., 1990a; Livingstone et al., 1992; Maffeis et al., 1994b; DeLany et al., 1995). Moreover, a significant correlation between the percentage of under-reporting of energy intake and body weight has also been observed, indicating that obese children tend to under-report more than the lean, paralleling several studies of obese adults (Bandini et al., 1990a; Maffeis et al., 1994b). Underestimation of self-reported food intake by obese children was demonstrated with dietary history and dietary records, as well as with a semi-quantitative food frequency questionnaire (Bandini et al., 1990a; Livingstone et al., 1992; Maffeis et al., 1994b). Prudence is recommended when interpreting data obtained from dietary interviews, especially those from obese children.

The potential inaccuracies in the available methods of estimating food intake and diet composition in obesity constitute important limitations to the use of total energy intakes as indications of children's energy requirements. Energy requirements seem more reliably estimated from TEE, if allowance can be made for the small contribution due to the energy costs of growth. Despite many methodological drawbacks in assessing energy intake, studies assessing the more qualitative aspects of the diet seem to show obese children prefer diets rich in lipid (Gazzaniga & Burns, 1993; Maffeis et al., 1996a). The higher energy density of fatty foods and their greater palatability compared with low-fat foods encourage high fat intakes (Rolls et al., 1994). Blundell et al. (1993) showed the satiety effect induced by food rich in fat is less than that obtained by isoenergetic food rich in protein or carbohydrate. Thus energy compensation at a meal is less accurately adjusted with high-fat meals than with low-fat/high-carbohydrate meals. Further, postprandial thermogenesis after the ingestion of fat is less ($\leq 3\%$ of the energy value of fat) than after the ingestion of carbohydrate or protein (5–8% and 20–25% of their energy content respectively). This, although quantitatively only a small effect, is a further contributing factor to fat gain.

Several energy balance studies have consistently demonstrated that TEE is significantly higher in obese than in nonobese children (Bandini et al., 1990b; Livingstone et al., 1992; Maffeis et al., 1994b; DeLany et al., 1995). The doubly labelled water technique ($^2H_2^{18}O$), which can be used to assess total energy output in unconstrained environments over prolonged periods of time, makes it possible to demonstrate potential errors in self-reporting methods of measuring energy intake. Assessing total daily energy expenditure for at least one week using $^2H_2^{18}O$, whilst simultaneously assessing total daily energy intakes, makes it possible to determine the relative error of the energy intake measurements. The method assumes that input and output data are representative of daily living conditions and that energy intakes slightly greater than energy expenditures are expected because of growth. However, the difference caused by growth is small and can be ignored, since the errors involved in the energy input/output variables outweigh this minute imbalance.

5.4 Components of total energy expenditure

If one excludes the energy costs of growth which (except in the first year of life and during puberty) only make a small fraction of energy expenditure, the different components of TEE have all been studied in schoolchildren and adolescents.

5.4.1 Basal metabolic rate

Basal metabolic rate (BMR or *resting energy expenditure*, REE) is the largest component of TEE in children, especially for those with sedentary and light activity behaviours. Long ago, it was reported that REE was more elevated in obese than in nonobese children (Brunch, 1939). More recent but very similar data on REE exist for both children (Elliot et al., 1989; Epstein et al., 1989; Maffeis et al., 1993a, 1996b) and adolescents (Bandini et al., 1990b; Molnár & Schutz, 1997).

Greater REE in the obese can be explained by larger amounts of metabolically active tissue (fat-free mass, FFM) in the obese. Using FFM as covariate in statistical comparisons between obese and nonobese children, Maffeis et al. (1992) showed REE was similar in both obese and nonobese, and in postobese and never-obese children. Many authors have indeed reported that REE in children is strongly correlated with FFM (Maffeis et al., 1993a, Goran et al., 1994). However, the slope of the regression line between REE and FFM is not constant over different ages in childhood probably because the proportion of muscle mass to organ mass within FFM increases as children mature (Weinsier et al., 1992).

Comparing the REE of Caucasian children with that of children in obesity-prone populations (such as Pima Indians or Mohawk Indians) demonstrates similar results if REE is adjusted for age, sex and body composition. This suggests that a reduced REE (BMR), *as such*, is not the risk factor for obesity in children (Fontvieille et al., 1993a; Goran et al., 1995b). A reduced absolute REE may be due simply to a reduced proportion of FFM. In black American children however, a relatively low REE has been recently reported (Yanovski et al., 1997). Further longitudinal studies are needed to assess the role of this finding on the risk of fat gain in this ethnic group. An REE which remains low after adjustment for FFM may be due to either different relative composition of FFM (muscle mass: non-muscle mass) since this is a very heterogeneous tissue, or to different metabolic activity in the tissues constituting the FFM.

5.4.2 Meal-induced thermogenesis

Meal-induced thermogenesis (MIT or postprandial thermogenesis) is another component of TEE. It represents the net rise in heat production when a food is ingested under standardized resting conditions, and is small in comparison with the REE component. Other thermogenic stimuli (e.g. caffeine; smoking; stress) are not considered here.

Few data are available on MIT in children. Findings vary but, in general, studies show inconsistent but small reductions in MIT in obese vs. nonobese children (Molnár et al., 1985; Maffeis et al., 1992; Tounian et al., 1993) confirming previous results from adult studies. Following weight loss, MIT rises to levels found in 'never-obese' children (Maffeis et al., 1992). There are no data on the magnitude of MIT in preobese children. Studies are needed to explore the potential role of MIT on subsequent fat gain in children, particularly in relation to meals of different macronutrient content.

5.4.3 Physical activity

Quantitatively, physical activity is the most variable component of TEE since it is largely dependent upon the activity behaviours of children. The definition of physical activity is rather vague. It could be subdivided into several components:

- occupational work/activity at school,
- household activity,
- leisure-time physical activity (leisure exercise and sport).

The type and nature of physical activity (recreational, occupational, discretionary movements and spontaneous movements, etc.) the intensity of activity, the duration of activity and its mechanical efficiency, have been little studied in children. Both the *quantitative* energy cost of work and the *qualitative* aspect (such as the nature of movements and type of physical activity) need assessing. In addition, the acute and chronic effects of exercise on the regulation of appetite and hunger have still to be determined in childhood.

In early work on physical activity and obesity, relatively simple techniques (such as activity meters and pedometers) were used to test whether obese children were less active than their lean counterparts. Using a cinematography method, the classical study of Mayer's group (Bullen et al., 1964) reported that the amount and duration of obese children's movements were frequently reduced. The key question however is whether low levels of physical activity are consequence or cause of obesity – or both.

The doubly labelled water technique, with the advantages of being a totally noninvasive technique, has enabled a number of novel studies of TEE. When combined with assessments of REE, the energy cost of physical activity can be calculated by the following equation:

TEE – REE = activity-related energy expenditure

This assumes that postprandial thermogenesis is either a fixed component or a negligible component of REE.

The energy expended in a physical activity depends largely upon body weight. The greater the body weight, the greater is the energy cost of a specific activity. This component is similar in obese and nonobese children (Bandini et al., 1990b; Maffeis et al., 1996b). The paradox of greater sedentary behaviour in obese children despite comparable energy expenditure to nonobese children, may be largely explained by the higher net energy cost of weight-bearing activities due to the heavier body that obese subjects have to move (Maffeis et al., 1993b). The same bodily movement in obese and lean children will involve a greater absolute energy cost in the obese children.

An alternative way of assessing the average daily level of physical activity is to assess it as a *multiple of REE*, that is to calculate the ratio of TEE to REE (Schutz et al., 2001):

TEE/REE = Physical Activity Level (PAL)

In studies of 9-year-old children we found PAL was slightly higher in obese (mean weight 46 kg) compared with lean (mean weight 31 kg) children but this difference was not significant (Maffeis et al., 1996b). The influence of excess adiposity on total energy expenditure and its components has also been examined in both Afro-American and Caucasian children (DeLany et al., 1995). There were no significant differences between the groups for physical activity related energy expenditures.

The effect of parental obesity on activity-related energy expenditure in offspring has been studied by Goran et al. (1995a). The results showed that the activity-related energy expenditure in children was not related to obesity in either mothers or fathers.

One shortcoming of the $^2H_2^{18}O$ method is that the day-to-day pattern of physical activity cannot be calculated. In addition, it fails to distinguish different types of physical activity (such as fidgeting, structured exercise, occupation-related activities) and provides no information on the pattern of physical activity. Finally, the greatest limitation of this method is that a significant fraction of the activity-related energy expenditure component is not only related to the PAL of an activity, and to the duration of physical activity as such, but also to body weight and body composition. For example, a given activity energy expenditure expressed in absolute terms could indicate low physical activity in the obese but high physical activity in the lean. Thus, adjustment of the physical activity-related energy expenditure component to allow for body weight is required. In addition, a given component can express two different situations: a long period of physical activity of low intensity or a short period of heavy activity, with very little activity over the remaining period.

Physical activity can be expressed in different ways: intensity, duration and frequency. When physical activity is expressed as the *proportion* of the day spent in various 'activities' rather than as the *level* of energy expenditure, obese children were judged as having consistently more sedentary behaviour than their lean counterparts (Maffeis et al., 1996b, 1997). Thus, a given proportion of energy expenditure attributed to physical activity gives no indication of the type or duration of physical activity since this represents the combined costs of duration, intensity and frequency of muscular exercise.

We still need to determine the optimal levels of physical activity needed to prevent or treat obesity in childhood. Practical advice on how to encourage physical activity is presented in Chapter 15.

5.5 Excess energy intake vs. low energy expenditure

The relative importance of excess energy intake and low energy expenditure as predictors of subsequent weight gain and/or obesity has generated much discussion (Campbell, 1998; Roberts & Leibel, 1998; Wells, 1998).

5.5.1 Reduced energy expenditure as a predictor of weight gain

Reduced physical activity due to a greater placidity and sedentary lifestyle are associated with low TEE (Fontvieille et al., 1993b; Goran et al., 1993; Davies et al., 1994). The extent to which a clear relationship exists between a low PAL and the accumulation of body fat in children, has been the object of a number of studies in both Caucasians (Roberts et al., 1988; Davies et al. 1995) and Pima Indians (Fontvieille et al., 1993b).

Evidence that reduced TEE (secondary either to reduced physical activity, low resting metabolic rate, or low postprandial thermogenesis) is a risk factor for subsequent weight gain has not been clearly demonstrated in children (Griffiths et al., 1987). Roberts et al. (1988) found that TEE at 3 months of age was 20% lower in infants who became overweight at 1 year, compared with infants who did not become obese. However, Davies et al. (1995), studying a larger group of infants ($n = 124$), were not able to confirm these findings. Goran (1997) reviewed the topic of energy expenditure and body composition in childhood obesity thoroughly.

A few studies from both Europe and USA have demonstrated significant relationships between sedentary behaviour in preobese children and subsequent fat gain over time (Raitakari et al., 1994; Klesges et al., 1995; Moore et al., 1995). PAL was assessed by questionnaire but, using this rather subjective tool, low PALs were associated with extra body fat gain in prepubertal children. More recently, Goran et al. (1998) reported that basal energy expenditure did not predict changes in body fatness over a 4-year period in children aged 4–7 years on entry to the study. The interpretation of this study is difficult and has been challenged by Dietz (1998) in particular because of the sophisticated multiple adjustments used in the analysis.

Although hard evidence is lacking for reduced levels of energy expenditure as powerful etiologic factors in the development of obesity in children, most hypotheses do accept that the PAL has an important role in children's weight regulation (Obarzanek et al., 1994).

A negative relationship between the amount of body fat and PAL has been demonstrated in a number of studies (Dietz & Gortmaker, 1985; Obarzanek et al., 1994; Bar-Or et al., 1998). In a recent study by Goran (1997) comprising 101 prepubertal children, the amount of body fat was inversely correlated with the duration of activity (in hours per week), determined by questionnaire. However, this was not the case with the activity-related energy expenditure assessed by the doubly labelled water method.

These results suggest that slight increases in physical activity over a long duration may be more appropriate for preventing body fat gain since aerobic activity favours fat oxidation, modest activity creates a smaller cardiac load than high-intensity activities of short duration, and high-intensity activity may be compensated by increased placidity during the recovery period (Goran & Poehlman, 1992).

In terms of future research, the high isotopic, manpower and technical costs required by the doubly labelled water technique prevent the use of this method for the studies of large numbers of children necessary for definitive conclusions on the interaction of various types of physical activity and subsequent fat gain. Further, only limited information is so far available on the effects of exercise intensity, duration, frequency, metabolic efficiency, and the types of physical activity (occupational, recreational, obligatory or spontaneous movement) on total energy expenditure and subsequent body fat gain.

5.5.2 The impact of television

In industrialized countries rapid technological development as well as extensive urbanization contribute to sedentary behaviours in adults and children. The lack of incentive to move about in our modern society suggests we need to 'cure the environment' as well as obese individuals.

Time spent watching television can be considered a potential marker of sedentary behaviour and inactivity amongst children and adolescents. The classical study by Dietz & Gortmaker (1985) showed that the amount of time spent watching television was directly related to the degree of obesity in childhood. Television viewing has been repeatedly identified as a risk factor due to its suppressive effect on physical activity (Gortmaker et al., 1996). In one study, watching television depressed the energy requirement so much through strict immobility whilst concentrating on the show that REEs were reduced compared with REE of non-television-related-activities (Klesges et al., 1993).

Television is also a powerful tool for promoting food consumption by attractive advertisements on food and snacks and through presentation of a variety of models and messages about eating (Taras et al., 1989). Enormous pressures from all the media, but particularly television, undoubtedly affect children's food preferences and food selection (Lewis & Hill, 1998).

In conclusion, the total energy expenditure of overweight children is greater than that of their lean counterparts largely because of greater fat-free mass as well as greater fat mass. There is no definite evidence that reduced energy expenditure in activity accounts for the excess body fat in obese children when results for obese and lean are expressed in absolute terms.

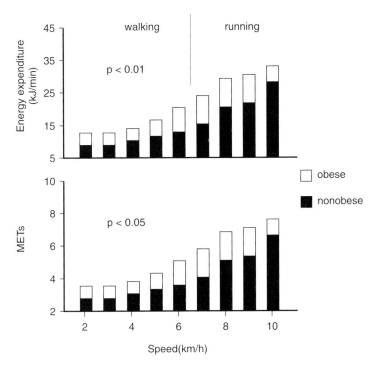

Figure 5.1   Effect of speed of locomotion on the rate of energy expenditure during walking and running on the treadmill in obese and control children, expressed in absolute value or in multiples of resting metabolic rate (METs) (from Maffeis et al., 1993b).

5.6 Aerobic capacity ($VO_{2\,max}$) in obesity

In adults, a high fat oxidation rate has been suggested as protecting against subsequent weight gain as well as against body weight gain following slimming (Froidevaux et al., 1993).

The metabolic activity of skeletal muscle has not been extensively studied in children. Indirect evidence suggests that maximal oxygen uptake ($VO_{2\,max}$) is not necessarily reduced in obese children since their excess weight can be considered as an 'obligatory' excess load keeping them physically fit (Fig. 5.1).

In a study of obese and nonobese children, $VO_{2\,max}$ expressed per unit fat-free mass was comparable in both groups (Maffeis et al., 1994a) confirming that obese children are not necessarily unfit. However, there are a number of additional factors, which may affect the level of physical activity of a child in daily life situations. Studies in adults have shown that family membership (a combination of the genetic and environmental effects of living together in the same family) accounted for about 60% of inter individual variability in the level of spontaneous physical activity amongst Pima Indians studied in a respiration chamber (Zurlo et al., 1992).

Exercise training is important for the obese since better fitness seems to encourage spontaneous physical activity in children. In a group of prepubertal nonobese boys, a 4-week training programme of five cycling sessions (of 1 hour each) increased TEE in comparison with pre-exercise measurements. More than half of the increase was accounted for by exercise itself but the remainder could be attributed to spontaneous increase in other activities (Blaak et al., 1992).

5.7 Substrate oxidation and substrate balance

Understanding substrate balance is based on the concept that protein, carbohydrate and fat are stored in their own macronutrient compartments. There is only very limited conversion of one macronutrient into another, except under unusual nutritional conditions. The conversion of carbohydrate into fat (de novo lipogenesis) occurs primarily in the liver and fat leaves this organ as very-low-density lipoprotein (VLDL) triglycerides. In adults, the total amount of fatty acid synthesis from glucose is approximately 10 g/day. We know of no quantitative information on the extent to which de novo lipogenesis occurs in children. The conversion of glucose into fatty acids is an energetically expensive process, with a net efficiency of conversion of approximately 75% indicating that 25% of the energy value of glucose converted to fat is dissipated as heat.

During growth, protein, lipid and carbohydrate balances are positive. The changes in carbohydrate stores can be ignored since they cannot be measured directly and, although varying from one day to the next, involve a relatively small component of the overall energy stores. In order to become obese, energy balance needs to be positive for a prolonged period of time. In the so-called 'preobesity' phase, average total energy intake must be greater than total energy expenditure. Development of a positive energy balance is usually by gradual build-up of an excess of energy intake over expenditure, which, on a day-to-day basis, may not be noticeable. A continuous energy imbalance of only 1% to 2% of total daily energy turnover (a small 'error' in the overall control of energy intake) can lead to significant increase in energy stores when accumulated over a long period of time. Currently, no techniques can detect such small differences in energy balance on a daily basis. The relative errors in measuring both energy input and output are substantially larger than the magnitude of this imbalance.

Fat gain (or excess fat storage such as in obesity) is the inevitable consequence of positive fat balance when fat intake is, on average, greater than fat oxidation.

Several factors, genetic and environmental, affect fat balance, promoting excess (or, alternatively, low) adiposity.

Increased fat in adipose tissue during the dynamic phase of the development of obesity is accompanied, at all ages, by increased rates of release of free fatty acids into the circulation, thus promoting fat oxidation.

Body fat accumulation may constitute an important factor for long-term equilibration of body fat balance because of its effects on fat oxidation. Schutz et al. (1992) have clearly shown a positive relationship between body fat mass and resting fat oxidation in a cross-sectional study of moderately to morbidly obese women maintaining stable body weight. Similar studies have been generated for children (Maffeis et al., 1995). Regression coefficients indicated that a 10 kg change in fat mass corresponded to a change in fat oxidation of about 20 g/day in adults (Schutz et al., 1992) and 18 g/day in prepubertal children (Maffeis et al., 1995). As a result, the equilibration of fat and energy balance after chronic exposure to excessive fat intakes may operate by enhanced fat oxidation in response to increased body fat mass.

Increased fat oxidation, as explained above, constitutes a long-term mechanism for altering substrate utilization. This is in contrast to the changes observed with carbohydrate oxidation. When an increase in the size of glycogen stores (e.g. consequent to a high carbohydrate diet) stimulates glucose utilization, it is the result of an acute phenomenon. Fat stores in adults are 50–100 times larger than glycogen stores, so the *relative* variation in substrate oxidation from day-to-day is much more limited for the former than for the latter.

The rate of resting fat oxidation is greater in obese than in lean children when expressed in absolute terms, that is when expressed as grams per hour or kilocalories per hour. When adjusted for body weight or FFM, the results are similar in both groups (Table 5.1).

We examined the proportion of exogenous fat oxidized by using lipids uniformly labelled with ^{13}C and found approximately 10% of the exogenous lipid was oxidized 'on-line', indicating that 90% was stored 'on-line' in adipose tissue, during the postprandial phase (Maffeis et al., 1999). The magnitude of exogenous vs. endogenous carbohydrate oxidation has also been studied in obese vs. nonobese children (Rueda-Maza et al., 1996). The results show that a decreased glycogen turnover may be operating at an early age in obese children.

The fuel mix oxidized can influence body weight regulation over a certain period of time. For example, as demonstrated in adults, a high level of sensitivity to insulin is associated with subsequent weight gain (Zurlo et al., 1990; Swinburn et al., 1991). By contrast, insulin resistance, consequent to substantial gain in body fat, promotes fat oxidation (shown by low respiratory quotient, RQ), thus moderating body fat gain and hence contributing to re-establishing fat balance.

Table 5.1. Differences in fat oxidation expressed in absolute and relative terms in lean and obese children (Maffeis et al., 1995)

Variable	lean	obese
Age (y)	9	9
Body weight (kg)	30	45
Body fat (%)	18	32
REE (kcal/d)	1090	1250
Respiratory quotient	0.88	0.86
Fat oxidation		
g/h	1.31	1.88
g/(h kg BW)	0.042	0.042
g/(h kg FM)	0.23	0.13
g/(h kg FFM)	0.054	0.063
g/h adjusted for FFM	1.5	1.7

REE: resting energy expenditure; BW: body weight; FM: fat mass; FFM: fat free mass.

5.8 Conclusions

The mechanisms controlling lipid oxidation appear of paramount importance in the regulation of body weight and body fat. Both excess fat intake and reduced fat oxidation favour fat gain and thus the development of obesity. From an energetic standpoint, obesity may be viewed as failure of regulation in energy and fat balances consequent to disturbances in the control of food (fat) intake accompanied (or not) by reduced relative TEE (especially due to reduced physical activity). The latter leads to deficient fat oxidation. Both situations probably coexist.

The measurement of physical activity is difficult in children as well as in adults. This is the main drawback for the assessment of the role of inactivity in the development and maintenance of obesity. Evidence that a reduced level of energy expenditure is a powerful aetiologic factor for the development of obesity in children is lacking, but there is evidence that absolute energy expenditure remains higher in overweight children than in their lean counterparts. This effect is primarily due to the greater amount of fat-free mass of the obese. Further studies, especially those with a longitudinal design, are needed to explore the potential relationships between several aspects of physical activity and TEE and subsequent body fat gain.

5.9 REFERENCES

Bandini, L.G., Schoeller, D.A., Cyr, H.D. & Dietz, W.H. (1990a). Validity of reported energy intake in obese and nonobese adolescents. *American Journal of Clinical Nutrition*, **52**, 421–5.

Bandini, L.G., Schoeller, D.A. & Dietz, W.H. (1990b). Energy expenditure in obese and nonobese adolescents. *Pediatric Research*, **27**, 198–203.

Bar-Or, O., Foreyt, J., Bouchard, C., Brownell, K.D., Dietz, W.H., Ravussin, E., Salbe, A.D., Schwenger, S., St Jeor, S. & Torun, B. (1998). Physical activity, genetic, and nutritional considerations in childhood weight management. *Medicine and Science in Sports and Exercise*, **30**, 2–10.

Blaak, E.E., Westerterp, K.S., Bar-Or, O., Wouters, L.J. & Saris, W.H. (1992). Total energy expenditure and spontaneous activity in relation to training in obese boys. *American Journal of Clinical Nutrition*, **55**, 777–82.

Blundell, J.E., Burley, V.J., Cotten, J.R., Wouters, L.J. & Saris, W.H. (1993). Dietary fat and the control of energy intake: evaluating the effects of fat on meal size and postmeal satiety. *American Journal of Clinical Nutrition*, **57(S)**, 772S–8S.

Brunch, H. (1939). Obesity in childhood. II Basal metabolism and serum cholesterol of obese children. *American Journal of Diseases of Children*, **58**, 1001–12.

Bullen, B.A., Reed, R.B. & Mayer, J. (1964). Physical activity of obese and nonobese adolescent girls appraised by motion picture sampling. *American Journal of Clinical Nutrition*, **14**, 211–23.

Campbell, L.V. (1998). A change of paradigm: obesity is not due to *either* 'excess' energy intake *or* 'inadequate' energy expenditure. *International Journal of Obesity*, **22**, 1137.

Davies, P.S.W., Coward, W.A., Gregory, J., White, A. & Mills, A.J. (1994). Total energy expenditure and energy intake in the pre-school child: a comparison. *British Journal of Nutrition*, **72**, 13–20.

Davies, P.S.W., Wells, J.C.K., Fieldhouse, C.A., Day, J.M. & Lucas, A. (1995). Parental body composition and infant energy expenditure. *American Journal of Clinical Nutrition*, **61**, 1026–29.

DeLany, J.P., Harsha, D.W., Kime, J.C., Kumler, J., Melancon, L. & Bray, G.A. (1995). Energy expenditure in lean and obese prepubertal children. *Obesity Research*, **3** (suppl 1), 67–72.

Dietz, W.H. (1998). Does energy expenditure affect changes in body fat in children? *American Journal of Clinical Nutrition*, **67**, 190–1.

Dietz, W.H. & Gortmaker, S.L. (1985). Do we fatten our children at the television set? Obesity and television viewing in children and adolescents. *Pediatrics*, **75**, 807–12.

Elliot, D.L., Goldberg, L., Kuhel, K.S. & Hanna, C. (1989). Metabolic evaluation of obese and nonobese siblings. *Journal of Pediatrics*, **114**, 957–62.

Epstein, L.H., Wing, R.R., Cluss, P.P., Fernstrom, M.H., Penner, B., Perkins, K.A., Nudelman, S., Marks, B. & Valoski, A. (1989). Resting metabolic rate in lean and obese children: relationship to child and parent weight and percent overweight change. *American Journal of Clinical Nutrition*, **49**, 331–6.

Fontvieille, A.M., Dwyer, J. & Ravussin, E. (1993a). Resting metabolic rate and body composition of Pima Indian and Caucasian children. *International Journal of Obesity*, **16**, 535–42.

Fontvieille, A.M., Harper, I., Ferraro, R., Spraul, M. & Ravussin, E. (1993b). Daily energy expenditure by 5-year old children measured by doubly-labelled water. *Journal of Pediatrics*, **123**, 200–7.

Froidevaux, F., Schutz, Y., Christin, L. & Jequier, E. (1993). Energy expenditure in obese women before and during weight loss, after refeeding and in the weight-relapse period. *American Journal of Clinical Nutrition*, **57**, 35–42.

Gazzaniga, J.M. & Burns, T.L. (1993). Relationship between diet composition and body fatness, with adjustment for resting energy expenditure and physical activity, in preadolescent children. *American Journal of Clinical Nutrition*, **58**, 21–8.

Goran, M.I. (1997). Energy expenditure, body composition, and disease risk in children and adolescents. *Proceedings of the Nutrition Society*, **56**, 195–209.

Goran, M.I. & Poehlman, E.T. (1992). Endurance training does not enhance total energy expenditure in healthy elderly persons. *American Journal of Physiology*, **263**, E950–7.

Goran, M.I., Carpenter, W.H. & Poehlman, E.T. (1993). Total energy expenditure in 4 to 6 year old children. *American Journal of Physiology*, **264**, E706–11.

Goran, M.I., Kaskoum, M.C. & Johnson, R.K. (1994). Determinants of resting energy expenditure in young children. *Journal of Pediatrics*, **125**, 362–7.

Goran, M.I., Carpenter, W.H., McGloin, A., Johnson, R., Hardin, J.M. & Weinsier, R.L. (1995a). Energy expenditure in children of lean and obese parents. *American Journal of Physiology*, **268**, E917–24.

Goran, M.I., Kaskoun, M.C., Martinez, C., Martinez, C., Kelly, B. & Hood, V. (1995b). Energy expenditure and body fat distribution in Mohawk Indian children. *Pediatrics*, **95**, 89–95.

Goran, M.I., Shewchuk, R., Gower, B.A. Nagy, T.R., Carpenter, W.H. & Johnson, R.K. (1998). Longitudinal changes in fatness in white children: no effect of childhood energy expenditure. *American Journal of Clinical Nutrition*, **67**, 309–16.

Gortmaker, S.L., Must, A. & Sobol, A.M. (1996). Television viewing as a cause of increasing obesity among children in the United States, 1986–1990. *Archives of Pediatric and Adolescent Medicine*, **150**, 356–62.

Griffiths, M., Rivers, J.P.W. & Payne, P.R. (1987). Energy intake in children at high and low risk of obesity. *Human Nutrition: Clinical Nutrition*, **41C**, 425–30.

Johnson, M.L., Burke, B.S. & Mayer, J. (1956). Relative importance of inactivity and overeating in the energy balance of obese high school girls. *American Journal of Clinical Nutrition*, **4**, 37–44.

Klesges, R.C., Shelton, M.L. & Klesges, L.M. (1993). Effects of televison on metabolic rate: potential implications for childhood obesity. *Pediatrics*, **91**, 281–6.

Klesges, R.C., Klesges, L.M., Eck, L.H. & Shelton, M.L. (1995). A longitudinal analysis of accelerated weight gain in preschool children. *Pediatrics*, **95**, 126–30.

Lewis, M.K. & Hill, A.J. (1998). Food advertising on British children's television: a content analysis and experimental study with nine-year olds. *International Journal of Obesity*, **22**, 206–14.

Livingstone, M.B.E., Prentice, A.M., Coward, W.A. Strain, J.J., Black, A.E., Davies, P.S., Stewart, C.M., McKenna, P.G. & Whitehead, R.G. (1992). Validation of estimates of energy intake by weighed dietary record and diet history in children and adolescents. *American Journal of Clinical Nutrition*, **56**, 29–35.

Maffeis, C., Schutz, Y. & Pinelli, L. (1992). Effect of weight loss on resting energy expenditure in obese prepubertal children. *International Journal of Obesity*, **16**, 41–7.

Maffeis, C., Schutz, Y., Micciolo, R., Zoccante, L. & Pinelli, L. (1993a). Resting metabolic rate in six- to ten-year-old obese and nonobese children. *Journal of Pediatrics*, **122**, 556–62.

Maffeis, C., Schutz, Y., Schena, F., Zaffanello, M. & Pinelli, L. (1993b). Energy expenditure during walking and running in obese and nonobese prepubertal children. *Journal of Pediatrics*, **123**, 193–9.

Maffeis, C., Schena, F., Zaffanello, M. et al. (1994a). Maximal aerobic power during running and cycling in obese and non-obese children. *Acta Paediatrica*, **83**, 113–16.

Maffeis, C., Schutz, Y., Zaffanello, M., Piccoli, R. & Pinelli, L. (1994b). Elevated energy expenditure and reduced energy intake in obese prepubertal children: paradox of poor dietary reliability in obesity? *Journal of Pediatrics*, **124**, 348–54.

Maffeis, C., Pinelli, L. & Schutz, Y. (1995). Increased fat oxidation in prepubertal obese children: A metabolic defense against further weight gain? *Journal of Pediatrics*, **126**, 15–20.

Maffeis, C., Pinelli, L. & Schutz, Y. (1996a). Fat intake and adiposity in 8- to 11-year-old obese children. *International Journal of Obesity*, **20**, 170–4.

Maffeis, C., Zaffanello, M., Pinelli, L. & Schutz, Y. (1996b). Total energy expenditure and patterns of activity in 8–10-year-old obese and nonobese children. *Journal of Pediatric Gastroenterology and Nutrition*, **23**, 256–61.

Maffeis, C., Zaffanello, M. & Schutz, Y. (1997). Relationship between physical inactivity and adiposity in prepubertal boys. *Journal of Pediatrics*, **131**, 288–92.

Maffeis, C., Armellini, F., Tato, L. & Schutz, Y. (1999). Fat oxidation and adiposity in prepubertal children: exogenous versus endogenous fat utilization. *Journal of Clinical Endocrinology and Metabolism*, **84**, 654–8.

Molnár, D. & Schutz, Y. (1997). The effect of obesity, age, puberty and gender on resting metabolic rate in children and adolescents. *European Journal of Pediatrics*, **156**, 376–81.

Molnár, D., Varga, P., Rubecz, I., Hamar, A. & Mestyan, J. (1985). Food induced thermogenesis in obese children. *European Journal of Pediatrics*, **144**, 27–31.

Moore, L.L., Nguyen, U.S. & Rothman, K.J. (1995). Preschool physical activity level and change in body fatness in young children. *American Journal of Epidemiology*, **142**, 1423–7.

Obarzanek, E., Schreiber, G.B., Crawford, P.B. et al. (1994). Energy intake and physical activity in relation to indexes of body fat: The National Heart, Lung, and Blood Institute Growth and Health Study. *American Journal of Clinical Nutrition*, **60**, 15–22.

Raitakari, O.T., Poekka, K.V. & Taimela, S. (1994). Effect of persistent physical activity and inactivity on coronary risk factors in children and young adults. *American Journal of Epidemiology*, **140**, 195–205.

Roberts, S.B. & Leibel, R.L. (1998). Excess energy intake and low energy expenditure as predictors of obesity. *International Journal of Obesity*, **22**, 385–6.

Roberts, S.B., Savage, J., Coward, W.A., Chew, B. & Lucas, A. (1988). Energy expenditure and intake in infants born to lean and overweight mothers. *New England Journal of Medicine*, **318**, 461–6.

Rolls, B.J., Kim-Harris, S., Fischman, M.W., Foltin, R.W., Moran, T.H. & Stoner, S.A. (1994). Satiety after preloads with different amounts of fat and carbohydrate: implications for obesity. *American Journal of Clinical Nutrition*, **60**, 476–87.

Rosenbaum, M. & Leibel, R.L. (1998). The physiology of body weight regulation: relevance to the etiology of obesity in children. *Pediatrics*, **101**, 525–39.

Rueda-Maza, C.L., Maffeis, C., Zaffanello, M. & Schutz, Y. (1996). Total and exogenous carbohydrate oxidation in obese prepubertal children. *American Journal of Clinical Nutrition*, **64**, 844–9.

Schoeller, D.A., Ravussin, E., Schutz, Y., Acheson, K.J., Baertschi, P. & Jequier, E. (1986). Energy expenditure by doubly labeled water: validation in humans and proposed calculation. *American Journal of Physiology*, **250**, R823–30.

Schutz, Y. & Deurenberg, P. (1996). Energy metabolism: overview of recent methods used in human studies. *Annals of Nutrition and Metabolism*, **40**, 183–93.

Schutz, Y., Tremblay, A., Weinsier, R.L & Nelson, K.M. (1992). Role of fat oxidation in the long-term stabilization of body weight in obese women. *American Journal of Clinical Nutrition*, **55**, 670–74.

Schutz, Y., Weinsier, R.L. & Hunter, G.R. (2001). Assessment of currently available and proposed new measures. *Obesity Research*, **9**, 368–79.

Schutz, Y., Weinsier, S., Terrier, P. & Durrer, D. (2002). A new accelerometric method to assess the daily walking practice. *International Journal of Obesity*, **26**, 111–18.

Swinburn, B.A., Nyomba, B.L., Saad, M.F. et al. (1991). Insulin resistance associated with lower rates of weight gain in Pima Indians. *Journal of Clinical Investigation*, **88**, 168–73.

Taras, H.L., Sallis, J.F., Patterson, T.L., Nader, P.R. & Nelson, J.A. (1989). Television's influence on children's diet and physical activity. *Development and Behavior in Pediatrics*, **10**, 176–80.

Tounian, P., Girardet, J.P., Carlier, L., Frelut, M.L., Veinberg F. & Fontaine, J.L. (1993). Resting energy expenditure and food-induced thermogenesis in obese children. *Journal of Pediatric Gastroenterology and Nutrition*, **16**, 451–7.

Troiano, R.P. & Flegal, K.M. (1998). Overweight children and adolescents: description, epidemiology, and demographics. *Pediatrics*, **101**, 497–504.

Weinsier, R.L., Schutz, Y. & Bracco, D. (1992). Re-examination of the relationship of resting metabolic rate to fat-free mass and to the metabolically active components of fat-free mass in humans. *American Journal of Clinical Nutrition*, **55**, 790–4.

Wells, J.C.K. (1998). Is obesity really due to high energy intake or low energy expenditure? *International Journal of Obesity*, **22**, 1139–40.

Wilkinson, P.W., Parkin, J.M., Pearlson, G., Strong, M. & Sykes, P. (1977). Energy intake and physical activity in obese children. *British Medical Journal*, **1**, 756.

Yanovski, C., Reynolds, J.C., Boyle, A. & Yanovski, J.A. (1997). Resting metabolic rate in African American and Caucasian children. *Obesity Research*, **5**, 321–5.

Zurlo, F., Lillioja, S., Esposito-Del Puente, A. et al. (1990). Low ratio of fat to carbohydrate oxidation as a predictor of weight gain: study of 24-h RQ. *American Journal of Physiology*, **259**, E650–7.

Zurlo, F., Ferraro, R.T., Fontvieille, A.M. & Ravussin, E. (1992). Spontaneous physical activity and obesity: cross-sectional and longitudinal studies in Pima Indians. *American Journal of Physiology*, **263**, E296–E300.

6

Psychosocial factors

Andrew J. Hill[1] and Inge Lissau[2]

[1]Academic Unit of Psychiatry and Behavioural Sciences, School of Medicine, University of Leeds. [2]National Institute of Public Health, Copenhagen

With obesity increasing in both adult and child populations, interest in the social context and psychological consequences of obesity has also risen. Accordingly, this chapter will overview some of the social and psychological issues pertinent to childhood obesity. The intention is not to review the topic exhaustively, but to illustrate the depth and complexity of the issues faced by children and their parents today.

6.1 Children's social background

One of the richer issues in terms of research publications still, and particularly contentious, is the relationship between obesity and socioeconomic status (SES). It is contentious because of questions of causality and because it is an example of the broader problem of the origins of health inequalities in populations, something of major social and political significance (Power & Matthews, 1997).

Sobal and Stunkard reviewed the literature on obesity and SES (some 144 studies) in 1989. They distinguished between studies conducted in developed and developing countries, those on women and men, and those that included children. Research conducted in developed countries showed that for women there was a strong inverse relationship between SES and obesity, with a higher proportion of obese women in low SES categories. This relationship was much weaker in studies that included girls. Indeed, only 40% of the latter studies showed this negative relationship. A quarter showed a direct positive relationship and a third no relationship at all. This mixed pattern was also apparent for boys. In contrast, research on children in developing societies showed a strong and consistent direct relationship, obesity being more prevalent in children from higher SES families.

A weakness of this literature has been the relative overabundance of cross-sectional studies and scarcity of longitudinal investigations. Highlighting British longitudinal data, Sobal & Stunkard (1989) noted that the inverse relationship between SES and obesity strengthened as girls became women (e.g. Peckham et al., 1983; Braddon et al., 1986; Power & Moynihan, 1988). In fact, age is an important issue in this relationship and is one of the factors identified as impairing the consistency in research outcome. The suggestion that adolescence is a time when SES could exert a large effect on obesity development is supported by a study of Belgian teenagers (De Spiegelaere et al., 1998). Information on parental SES was collected together with children's body mass index (BMI) at age 12 and 14 years. Over the space of 2 years the inverse relationship between SES and obesity in girls strengthened. This was the result of an increase in new cases in lower SES girls and the failure of obese low SES girls to lose weight. In addition, for boys this inverse relationship started to become apparent at age 15 years.

Other longitudinal studies have followed Sobal and Stunkard's review. For example, Lissau & Sørensen (1992) conducted a 10-year follow-up of Danish 9- and 10-year-olds. As expected, parental education and occupation was inversely related to their offspring's overweight in adulthood. However, the most important risk factor was the quality of housing in the area children were brought up in. This effect persisted even when controlling for parental education and occupation, degree of fatness in childhood, and children's gender. Being brought up in deprived city areas increased the risk of becoming overweight by over three times that of being brought up in more affluent areas.

Further analysis of this Danish cohort has given some insight into the potential mechanisms underlying the relationship between SES and obesity. Teacher's ratings of parental support for the child, together with school medical service data on the child's state of cleanliness, were used to define parental neglect (Lissau & Sørensen, 1994). Dirty and unsupported children were at much greater risk of adult obesity than supported and well-groomed children. Furthermore, risk of overweight was significantly increased if mothers reported little knowledge of their offspring's sweet eating habits (Lissau et al., 1993). Again, this increased risk was apparent even when controlling for childhood obesity, gender and social background.

These latter findings are consistent with popular assumptions about the relationship between SES and obesity. Socially disadvantaged families have low nutritional knowledge and interest, poor nutrition overall, and fewer opportunities for physical exercise and activity. In other words, the arguments for low SES causing obesity in children (as well as adults) are compelling. Unfortunately, the relationship is not this simple (Stunkard & Sørensen, 1993). There are two other possible causal models. Obesity may promote a reduction in SES. Alternatively, low SES and obesity may share causes that lead to both. It has been argued that many of the findings that support the simple models also allow for the possibility that both obesity and low SES have common causes. The likelihood is that their relationship is too complex to attribute simple cause–effect relationships (Sørensen, 1995).

6.2 Attitudes to obesity

6.2.1 Children's perception of obesity

In their discussion of moderators of the relationship between social background and obesity Sobal & Stunkard (1989) place likely candidates such as social mobility, physical activity and dietary restraint within a context of societal attitudes to obesity. Overwhelmingly negative, these attitudes have repercussions for children as well as adults. Research into children's perception and attitudes to overweight and obesity has its origins in studies of the stereotyping of disability and of the personality attributes associated with particular body shapes. Children have figured prominently since a developmental perspective in these areas is useful. There is also an element of 'naive psychology', in that their appraisal is believed to be more honest and less contaminated by adult knowledge and experiences. The methodologies used fall into two broad types.

Richardson et al. (1961) used a picture-rating task. Six line drawings showed a child as physically normal and with each of five physical disabilities, one of which was obvious overweight. These drawings were presented to the respondent who was asked to choose the one he or she liked best. The selected picture was put to one side and the question repeated to give a rank order of preference. The 10- and 11-year-olds in Richardson et al.'s study consistently preferred the child with no physical handicap. The second most preferred drawing was the child with crutches and leg brace, followed by the child sitting in a wheelchair, the child missing his/her left hand, and the child with a facial disfigurement. The overweight child was ranked bottom.

In a review of the research that followed, DeJong & Kleck (1986) noted the constancy of this rank ordering, with American children almost always placing the overweight child last or next to last. They also drew the following conclusions from the mass of replications and extensions to this now famous study. First, the least accepting attitudes to overweight peers are found in industrialized, Western cultures. Second, girls are less accepting of overweight same-sex peers than are boys.

The other principal research strategy has been to present children with full-body silhouettes of a thin, muscular and fat body figure. Staffieri (1967), for example, asked 6- to 10-year-old boys to assign each of 39 adjectives to the silhouette they best described. The fat body shape was more frequently labelled lazy, stupid, sloppy, dirty, naughty, mean, ugly and gets teased and, least frequently, best friend and has lots of friends. Research that has followed has adapted the stimulus materials using photographs, written descriptions or ratings as alternatives to the forced choice of adjectives. Consequently, there is some variation in outcome. DeJong & Kleck (1986) summarize the main findings as follows. For some traits, the fat and thin figures are similar in receiving far fewer endorsements than the muscular or medium body shape. Some children reject any deviation from normal body shape. Yet, amidst this, the specific rejection of fatness is clear. The three labels most commonly attached to fat figures are low intelligence, laziness and social isolation (lonely, shy, least often chosen as a friend). This negative picture is compounded by the general failure of studies to document the 'fat but happy' trait, which is believed to be the single, consistently positive feature of the overweight stereotype.

Both DeJong & Kleck (1986) and Jarvie et al. (1983) have detailed the methodological failings of research in this area. The generalizability of drawings to real life people and situations, confounding of facial attractiveness, the use of ranking and forced choice methods of assessment, failure to check children's perception of the degree of overweight depicted, or of their basis for selecting a picture, have all been raised. Against this, the overall research outcome is consistent with many people's world view regarding the stereotyping of overweight. Moreover, children's views are routinely accepted as barometers of the prevailing social climate.

6.2.2 Attributions of health and social class effects

Although there has been a relative decline in research interest into children's attitudes, two recent observations are worthy of comment. The first examined attributions of health. Hill & Silver (1995) presented 188 9-year-old girls and boys with four face-on and profile silhouette pictures depicting slim or fat children (Fig. 6.1). The girl and boy shapes were distinguishable by the shape of their hair and the label underneath the picture, 'This girl . . .' or 'This boy . . .'. Each panel was placed at the top of a single page followed by eight rating scales describing different personal attributes. Several were taken from previous research (e.g. has many friends, liked by her/his parents, does extremely well at school). Others addressed the perceived health and fitness of the pictured children, a relatively neglected issue.

Children's ratings of the four silhouette variations were dominated by the size of the figure being judged. The fat figures were rated to have far fewer friends, to do less well at school and to be less content with their appearance. Gender had a comparatively mild impact on the ratings with, for example, general agreement that the girl figures would perform better academically and be more content with their appearance, the latter most pronounced for the thin girl figure. In children's appraisal of health, again the overriding factor in their judgements was figure size. The fat figures were seen as extremely unhealthy, unfit and extremely unlikely to

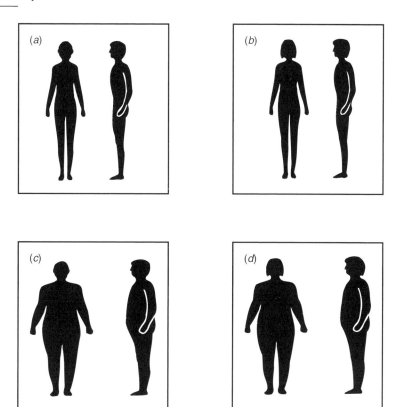

Figure 6.1   Body shape silhouettes of (*a*) thin boy, (*b*) thin girl, (*c*) overweight boy, and (*d*) overweight girl, as used by Hill & Silver (1995).

eat healthily, this appraisal being in stark contrast with the superior health state of the thin figures. Nine-year-old children appear to have received health professionals' warnings of the association between obesity and future poor health.

Wardle et al. (1995) used a similar methodology to Staffieri (1967) and asked children to assign 18 adjectives to one of three body shapes (Fig. 6.2). By selecting half of their 4- to 11-year-olds from private (fee-paying) schools and half from state schools they were able to evaluate the impact of social class background on children's judgements. The fat figure was assigned significantly more negative characteristics than either the medium or thin figure and fewer positive characteristics than the medium (but not the thin) figure. Younger children ascribed more positive adjectives to the fat figures than older children did. Similarly, children from higher SES schools assigned fewer positive characteristics to fat figures than those from low SES schools. Looking at specific attributes, high SES schoolchildren selected the fat figures as less happy, less pretty/handsome, would like to play

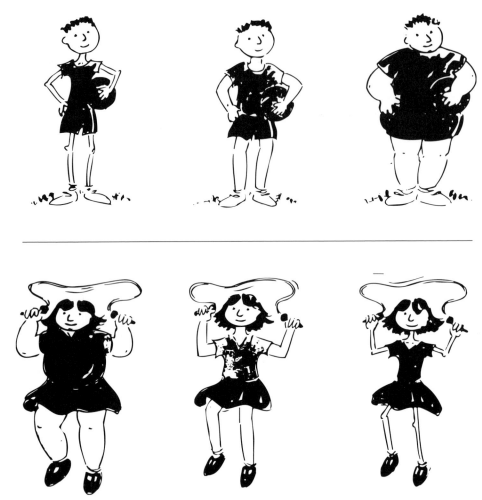

Figure 6.2   Body shape drawings of thin, average and obese children, as used by Wardle et al. (1995). Reproduced with permission.

with least, and unhealthy. Furthermore, they were significantly more likely than low SES children to label the fat figures as, 'eats the most'.

6.2.3 Stereotyping

Research into stereotypes is important because stereotypes represent a way in which people integrate information about others (Zebrowitz, 1990). As such, they should shape future behaviour, biasing attitudes and responses to individuals who display the principal feature of the stereotype. In addition, personality traits bound together within a single stereotype have an affinity, in that many positive attributes are assumed of a positive stereotype and many negative attributes of a negative stereotype. This aggregation of characteristics is known as the 'halo effect'. The stereotypes of fatness and thinness are commonly held as logical opposites and value laden in that 'thin is good' and 'fat is bad.' The above research shows that preadolescent children have accepted the prevalent 'health halo' associated with thinness which in addition to personal and social edification includes the positive attributes of well-being, healthy eating and physical fitness. Moreover, this is more likely to be voiced by those from a higher SES background, and so less likely themselves to be overweight or obese.

However, what of those children who are overweight? Are their stereotyped views any different to their leaner peers? Unsurprisingly, given the above commentary few studies have given a voice to overweight children. Those that have report few, if any, differences. Counts et al. (1986) contrasted the perception of fat and thin photograph stimuli by obese and nonobese preadolescents. The two groups of children did not differ in their assignment of positive characteristics to the thin person and negative characteristics to the fat person. Nor did children's BMI have any impact on the pattern of attributions described by Wardle et al. (1995). Hill & Silver (1995) observed some moderating effects of BMI in their study of stereotyped perception. For example, the heaviest children judged all the figures (fat and thin) to be more fit than did the lighter children. In addition, the heavy girls judged all figures to be more liked by their parents than did the lighter girls, the reverse being true for the boys. Overall, however, the heaviest children shared the extremely negative perception of the fat figures.

6.3 Children's self-worth

6.3.1 Self-perception and self-esteem

What about obese children's self-perception? There are good reasons to expect that this should not follow the pattern of judgements made of impersonal line drawings. Indeed, there is evidence that children do not generalize stereotyped figure traits to judgements of fat and thin classmates, let alone to themselves (Lawson, 1980). So what do children feel about their body shape and their self-worth generally?

Body shape discontent is clearly evident. Amidst the tendency for preadolescent (Collins, 1991) and adolescent girls (Cohn et al., 1987) to express a preference for a slimmer figure, there is a marked effect of actual weight. Using a graded scale of body shape drawings for children to indicate their current and preferred body shapes, overweight children's desire to be thinner is almost unanimous. In one study, none of the overweight preadolescents placed their preferred body figure as broader than their current shape (Hill et al., 1994). In contrast, nearly 80% of overweight and obese girls and boys desired a thinner body shape. It is hardly surprising that overweight adolescents also express the greatest dissatisfaction with their weight and figure (Wadden et al., 1989).

Alongside overweight children's discontent with appearance come questions about their self-esteem and general psychological well-being. Research on the impact of obesity on children's self-esteem has been reviewed by French et al. (1995b). These authors found 35 studies on self-esteem and obesity in this age-group but no clear and consistent outcome. Only 13 of the 25 cross-sectional studies revealed significantly lower self-esteem in obese youngsters. Adolescents aged 13–18 years showed the clearest effects, but no pattern was apparent in those aged 7–12 years. Even when detected, low self-esteem amounted to a moderate impairment that rarely fell below the normal range. Moreover, neither prospective studies nor weight-loss treatment programmes assisted in showing a close correspondence between changes in either measure. It is notable that the adult literature is equally deficient in documenting low self-esteem associated with obesity (Friedman & Brownell, 1995).

Several features of the research literature contribute to the inconsistency in outcome. One is sample size, with 16 of the 35 studies reviewed by French et al. (1995b) including fewer than 100 participants. A second is the definition of overweight used by researchers. This has ranged from 120% of ideal weight (Wadden et al., 1984), or above the 67th centile of relative BMI (Kaplan & Wadden, 1986), to using weight as a continuous variable in correlation and regression analyses (Mendelson et al., 1995a; French et al., 1996). Their variety compromises direct comparison between studies. Furthermore, the relationship between BMI and self-esteem is unlikely to be linear since both over- and underweight children express body shape dissatisfaction.

A third problem lies in the assessment of self-esteem. Most established measures aggregate responses to yield a single global score. The likely insensitivity of a global measure is revealed when self-esteem and body-esteem are measured concurrently. Finding reduced body-esteem but preserved global self-esteem in overweight young children (Mendelson & White, 1985; Hill et al., 1994) suggests a developmental lag in the effects of obesity on self-esteem relative to body-esteem.

6.3.2 Self-esteem conceptualization and assessment

Until relatively recently the assessment of self-esteem has been only weakly related to any conceptual framework. In response, Harter (1993) has found it useful to return to the contrasting views of William James and Charles Cooley. Both of these theorists concurred that a person holds a global concept of self over and above more specific self-evaluations. Where they differ is in how this global sense of self-worth is derived. According to Harter, the Jamesian approach holds that global self-esteem is the ratio of one's successes to one's pretensions. Individuals focus their self-appraisal on their abilities in domains they judge as important. Conversely, lack of competence in an area not perceived as important should not adversely affect self-esteem. Cooley's approach to the origins of self-esteem was primarily social in nature. For Cooley, self-esteem is constructed by reviewing the opinions of significant others towards oneself. This 'looking glass self' therefore relies on others' views and behaviours to determine self-regard. These contrasting theoretical perspectives usefully point to two directions for future investigation of self-esteem: in domain-specific competencies, and in the social behaviour and perception of others.

The Self-Perception Profile for Children was developed by Harter (1985) to measure domain-specific competence and global self-worth. Using a version of this questionnaire for adolescents, French et al. (1996) found that a higher BMI in teenage girls was associated with lower global self-worth and reduced self-competence in the areas of physical appearance, close friendship and behavioural conduct. For adolescent boys, higher BMI was associated with reduced self-competence in physical appearance, athletic competence and romantic appeal. In a second study and using a younger children's version of the assessment, Phillips & Hill (1998) found that both overweight and obese 9-year-old girls scored significantly lower than their normal-weight peers on athletic competence and physical-appearance self-esteem. There were no weight-related differences in other competencies or in perceived domain importance. The latter suggests that by age 9 years, overweight had limited effects on perceived self-competence but did not markedly influence girl's aspirations to succeed in any measured domain.

The study by Phillips & Hill (1998) also casts some light on girls' peer-group appraisal. The self-perceived social acceptance of overweight and obese preadolescent girls was similar to that of their normal-weight peers. This was confirmed by a sociometric analysis of peer-nominated popularity. The heaviest girls received a similar number of classmate choices as a friend, compared with lighter girls. However, two notes of caution are necessary to this conclusion of equal popularity. First, obese girls were significantly less likely to endorse the high importance of being socially accepted. Denying the importance of being liked by one's friends could represent a form of self-protection following occasions of past social rejection (see the commentary on teasing below). Second, their peer group confirmed the heavier girl's self-perception of unattractiveness. Overweight and obese girls received significantly fewer nominations from their peers as the 'prettiest girl in the class'. Indeed, 50% of obese and 35% of overweight girls received no attractiveness nominations at all.

The observation that overweight preadolescent and teenage girls (and some boys) express low physical-appearance self-esteem is of note. Research shows that self-evaluations of physical appearance are inextricably linked to global self-esteem, albeit from teenage years onwards, and remain so across the life span (Harter, 1993). The evaluation of one's appearance takes precedence over every other feature of self-perception as the number-one predictor of self-esteem. Western society heavily promotes image and the physical or outer self is an omnipresent feature constantly on display for oneself and others to observe. While overweight is synonymous with unattractiveness, self-observed or socially derived self-worth will always be under threat. This will apply at any and all ages.

6.3.3 Psychological health

Allied to concerns about damaged self-esteem is the general psychological health of obese children. Unfortunately, there is only limited research evidence on this beyond the assessment of self-esteem. Wadden et al. (1989) included measures of anxiety and depression in their study of 15-year-old girls. Overweight girls scored no differently on these assessments than normal or underweight girls. A broader measure of psychological functioning, the Symptom Checklist-90, was used by Friedman et al. (1995) in a community sample of older adolescent girls. Again, the heaviest girls scored no differently on any of the sub-scales of this measure. Excess weight was, however, associated with higher scores on three scales of the Eating Disorders Inventory: body dissatisfaction, drive for thinness and bulimia.

The association between overweight, body dissatisfaction and dieting has been amply demonstrated, albeit with a focus on girls rather than boys (Hill, 1993). This association is apparent by the age of 8 years and possibly earlier (Hill & Pallin, 1998). Heavier teenage girls are more likely to use both healthy weight-loss methods and more extreme behaviours such as fasting and vomiting (French et al., 1995a). Moreover, premorbid (childhood) overweight and family weight problems are recognized risk factors for bulimia nervosa (Fairburn et al., 1997). Therefore, the only currently demonstrable consequence of childhood overweight on psychological well-being appears to be an enhanced risk of certain eating disorders. This is unlikely to be the case for boys. Generally, this area is in need of major development of research strategies. Accordingly, Friedman & Brownell (1995) have argued that attention must turn from whether obese persons suffer psychological problems to who will suffer and in what ways.

6.4 Parents and peers

Children's relationships with their parents and peers are cornerstones of the process of socialization. Since body weight and physical appearance are such potent moderators of social behaviour, overweight will surely have some impact on children's social relationships. This literature is far from integrated. However, examples are presented below of how parents respond to their overweight children, of the styles of interaction in families with overweight children, and of peer-group teasing and victimization.

6.4.1 Parental control of eating

Parental overweight is a useful starting point. Striegel-Moore & Rodin (1985) describe a study by Susan Wooley and colleagues in which they questioned mothers of new-borns about their own weight and dieting, and their infant feeding practices. The researchers statistically separated the effects of mother's weight and their tendency to diet. Being overweight was associated with a preference for thinner babies and an unwillingness to feed their own infants much food. In contrast, a mother's tendency to diet and dissatisfaction with her own weight was associated with overinterpretation of baby's hunger, preference for a fatter baby, and a greater willingness to provide food.

The dynamic described above between mother's weight and self-perception and her attitude to infant feeding is complex. However, parental control of children's eating is relevant to both over- and undereating. For example, Stein et al. (1994) have shown that mothers with an eating disorder differ from non-eating-disordered controls in their interaction with their 12-month-old infants. Eating-disordered mothers were found to be more intrusive during mealtimes, expressed more negative emotion and had more conflict at mealtimes. Furthermore, infant weight was inversely related to the extent of mothers' concern about their own body shape. Other studies have described a correspondence between the dieting behaviour of mothers and that of their preadolescent (Hill et al., 1990; Ruther & Richman, 1993) and adolescent daughters (Pike & Rodin, 1991). There is also evidence of direct parental involvement in their daughters' weight control (Thelen & Cormier, 1995), with comments to the child about their weight especially influential between mother and daughter (Smolak et al., 1999).

One of the issues of concern regarding parental regulation of children's eating is that it may undermine the acquisition of self-regulatory skills. Bruch (1973) was one of the first to suggest that early-onset obesity may stem from faulty learning in infancy. She suggested that some mothers fail to differentiate their child's need for food from signals regarding other aversive states and so feed the child indiscriminately. This faulty learning process causes the infant to confuse hunger with other internal sensations, a confusion that persists and contributes to overeating and overweight.

Johnson & Birch (1994) have promised experimental support for this. Building on Birch's laboratory investigations of the determinants of food preferences, they tested 3- to 5-year-old children's ability to adjust food intake in response to changes in the caloric density of their diet. The best predictor of this ability was parental control of the feeding situation. Those parents who were more controlling (for example, using bribes, threats and food rewards to control food intake) had children who showed less ability to self-regulate energy intake, a deficit most apparent in the girls. Furthermore, overcontrolling mothers were more likely themselves to be dieting. This parental overcontrol is also reported by young adolescent girls (Edmunds & Hill, 1999). In particular, those 12-year-olds most concerned with dieting reported a greater parental control of eating, especially perceived overeating.

In an analysis of proneness to obesity, Costanzo & Woody (1985) have argued that parents are especially controlling in areas of their children's development in which they perceive the child to be at risk, or in areas in which parents have high personal investment. So, an obese or chronically dieting parent may be particularly concerned about their children's eating habits and see the child at risk of obesity. Persistent parental attempts at regulating their child's food intake will therefore deprive the child of opportunities to learn to control his/her own eating behaviour. Again, gender may moderate this influence with parents responding differently to overweight sons and daughters. For example, parents of an overweight son were unlikely to blame him for his weight status (Woody & Costanzo, 1982), thus sparing boys from internalizing their weight problem as a personal failure. There was a very different response for obese girls. Parents saw their daughters as liable to eat in response to both negative and positive moods. The conceptualization of their daughter's obesity was in terms of problematic eating and so they were more inclined to take an active role in restraining food intake in obese girls than in obese boys.

6.4.2 Family interaction and functioning

With such a focus on food and overeating it is reasonable to expect other areas of family functioning to be affected by the presence of an obese child or adolescent. Both interview and questionnaire studies have supported the idea that obese families are dysfunctional in comparison with families with no obese children. Using the Family Environment Scale to record perceptions of family functioning, families with obese preadolescent children have described themselves as less cohesive, less independent and as less interested in social and cultural activities (Beck & Terry, 1985; Banis et al., 1988). In an interview study, Kinston et al. (1988) observed that obese families more often wanted their needs and problems to be covered up and hidden. Additionally, within obese families there was a weak marital alliance (often with interparental hostility), direct criticism of the obese child, a differential handling of children in the family, and persistent attempts by the obese child to make parental contact interspersed with and finally leading to withdrawal.

Consistent with the findings of Woody & Costanzo (1982) above, the child's gender also influences family functioning. Kinston et al. (1990) reported that families of obese girls showed worse family functioning and a more intense and ambivalent orientation towards the obesity than did families of obese boys. Looking exclusively from the child's perspective, Mendelson et al. (1995b) found that overweight and obese girls reported lower cohesion, expressiveness, and democratic style in their families. Overweight and obese adolescent boys reported no such differences. Rather, there was a tendency for underweight boys to express the same family characteristics reported by the overweight girls. Pierce & Wardle (1993) have also observed shared parental dissatisfaction with overweight in preadolescent girls and underweight in boys.

What this small literature has so far failed to address is the direction of causality. Do dysfunctional families contribute to the development of a child's obesity (as suggested by Bruch, 1973), or are family members' expressions of discontent a consequence of the child's overweight? The latter appears more likely. However, family dynamics are complex and reciprocal, and it is possible to envisage circumstances that undermine children's self-regulation and facilitate weight gain. Likewise, it is possible that parents who 'want to help' their daughters may become intrusive about eating behaviour, assistance that is viewed negatively by their adolescent daughters (Mendelson et al., 1995b).

The literature on family functioning is useful in broadening our perspective. A child's obesity may be important for the family and have consequences for how the family interacts and self-appraises on weight- and non-weight-related issues. However, it will not be the most important or continuously important issue for all. For adolescents generally, worries about looks, figure and weight coexist with concerns about a multitude of other issues. Obesity increases their salience but does not necessarily inflate other concerns or generalize to overall anxiety (Wadden et al., 1991). In addition, the problems exhibited by obese children appear better related to parental psychological problems than either child or parental obesity (Epstein et al., 1994, 1996). In other words, the child's obesity cannot be blamed for all manner of individual and family problems.

6.4.3 Peer behaviour

Early adolescence sees a change in the balance of children's social support from parents to peers. From the age of 12 years onwards parents become less important as support providers, although they rarely become unimportant (Berndt & Hestenes, 1996). Simultaneously, the nature of peer relationships changes from a platform of companionship to include loyalty and intimacy. With this change children are increasingly vulnerable to the vagaries of peer behaviour, and while social support generally acts as a buffer against the negative effects of life stress, teasing and bullying by peers can be very hurtful.

A common but false belief is that teasing is a mainly light-hearted form of interaction. For some, being teased can be a very negative experience (Shapiro et al., 1991), especially when the focus is on a sensitive personal feature such as body size or weight. In a survey, Cash et al. (1986) found that women who had been teased about their appearance during childhood were more likely to report dissatisfaction with their appearance as adults. Similarly, Thompson & Psaltis (1988) found that the frequency of previous weight-related teasing and the degree to which it caused upset were positively correlated with current levels of body dissatisfaction and eating disturbance in college-age women. Studies with adolescent girls have shown similar results. For example, Brown et al. (1989) reported that adolescents with eating disorders had a greater history of being teased about their appearance than those without eating problems.

Past experiences of weight-related teasing have been investigated in adult obese women using the Physical Appearance Related Teasing Scale (PARTS; Thompson et al., 1991). Grilo et al. (1994) examined a small group of women from an obesity treatment clinic. Those with early-onset obesity reported a significantly greater frequency of being teased about their weight/size and about general appearance while growing up than did women with adult-onset obesity. Furthermore, the frequency of past teasing about weight/size was significantly associated with current body dissatisfaction and self-esteem. There are, however, few data on the extent, nature and severity of weight-related teasing and other forms of victimization among obese children. Wilfley et al. (1998) examined obese children attending a fitness and weight-loss camp. Eighty-one per cent had been either teased or criticized about their weight, a majority saying that they were at least moderately upset by it. Far more information is needed on weight-related victimization than we have at present. Key questions include how these experiences influence social adjustment and self-esteem, and how children respond behaviourally, especially in terms of their eating behaviour.

6.5 Conclusions

It is becoming recognized that psychosocial problems are the most prevalent form of morbidity associated with childhood obesity (Dietz, 1998). Research is confirming what some have long suspected about the repercussions of growing up in a society that stigmatizes overweight. Data on social achievement, such as those gathered by the National Longitudinal Survey of Youth in the US, provide invaluable quantification of this process (Gortmaker et al., 1993). Girls overweight at age 16 years (BMI > 95th centile) were compared with their lean peers 7 years later. They were found to have completed fewer years of school, earned less, had higher rates of household poverty and were less likely to be married. All of these difficulties were independent of their teenage SES. The same adult financial penalties of adolescent overweight have been found in British women (Sargent & Blanchflower, 1994).

The evidence presented in this chapter suggests that the psychosocial consequences of obesity are apparent in advance of adolescence. Some effects may be relatively subtle. For example, the observation that overweight children are often taller than their lean peers has led Dietz (1998) to suggest that they will often be viewed as more mature than their true chronological age. Failure to live up to adult expectations may therefore impair confidence and socialization. In contrast, weight-related teasing and bullying are blatant expressions of this stigmatization. It is also important to recognize that girls bear more of these effects than boys. Male adolescents express more reluctance with regard to dating overweight partners than female adolescents (Sobal et al., 1995). In the study by Gortmaker et al. (1993), the only consequence of overweight during adolescence for men was that they were less likely to be married. There was no educational or economic penalty attached to their earlier obesity.

Crandall (1994), in research with college-age adults, has concluded, 'antifat attitudes appear to be currently at the same stage that racism was some 50 years ago: overt, expressible and widely held'. Our lives and those of our children are influenced by this prejudice. It is right to recognize the psychosocial needs of obese children. It is right to include these, alongside weight loss, as legitimate treatment goals. However, our children need more. Ultimately, they need their parents and other adults around them to marginalize antifat attitudes and to establish a climate of tolerance.

6.6 REFERENCES

Banis, H.T., Varni, J.W., Wallander, J.L., Korsch, B.M., Jay, S.M., Adler, R., Garcia-Temple, E. & Negrete, V. (1988). Psychological and social adjustment of obese children and their families. *Child: Care, Health and Development*, **14**, 157–73.

Beck, S. & Terry, K. (1985). A comparison of obese and normal weight families' psychological characteristics. *American Journal of Family Therapy*, **13**, 55–9.

Berndt, T.J. & Hestenes, S.L. (1996). The developmental course of social support: Family and peers. In *The Developmental Psychopathology of Eating Disorders*, eds. L. Smolak, M.P. Levine & R. Striegel-Moore, pp. 77–106. Mahwah, NJ: Lawrence Erlbaum.

Braddon, F.E.M., Rodgers, B., Wadsworth, M.E.J. & Davies, J.M.C. (1986). Onset of obesity in a 36 year birth cohort study. *British Medical Journal*, **293**, 299–303.

Brown, T.A., Cash, T.F. & Lewis, R.J. (1989). Body image disturbance in adolescent binge-purgers: A brief report of a national survey in the USA. *Journal of Child Psychology and Psychiatry*, **30**, 605–13.

Bruch, H. (1973). *Eating Disorders: Obesity, Anorexia Nervosa and the Person Within*. New York: Basic Books.

Cash, T.F., Winstead, B.W. & Janda, L.H. (1986). The great American shape-up: body image survey report. *Psychology Today*, **20**, 30–7.

Cohn, L.D., Adler, N.E., Irwin, C.E., Millstein, S.G., Kegeles, S.M. & Stone, G. (1987). Body figure preferences in male and female adolescents. *Journal of Abnormal Psychology*, **96**, 276–9.

Collins, M.E. (1991). Body figure perceptions and preferences among pre-adolescent children. *International Journal of Eating Disorders*, **10**, 199–208.

Costanzo, P.R. & Woody, E.Z. (1985). Domain-specific parenting styles and their impact on the child's development of particular deviance: the example of obesity proneness. *Journal of Social and Clinical Psychology*, **3**, 425–45.

Counts, C.R., Jones, C., Frame, C.L., Jarvie, G.J. & Strauss, C.C. (1986). The perception of obesity by normal weight versus obese school-age children. *Child Psychiatry and Human Development*, **17**, 113–20.

Crandall, C.S. (1994). Prejudice against fat people: ideology and self-interest. *Journal of Personality and Social Psychology*, **66**, 882–94.

DeJong, W. & Kleck, R.E. (1986). The social psychological effects of overweight. In *Physical Appearance, Stigma, and Social Behaviour: The Ontario Symposium*, eds. C.P. Herman, M.P. Zanna & E.T. Higgins, pp. 65–87. Hillsdale, NJ: Lawrence Erlbaum.

De Spiegelaere, M., Dramaix, M. & Hennart, P. (1998). The influence of socio-economic status on the incidence and evolution of obesity during early adolescence. *International Journal of Obesity*, **22**, 268–74.

Dietz, W.H. (1998). Health consequences of obesity in youth: childhood predictors of adult disease. *Pediatrics*, **101**, 518–25.

Edmunds, H. & Hill, A.J. (1999). Dieting and the family context of eating in young adolescent children. *International Journal of Eating Disorders*, **25**, 435–40.

Epstein, L.H., Klein, K.R. & Wisniewski, L. (1994). Child and parent factors that influence psychological problems in obese children. *International Journal of Eating Disorders*, **15**, 151–8.

Epstein, L.H., Myers, M.D. & Anderson, K. (1996). The association of maternal psychopathology and family socioeconomic status with psychological problems in obese children. *Obesity Research*, **4**, 65–74.

Fairburn, C.G., Welch, S.L., Doll, H.A., Davies, B.A. & O'Connor, M.E. (1997). Risk factors for bulimia nervosa: a community-based case-control study. *Archives of General Psychiatry*, **54**, 509–17.

French, S.A., Perry, C.L., Leon, G.R. & Fulkerson, J.A. (1995a). Dieting behaviours and weight change history in female adolescents. *Health Psychology*, **14**, 548–55.

French, S.A., Story, M. & Perry, C.L. (1995b). Self-esteem and obesity in children and adolescents: a literature review. *Obesity Research*, **3**, 479–90.

French, S.A., Perry, C.L., Leon, G.R. & Fulkerson, J.A. (1996). Self-esteem and changes in body mass index over 3 years in a cohort of adolescents. *Obesity Research*, **4**, 27–33.

Friedman, M.A. & Brownell, K.D. (1995). Psychological correlates of obesity: moving to the next research generation. *Psychological Bulletin*, **117**, 3–20.

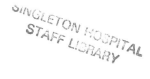

Friedman, M.A., Wilfley, D.E., Pike, K.M., Striegel-Moore, R.H. & Rodin, J. (1995). The relationship between weight and psychological functioning among adolescent girls. *Obesity Research*, **3**, 57–62.

Gortmaker, S.L., Must, A., Perrin, J.M., Sobol, A.M. & Dietz, W.H. (1993). Social and economic consequences of overweight in adolescence and young adulthood. *New England Journal of Medicine*, **329**, 1008–12.

Grilo, C.M., Wilfley, D.E., Brownell, K.D. & Rodin, J. (1994). Teasing, body image, and self-esteem in a clinical sample of obese women. *Addictive Behaviours*, **19**, 443–50.

Harter, S. (1985). *Manual for the Self-Perception Profile for Children*. Denver, CO: University of Denver.

Harter, S. (1993). Causes and consequences of low self-esteem in children and adolescents. In *Self-Esteem: The Puzzle of Low Self-Regard*, ed. R.F. Baumeister, pp. 87–116. New York: Plenum Press.

Hill, A.J. (1993). Pre-adolescent dieting: Implications for eating disorders. *International Review of Psychiatry*, **5**, 87–100.

Hill, A.J. & Pallin, V. (1998). Dieting awareness and low self-worth: related issues in 8-year old girls. *International Journal of Eating Disorders*, **24**, 405–13.

Hill, A.J. & Silver, E. (1995). Fat, friendless, and unhealthy: 9-year old children's perception of body shape stereotypes. *International Journal of Obesity*, **19**, 423–30.

Hill, A.J., Weaver, C. & Blundell, J.E. (1990). Dieting concerns of 10-year old girls and their mothers. *British Journal of Clinical Psychology*, **29**, 346–8.

Hill, A.J., Draper, E. & Stack, J. (1994). A weight on children's minds: body shape dissatisfactions at 9-years old. *International Journal of Obesity*, **18**, 383–9.

Jarvie, G.J., Lahey, B., Graziano, W. & Framer, E. (1983). Childhood obesity and social stigma: what we know and what we don't know. *Developmental Review*, **3**, 237–73.

Johnson, S.L. & Birch, L.L. (1994). Parents' and children's adiposity and eating style. *Pediatrics*, **94**, 653–61.

Kaplan, K.M. & Wadden, T.A. (1986). Childhood obesity and self-esteem. *Journal of Pediatrics*, **109**, 367–70.

Kinston, W., Loader, P., Miller, L. & Rein, L. (1988). Interaction in families with obese children. *Journal of Psychosomatic Research*, **32**, 513–32.

Kinston, W., Miller, L., Loader, P. & Wolff, O.H. (1990). Revealing sex differences in childhood obesity by using a family systems approach. *Family Systems Medicine*, **8**, 371–86.

Lawson, M.C. (1980). Development of body build stereotypes, peer ratings, and self-esteem in Australian children. *Journal of Psychology*, **104**, 111–18.

Lissau, I. & Sørensen, T.I.A. (1992). Prospective study of the influence of social factors in childhood on risk of overweight in young adulthood. *International Journal of Obesity*, **16**, 169–75.

Lissau, I. & Sørensen, T.I.A. (1994). Parental neglect during childhood and increased risk of obesity in young adulthood. *Lancet*, **343**, 324–7.

Lissau, I., Breum, L. & Sørensen, T.I.A. (1993). Maternal attitude to sweet eating habits and risk of overweight in offspring: a ten-year prospective population study. *International Journal of Obesity*, **17**, 125–9.

Mendelson, B.K. & White, D.R. (1985). Development of self-body-esteem in overweight youngsters. *Developmental Psychology*, **21**, 90–6.

Mendelson, B.K., White, D.R. & Mendelson, M.J. (1995a). Children's global self-esteem predicted by body esteem but not by weight. *Journal of Clinical Investigation*, **80**, 97–8.

Mendelson, B.K., White, D.R. & Schliecker, E. (1995b). Adolescent's weight, sex, and family functioning. *International Journal of Eating Disorders*, **17**, 73–9.

Peckham, C.S., Stark, O., Simonite, V. & Wolff, O.H. (1983). Prevalence of obesity in British children born in 1946 and 1958. *British Medical Journal*, **286**, 1237–42.

Phillips, R.G. & Hill, A.J. (1998). Fat, plain, but not friendless: self-esteem and peer acceptance of obese pre-adolescent girls. *International Journal of Obesity*, **22**, 287–93.

Pierce, J.W. & Wardle, J. (1993). Self-esteem, parental appraisal and body size in children. *Journal of Child Psychology and Psychiatry*, **34**, 1125–36.

Pike, K.M. & Rodin, J. (1991). Mothers, daughters, and disordered eating. *Journal of Abnormal Psychology*, **100**, 198–204.

Power, C. & Matthews, S. (1997). Origins of health inequalities in a national population sample. *Lancet*, **350**, 1584–9.

Power, C. & Moynihan, C. (1988). Social class and changes in weight-for-height between childhood and early adulthood. *International Journal of Obesity*, **12**, 445–53.

Richardson, S.A., Hastorf, A.H., Goodman, N. & Dornbusch, S.M. (1961). Cultural uniformity in reaction to physical disabilities. *American Sociological Review*, **26**, 241–7.

Ruther, N.M. & Richman, C.L. (1993). The relationship between mothers' eating restraint and their children's attitudes and behaviours. *Bulletin of the Psychonomic Society*, **31**, 217–20.

Sargent, J.D. & Blanchflower, D.G. (1994). Obesity and stature in adolescence and earnings in young adulthood. Analysis of a British birth cohort. *Archives of Pediatrics and Adolescent Medicine*, **148**, 681–7.

Shapiro, J.P., Baumeister, R.F. & Kessler, J.W. (1991). A three-component model of children's teasing: aggression, humour, and ambiguity. *Journal of Social and Clinical Psychology*, **10**, 459–72.

Smolak, L., Levine, M.P. & Schermer, F. (1999). Parental input and weight concerns among elementary school children. *International Journal of Eating Disorders*, **25**, 263–71.

Sobal, J. & Stunkard, A.J. (1989). Socioeconomic status and obesity: a review of the literature. *Psychological Bulletin*, **105**, 260–75.

Sobal, J., Nicolopoulos, V. & Lee, J. (1995). Attitudes about overweight and dating among secondary school students. *International Journal of Obesity*, **19**, 376–81.

Sørensen, T.I.A. (1995). Socio-economic aspects of obesity: causes or effects? *International Journal of Obesity*, **19** (Suppl. 6), S6–S8.

Staffieri, J.R. (1967). A study of social stereotype of body image in children. *Journal of Personality and Social Psychology*, **7**, 101–4.

Stein, A., Wooley, H., Cooper, S.D. & Fairburn, C.G. (1994). An observational study of mothers with eating disorders and their infants. *Journal of Child Psychology and Psychiatry*, **35**, 733–48.

Striegel-Moore, R. & Rodin, J. (1985). Prevention of obesity. In *Prevention in Health Psychology*, eds. J.C. Rosen & L.J. Solomon, pp. 72–110. Hanover, PA: University Press of New England.

Stunkard, A.J. & Sørensen, T.I.A. (1993). Obesity and socioeconomic status – a complex relation. *New England Journal of Medicine*, **329**, 1036–7.

Thelen, M.H. & Cormier, J.F. (1995). Desire to be thinner and weight control among children and their parents. *Behaviour Therapy*, **26**, 85–99.

Thompson, J.K. & Psaltis, K. (1988). Multiple aspects and correlates of body figure ratings: a replication and extension of Fallon and Rozin. *International Journal of Eating Disorders*, **7**, 813–18.

Thompson, J.K., Fabian, L.J., Moulton, D.O., Dunn, M.E. & Altabe, M.N. (1991). Development and validation of the Physical Appearance Related Teasing Scale. *Journal of Personality Assessment*, **56**, 513–21.

Wadden, T.A., Foster, G.D., Brownell, K.D. & Finley, E. (1984). Self-concept in obese and normal weight children. *Journal of Consulting and Clinical Psychology*, **52**, 1104–5.

Wadden, T.A., Foster, G.D., Stunkard, A.J. & Linowitz, J.R. (1989). Dissatisfaction with weight and figure in obese girls: discontent but not depression. *International Journal of Obesity*, **13**, 89–97.

Wadden, T.A., Brown, G., Foster, G.D. & Linowitz, J.R. (1991). Salience of weight-related worries in adolescent males and females. *International Journal of Eating Disorders*, **10**, 407–14.

Wardle, J., Volz, C. & Golding, C. (1995). Social variation in attitudes to obesity in children. *International Journal of Obesity*, **19**, 562–9.

Wilfley, D.E., Stein, R.I., Hayden, H.A., Dounchis, J.Z. & Zabinski, M.F. (1998). Social consequences of childhood obesity. *International Journal of Obesity*, **22** (Suppl 4), S15.

Woody, E.Z. & Costanzo, P.R. (1982). The socialisation of obesity prone behaviour. In *Developmental Social Psychology*, eds. S. Brehm, S. Kassin & R. Gibbons. London: Oxford University Press.

Zebrowitz, L.A. (1990). *Social Perception*. Milton Keynes: Open University Press.

Part II

Consequences

7

Clinical features, adverse effects and outcome

Karl F.M. Zwiauer,[1] Margherita Caroli,[2] Ewa Malecka-Tendera[3] and Elizabeth M.E. Poskitt[4]

[1]Department of Paediatrics, General Hospital, Saint Poelten. [2]Preventive Medicine, Francavilla Fontana (Brindisi). [3]Department of Pathophysiology, Silesian School of Medicine, Katowice. [4]International Nutrition Group, London School of Hygiene and Tropical Medicine

7.1 Clinical findings and immediate adverse effects

Obesity is one of the few conditions often diagnosed as easily by the layperson – even from a distance – as by the clinician. However, distinguishing normal fatness from abnormal fatness can be extremely difficult. This has been discussed in earlier chapters. Once obesity has been diagnosed, it is important to recognize the small proportion of obese children who have specific syndromes or pathology underlying their obesity. The vast majority of obese children remain those whose obesity does not seem associated with any underlying medical cause: simple, exogenous or nonpathological obesity. It is important to distinguish the obese children with underlying clinical disease or syndrome, but children with simple obesity also have specific problems and clinical signs. Tables 7.1 and 7.2 list the particular points to elicit in the clinical history and in clinical examination of children with simple obesity. Assessment is not easy. Too often, the subjective assumption – not totally unjustified – is that any symptomatology in these children must be secondary to their overweight and can therefore be cured by weight reduction alone. Further, the examination of grossly obese children, even when they are happy to be examined thoroughly, which is not always the case, is clinically difficult. Signs have to be elicited through the mass of fat. Equipment such as sphygmomanometers are not designed for use with the grossly obese. Thus, important symptoms and signs can easily be missed or ignored. Health-care workers should approach the assessment of obese children with their greatest clinical skill and objectivity.

Table 7.1. Clinical history in childhood obesity

Perinatal history

    Pregnancy: gestational diabetes

                      fetal movement

    Infant feeding: breast or bottle

                      age at weaning

                      weaning dietary history

Growth

    Birth weight and gestation

    Obesity as infant

    Obesity as young child

    History of slimming

Family

    Age and sex of other children

    Parental status: married, divorced, absent parent

    Parental employment

    Familial obesity

    Familial slimming

    Coping style dealing with child's obesity

Diet

    Detailed diet history

    Likes and dislikes

    School meals

    Meals/snacks outside the home

Physical activity

    Travel to school

    At school and during leisure hours

    At home: leisure/hobbies

               domestic

Inactivity

    Television watching

    Sleep habits

Psychosocial

    Peer group relationships

    Parent–child relationships

    Teacher–child relationships

    School progress

Table 7.2. Clinical examination in childhood obesity

General
    Facies: signs of congenital obesity syndrome
                  signs of endocrine disorder
    Skeletal: presence of congenital abnormality
                  hands: signs of obesity syndrome
                  legs: evidence of Blount's disease
                  signs of SCFE
    Blood pressure: elevated
    Cardiorespiratory function: impaired
    Pubertal staging: evidence of abnormality or hypogonadism
    Skin: striae: purple or white
             intertrigo in fat folds
             acanthosis nigricans
             excessive hirsuties
    Neuromuscular system: evidence of abnormality
    IQ: low

Anthropometry
    weight, height, waist and hip circumferences
    triceps, biceps, suprailiac and subscapular skinfold thicknesses

Biochemical
    urinary glucose
    fasting blood glucose
    lipid profile
    random cortisol
    thyroid function

Karyotype

IQ: intelligence quotient; SCFE: slipped capital femoral epiphysis.

7.1.1 Growth

Height for age

Obese children are usually above average height for age (Dietz, 1993). Relatively tall stature is helpful in distinguishing children with simple obesity since many of the congenital and endocrine conditions in which obesity is a common associated problem – hypothyroidism, Cushing's syndrome, growth hormone deficiency and pseudohypoparathyroidism – are associated with short stature. This association of obesity with tall stature is particularly marked prepubertally (Beunen et al., 1994). Height may be above the 95th centile for age, particularly if the children's midparental heights are also above average. However as children mature, tall stature is less marked. In the National Collaborative Perinatal Survey, obese 15-year-old children were not taller than their nonobese peers (Johnston & Mack, 1980) but the children who had been overweight at 1 year of age were taller at age 15 years than those who had been normal weight in infancy. It is thus possible that childhood and preadolescent fatness are associated with size differences because of advanced biological maturity. However the 'overweight for age' infants in the Johnston & Mack (1980) study might have been the 'long for age infants' with high lean body, rather than fat, mass and this high lean mass persisted. Tall stature is usually accompanied by increased lean body mass: increased skeletal size and muscle mass with, often, advanced bone age as well. This latter reflects rapid skeletal maturation which has been shown to correlate with the degree of over-weight.

Pubertal development

The age of puberty for boys and girls in Western Europe and North America has been dropping steadily during the last century in parallel with increasing average body fat. Polito et al. (1995) demonstrated a significant relation between advanced maturation of radius, ulna and carpal bones and height Z-scores in prepubertal obese children. However, advanced bone age and obesity are also associated with early sexual maturity. Obese girls have, on average, lower age at menarche compared with nonobese girls (Dietz, 1993). The hypothesis that the timing of menarche depends on a critical mass of body fat is supported by this and by the finding that mice treated with leptin develop earlier fertility than untreated controls (Chehab et al., 1997). Thus, advanced maturity in obese adolescents could reflect increased leptin concentrations due to high body fat.

The onset of puberty can be difficult to judge in obese girls since collections of subcutaneous fat in the mammary region (steatomastia) in prepubertal, tall-for-age, obese girls may be confused with true (precocious) puberty. Differentiation is by palpation for the presence or absence of glandular tissue in the 'breasts' and by examination for other evidence of puberty. Hand/wrist X-ray is helpful since bone age is never as advanced in simple obesity as in true precocious puberty and is rarely more than 1–1.5 years ahead of chronological age (Beunen et al., 1994). Likewise, stature, although often in the region of the 97th centile, does not show the acceleration in growth rate expected in early puberty.

Longitudinal studies show height gain can accelerate with weight gain (Forbes, 1977). Early maturation shown by early peak height velocity and age of menarche is also associated with increased fatness in adulthood and with increased abdominal obesity in women. These associations are still demonstrable after adjustment for greater fatness at the same chronological age. Early maturation seems to be a biological determinant of later obesity.

7.1.2 Cosmetic problems

Excess tissue

For obese boys the most troubling problems are often pseudo-gynaecomastia and pseudo-hypogenitalism. 'Breasts' may be very prominent. If some glandular tissue is palpable within the huge pad of fat, benign pubertal gynaecomastia is the most likely cause, although conditions such as Klinefelter's syndrome, testicular tumours, defects in testosterone production and drug reactions need excluding (Styne, 1996). Apparent hypoplasia of the genitalia may accompany the gynaecomastia suggesting hormonal abnormalities. Usually the apparent hypoplasia is due to external genitalia being buried by lower abdominal fat and thus appearing disproportionately small considering the boys' overall size. These perceived abnormalities can lead to obese boys being referred for further investigation when thorough clinical examination and gently pushing aside the fat shows normal penile size together with testicular volumes appropriate for age.

In both sexes, gross obesity is very disfiguring. In central obesity the abdomen is often pendulous. White or purplish striae on the abdomen and around the breasts are unattractive. In gluteal obesity, common in adolescent girls, striae are present on hips and thighs. Striae may become paler with time but do not disappear with weight reduction.

In obese girls, particularly, hirsutism and acne are often obvious and distressing. Precise data on the prevalences of these problems do not exist since the experiences of obesity clinics are unlikely to reflect true population prevalence.

Intertrigo infected with *Candida* spp. can be irritating and painful when it develops to red, raw and weeping lesions in the folds of fat, particularly under the breasts and in abdominal fat folds.

Acanthosis nigricans (AN)

This is a rare skin condition occurring in association with a wide variety of clinical pathology. There is thickening and pigmentation in skin folds, particularly at the back of the neck, in axillae and groins, under the breasts and the anogenital folds. A high proportion of children with AN are obese. The prevalence of AN in childhood obesity is unknown. The importance of AN is its association with some obesity syndromes and with glucose intolerance, making it a clinical marker of insulin resistance (Richards et al., 1985).

These cosmetic problems are of little *clinical* significance but they can have a very negative impact on the body image and the daily life of both boys and girls with obesity. The embarrassment of taking part in sports and swimming is often considerable and can interfere with normal social life.

7.1.3 Hormonal problems

Polycystic ovary (Stein–Leventhal) syndrome

The prevalence of polycystic ovary syndrome – oligomenorrhoea or amenorrhoea, acne and acanthosis nigricans – in obese adolescents is unknown. Nevertheless, obesity appears to play a major role in pathogenesis. Hirsutism and menstrual abnormalities are more common in obese than in lean adolescent girls and are features heralding polycystic ovary syndrome in adult life. High androgen activity was documented in overweight girls with abdominal pattern of fat distribution together with correlations between free androgen index and weight/height (W/H) ratio (Wabitsch et al., 1995) and between testosterone level and body mass index (BMI) (Malecka-Tendera et al., 1998). Hormonal patterns typical of polycystic ovary syndrome, however, have also been described in other obese adolescents (Richards et al., 1985; Lazar et al., 1995).

7.1.4 Orthopaedic problems

Immature cartilage, unfused growth plates and softer cartilaginous bones which have not evolved to carry substantial body mass, contribute to the variety of orthopaedic complications of childhood and adolescent obesity. Two specific conditions seem particularly associated with obese children: Blount's disease in younger children and slipped femoral epiphysis in early adolescence.

Blount's disease

In Blount's disease there is abnormal growth of the medial aspect of the proximal tibial epiphysis resulting in progressive varus angulation of the leg below the knee. It is commonly bilateral. The condition may have infantile (1–3 years), juvenile (4–10 years) or adolescent (11 + years) onset with both the latter two conditions described as late-onset Blount's disease. It is suggested that the condition results from growth suppression due to increased compressive forces across the medial aspect of the knee (Thompson & Carter 1990; Behrman et al., 2000). The condition is not common and its prevalence in childhood obesity is not known, but 60–80% of children with Blount's disease, both early- and late-onset, are obese (Dietz et al., 1982).

Orthotic management can be considered for younger children. Surgery is often used to correct deformity in older children but surgical intervention should not be undertaken lightly. One-third of infantile cases have achieved straight knees, even without surgery, by the age of 40 years (Ingvarsson et al., 1998). Even in late-onset Blount's disease, despite the shorter growing period left to the child, Ingvarsson et al. (1997) found 25% of children who received no surgery had straight legs at age 40 years. Recurrence after orthopaedic surgical intervention is common. Vigorous attempts to reduce the children's weights would seem important aspects of any management programme.

Slipped capital femoral epiphysis (SCFE)

This condition of unknown aetiology affecting children in early adolescence is often suggested to have an endocrine basis since it is also associated with hypothyroidism and growth hormone deficiency as well as simple obesity. Increased weight on the cartilaginous growth plate of the hip appears to be one of the major reasons for SCFE. The incidence is approximately 3.4 per 100 000 children (Kelsey et al., 1972). However, 50–70% of patients with SCFE are obese (Sørensen, 1968; Kelsey et al., 1972; Wilcox et al., 1988), and two-thirds of patients with bilateral SCFE are obese (Loder et al., 1993). Children occasionally present with acute slippage but usually the condition develops insidiously with pain in the hip (occasionally referred pain in the knee) and limping. Orthopaedic treatment is urgent to prevent further slippage so as to minimize later complications to the damaged hip. Occasionally, avascular necrosis of the femoral head or degeneration of the articular cartilage of the hip complicate the problem.

The condition affects adolescents before fusion of the proximal femoral epiphyses. Children presenting with SCFE before the age of 10 years should have thyroid function checked and be reviewed for other endocrine disorders. Checking thyroid function is so simple that it is probably advisable in all cases of SCFE associated with any degree of obesity.

7.1.5 Gastrointestinal problems

Elevated concentrations of liver enzymes are another common obesity-related finding in children and adolescents (Kinugasa et al., 1984; Noguchi et al., 1995). More than 10% of Japanese children attending a general obesity clinic had modestly elevated circulating liver enzymes and high levels were associated with fatty liver, fatty hepatitis, fatty fibrosis and cirrhosis. Fatty liver is a common finding in morbidly obese children, particularly boys with abdominal obesity (Moran et al., 1983; Frelut et al., 1995, 1996), indicating either increased storage or reduced delivery of triglycerides to the blood stream. Mild elevations of alanine aminotransferase correlating positively with waist on hip ratio have been reported in obese children with fatty liver (Frelut et al., 1996). All these hepatic abnormalities seem to regress with slimming (Vajro et al., 1994).

The proportion of cholesterol excreted into the bile is elevated in obesity in comparison with the excretion of bile acids and phospholipids, increasing the likelihood of gallstones (Shaffer & Small, 1977). Obesity is associated with 8–50% of all gallstones diagnosed in children (Crichlow et al., 1972; Halcomb et al., 1980; Friesen & Roberts, 1989) but accounts for the majority of gallstones in children and adolescents without underlying diseases such as haemolytic disease, congenital heart disease or prolonged parenteral nutrition. The relative risk of gallstones in adolescent girls above 110% ideal body weight compared with normal-weight girls has been estimated as approximately 4.2 (Honore, 1980). A prospective study of obese adolescent female Pima Indians demonstrated that from the age of 13 years the bile becomes supersaturated with cholesterol. The prevalence of gallstones rises dramatically from 17 years old, affecting 70% of individuals at 30 years (Sampliner et al., 1970; Bennion et al., 1979). In obese adults, the risks of clinically symptomatic and asymptomatic gallstones are doubled (Acalivschi et al., 1997) and risks are even greater in individuals with a history of weight reduction (Liddle et al., 1989).

7.1.6 Respiratory and sleep-related problems

Obesity in childhood contributes to respiratory disease in a number of ways. Overweight has been associated with significantly more severe symptomatology in asthmatic subjects (Luder et al., 1998). Asthmatic children with high BMI had significantly lower peak expiratory flow rates than those with lower BMIs. Further, obese asthmatic children missed more school days and had more medication prescribed than their nonobese asthmatic peers. At the same time, asthma may be a risk factor for low levels of physical activity in obese asthmatic children, particularly for those with exercise-induced bronchospasm (Gennuso et al., 1998).

Pulmonary-function tests show a high incidence of mild obstructive lung disease in obese children and this may predispose to the obesity–hypoventilation syndrome in adulthood. Nonasthmatic obese children showed more severe bronchial hyper-reactivity after exercise than their lean nonasthmatic peers with greater falls in forced expiratory flow rate in 1 second and lower peak expiratory and mid-expiratory flow rates (Kaplan & Montana, 1993). In Chinese children, however, positive correlations between lung function and BMI were demonstrated in normal-weight children and in overweight girls but not in overweight boys (Fung et al., 1990).

Sleep disorders

The prevalence of sleep disorders in childhood obesity seems to relate to the degree of obesity. In the majority of affected children problems are manifest as snoring but episodes of obstructive sleep apnoea syndrome (OSAS) also occur. Mallory et al. (1989) found that one-third of 41 children with severe obesity reported symptoms of OSAS and one-third had some form of sleep disorder. There was evidence of severe OSAS in 5%. Polysomnography studies show that in a group of severely obese children (> 200% relative body weight; RBW) with sleep-associated breathing disorders, 94% had abnormal sleep patterns and oxygen saturation below 90% for half the total sleep time. Approximately 40% had evidence of central hypoventilation (Silvesti et al., 1993). In 3671 obese Singaporean children, with OSAS defined as apnoea/hypoxia indices above 5 per hour, 0.7% had evidence of OSAS. However amongst those with greater than

180% ideal body weight, the prevalence of OSAS was 13.3%. OSAS was more common in children with adeno-tonsillar hypertrophy and in those who slept sitting up (Chay et al., 2000).

Pickwick syndrome

In this rare condition which occurs with extreme obesity, there is severe cardiorespiratory distress with alveolar hypoventilation. Symptoms include hypoventilation, somnolence, right ventricular hypertrophy, cyanosis, polycythaemia and evidence of congestive cardiac failure. The respiratory drive may be dependent on hypoxaemia and thus the administration of oxygen can be disastrous. Pulmonary embolus may be a further complication. Death from cardiac failure or sudden respiratory failure is common unless aggressive attempts to reduce weight are instigated (Riley et al., 1976) – and are successful.

7.1.7 Neurological problems

Pseudotumor cerebri (PTC)

This rare condition occurs in association with a wide variety of disorders including severe obesity. Up to 50% of all children with PTC are obese. In obese children PTC usually develops before adolescence (Dietz, 1998). Symptoms are those of raised intracranial pressure: severe (occipital) headache, pulsatile tinnitus, vomiting and visual problems. Papilloedema is usual. Sixth nerve palsy leading to diplopia and paralytic squint are common. Cerebrospinal fluid (CSF) pressure is raised, but brain scan findings are usually normal. Visual damage can lead to blindness (Weisberg & Chutorian, 1977). Unlike other causes of raised intracranial pressure, the children are usually mentally alert. It has been suggested that the raised CSF pressure is secondary to raised intra-abdominal pressure leading to raised intrathoracic pressure (Sugerman et al., 1999). Obesity associated with PTC should be treated promptly and aggressively by VLCD (very-low-calorie diet) or protein-sparing modified fast (PSMF).

7.1.8 Immunological problems

Some studies have shown that obese infants have more frequent respiratory infections than expected (Tracy et al., 1971). These studies, which were retrospective and without controls, took place at a time when infant feeding practices were contributing to a high prevalence of obesity in early infancy. Thus the current value of their findings can be questioned. More recently, obese children have been shown to suffer more from common infectious episodes than their normal-weight peers. Episodes of infection do not occur more often but are more severe and last longer (Caroli & Chandra, unpublished data).

The higher morbidity of obese children has recently been linked to hyperinsulinaemia which reduces lymphocyte-mediated cytotoxicity (Koffler et al., 1991), and to leptin which modulates T-cell immune function through its lymphocyte receptors (Lord et al., 1998).

Obese children, even when in good health, commonly have elevated erythrocyte sedimentation rates (ESR) without other evidence of infection or inflammation (Kasapçopur et al., 1991). This is important to recognize so as to avoid obese children undergoing unnecessary investigations for elevated ESR in the absence of other symptoms or signs.

7.1.9 Metabolic problems

Childhood obesity is associated with a variety of metabolic and endocrine alterations, which do not become apparent for a long time but can be demonstrated biochemically before they cause clinical symptoms. These metabolic and endocrine disturbances are perceived as precursors of conditions associated with increased morbidity and mortality in adult life. Childhood obesity is, for example, an important factor in the evolution of cardiovascular risk (Chapter 11). Coronary atherosclerosis is more likely to be present in young adults with excess adipose tissue, independent of other risk factors (McGill et al., 1995). Increased cardiovascular risk factors and other adverse consequences for physical health, in particular hyperinsulinaemia, are already present in obese children and adolescents and herald significant morbidity in adult life (Mossberg, 1989; Must et al., 1992; Gunnell et al., 1998). As children progress from childhood to adult life with the complications of high blood pressure, elevated low-density-lipoprotein (LDL)-cholesterol, low high-density-lipoprotein (HDL)-cholesterol and increased risk for non-insulin-dependent diabetes mellitus (NIDDM), the accumulation of even more excess body fat becomes the major predictor of further increased health risk (Lauer & Clarke, 1984; Lauer et al., 1988; Manolio et al., 1990).

Hyperinsulinaemia

Hyperinsulinaemia and impaired glucose tolerance are also associated with obesity in childhood (Chapter 3). Existing data indicate that hyperinsulinaemia, insulin resistance and hyperandrogenaemia are common findings (Richards et al., 1985; Zwiauer et al., 1989; Molnar, 1990). Even in children below 10 years, significant insulin resistance has been noted and obese prepubertal children show 20–45% reduction in insulin-stimulated glucose uptake (Caprio et al., 1996a). The importance of severe insulin resistance for the development of NIDDM is underlined by several large population studies: in the Bogalusa Heart Study, 2.4% of overweight adolescents, but no lean adolescents, developed NIDDM by the age of 30 years (Srinivasan et al., 1996). Another study from Cincinnati (Pinhas-Hamiel et al., 1996) found one-third (19 of 58) of all new cases of diabetes presenting in 1994 aged 10–19 years had NIDDM and over 90% of new diabetics had BMI above the 90th centile. The average BMI amongst the new patients with diabetes was $37 \, kg/m^2$ and approximately 40% had BMI above $40 \, kg/m^2$. The incidence of NIDDM in adolescence had increased ten-fold between 1982 and 1994, reflecting the increase in the prevalence of childhood obesity.

The underlying mechanisms for the relationship between obesity and NIDDM are probably similar to those observed in adults: basal insulin secretion, stimulated insulin secretion and insulin resistance relate directly to visceral fat mass and total body fat (Wabitsch et al., 1994; Caprio et al., 1995, 1996b). Whether visceral fat influences glucose and insulin metabolism independent of the effects of total body fat is not known. Nevertheless, the accumulation of excessive fat at adolescence is critical in the development of insulin resistance. As mentioned earlier, when present, AN acts as a clinical marker of insulin resistance.

Dyslipidaemia

The typical abnormalities in the lipid profile of obese children are high total serum cholesterol, LDL-cholesterol and triglycerides but low HDL-cholesterol levels (Zwiauer et al., 1992; Caprio et al., 1996b). Such a negative lipoprotein profile is found most commonly in obese adolescent boys (Lauer et al., 1988). The degree of obesity is consistently more strongly associated with high total cholesterol and abnormal lipoprotein profile in male than in female adolescents (Fredrichs et al., 1978; Glueck et al., 1980). In the Bogalusa Heart Study, overweight during adolescence was associated with a 2.4-fold increase in the prevalence of total cholesterol above 240 mg/dl, a three-fold increase in LDL levels above 160 mg/dl, and an eight-fold increase in HDL levels below 35 mg/dl in young adults (27–31 years) (Srinivasan et al., 1996). Recent data suggest that visceral fat distribution is associated not only with hyperinsulinaemia but also with an unfavourable lipid profile (Freedman et al., 1987, 1989a,b). However, weight reduction can decrease, or even normalize, risk factor levels (Wabitsch et al., 1992, 1994, 1995). Positive effects of weight reduction are more pronounced in patients with abdominal body fat distribution. Girls with abdominal fat distribution lose more body fat in the abdominal region with slimming than those with more gluteo-femoral fat distribution (Wabitsch et al., 1992). The role of fat distribution as a risk factor for the complications of obesity in children and adolescents has been discussed extensively (Zwiauer et al., 1990, 1992; Wabitsch et al., 1994; Dietz, 1998).

Intra-abdominal, or visceral, fat begins to accumulate in early childhood and, even before puberty, there is considerable variation in fat distribution in obesity. Recent data show that a predominantly abdominal fat distribution in adolescent girls is associated with an adverse risk factor profile (hyperinsulinaemia and lipid risk factors) and hyperandrogenaemia. The relationships of body fat distribution and risk factors in obese boys and in younger girls are less evident. Rapidly changing body fat distribution between the ages of 8 and 12 years and changes at puberty can explain these age and sex differences.

The significance of lower circulating levels of growth hormone and increased levels of growth hormone binding protein in the pathogenesis of the multi-metabolic syndrome is not clear. Several studies have shown that the observed metabolic disturbances seem directly related to the metabolic effects of growth hormone (Kratzsch et al., 1997). In vitro studies of cultured human adipocytes under chemically defined conditions strengthen this hypothesis (Wabitsch et al., 1996).

7.1.10 Psychosocial problems

Psychological problems are common in obese children and vary widely in severity. Some obese children, especially those from families in which obesity is a common problem affecting several members, show few psychological problems. Since obesity is considered to be characteristic of their family, they appear active, happy, and without negative adverse psychological effects from their obesity (Doherty & Harkaway, 1990).

On starting school, and even more dramatically during adolescence, obese children have to face a society which perceives the obese as lazy and stupid. In peer-group ranking of friends, obese children are liked less even than children affected by very severe handicaps (Richardson et al., 1961). Not surprisingly, it is at this stage in life that these children often seem to become more lonely, depressed and passive. They have low self-esteem and difficulties in peer-group relationships (Isnard-Mugnier et al., 1993; Wardle et al., 1995). Consequently, obese children and particularly obese adolescents demonstrate high levels of anxiety, and disturbed body image (Kimm et al., 1991). These aspects are discussed elsewhere in this book (Chapter 6).

7.2 Intermediate medical consequences

Many of the medical problems listed in the sections above persist through childhood and adolescence. Cardiovascular risk factors and psychosocial problems represent considerable burdens to overweight and obese children and adolescents. The persistence of obesity in many children and adolescents into adult life represents a significant consequence in itself, since obesity in adults is a well-established independent risk factor for NIDDM, cardiovascular disease (CVD), hyperlipidaemia, osteoarthritis, gallbladder disease and cancer (Burton et al., 1985).

7.2.1 Persistence of obesity

In evaluating the long-term outlook for child and adolescent obesity, it needs to be recognized that studies on this topic have tended to use different definitions for obesity, to present a range of time intervals between childhood and adult measurements, to vary in their criteria for persistence and to use different statistical methods for analysis (Charney et al., 1976; Freedman et al., 1987; Guo et al., 1994; Power et al., 1997). Further, the time intervals of most studies which compare childhood obesity with adult nutritional status rarely exceed 10 years. Nevertheless, these studies indicate that the probability of obesity persisting into adult life is related to the severity of obesity and the age when initially studied.

The likelihood of obesity persisting from early childhood into adult life is only moderate. However, prospective studies show that 20–50% of obese adolescents remain obese in adulthood although only 17–18% of 33-year-old obese adults were obese in childhood (Charney et al., 1976; Garn, 1985; Whitaker et al., 1997). The risks of obese children being obese as adults are two to 11 times higher (depending particularly on the ages studied) than for nonobese children. Probably the majority of obese children slim and become normal-weight adults. One prospective study with long-term follow-up found that the odds ratio for obesity at age 35 years increased from approximately 2 for girls and boys obese aged 1–6 years to 5–10 for those obese at ages 10–14 years (Guo et al., 1994). The odds ratios for adolescents obese at 15–18 years ranged from 8–57 for males and from 6–35 for females, indicating a relatively high risk for the persistence of adolescent obesity. The probability of being obese at age 35 years was estimated as 78% for male and 66% for female obese adolescents (Guo et al., 1994).

7.2.2 Psychosocial problems

The intermediate and long-term consequences of the accumulation of complex psychosocial problems during childhood and adolescence, as well as the resulting changes in the development, of obese children have been shown by a large prospective study from the USA (Gortmaker et al., 1993). This study demonstrated clearly the importance of obesity in changing socioeconomic status from late adolescence into adult life. Women who were obese in late adolescence and early adult life were more likely to have lower family incomes, higher rates of poverty and lower rates of marriage, than women with other chronic physical disabilities who were not obese in childhood (Gortmaker et al., 1993). Goldblatt et al. (1965) described the greater likelihood of obese women experiencing downward social and economic mobility than their nonobese peers. Obese adolescents have worse school performance, fewer academic qualifications and lower college acceptance rates to elite universities than their normal-weight peers with similar achievement scores (Canning & Mayer, 1966, 1967; Gortmaker et al., 1993). Lower household income, less schooling and higher rates of poverty were found amongst women becoming obese, compared with normal-weight women staying slim, over a 7-year period. Observations on obese men found differences between obese and nonobese individuals, but less than those amongst women (Gortmaker et al., 1993). Similar results were found for a British cohort of 23-year-old men and women. These studies suggest the persistent effects of obesity are the cause rather than the effect of low socioeconomic status (Sargent & Blanchflower, 1994). Obesity may be the worst socioeconomic handicap that women suffer. It is not only a serious problem in childhood and adolescence but, when it persists into adult life, it also has major negative long-term impact on affected subjects.

This psychosocial aspect of childhood obesity seems poorly recognized by health professionals. Research is needed to address the role of physicians and paediatricians, for example, in counteracting the complex psychosocial problems affecting obese children and adolescents (Chapter 16).

7.2.3 Cardiovascular consequences

Hypertension affects about 1% of obese children between 5 and 18 years of age but data show that almost 60% of children with persistently elevated blood pressure have relative body weight above 120% (Rames et al., 1978). Hypertension also occurs approximately nine times more frequently amongst obese than nonobese children (Lauer et al., 1975) with elevated systolic or diastolic blood pressures in 20–30% of obese children (weight $>$ 120% of ideal body weight) (Figueroa-Colon et al., 1997).

The metabolic and hormonal changes and risk factor profiles amongst obese children do not present morbidity per se, but do indicate increased likelihood of the development of cardiovascular disease – or other complications – later. Blood pressure levels track from childhood to adulthood. Thus increased systolic blood pressure during childhood may lead to hypertension in adulthood if the obesity persists or becomes more severe (Bao et al., 1994; Raitakari et al., 1994).

Prospective data from the Muscatine and Bogalusa Heart Studies indicate that obese children and adolescents (BMI $>$ 90th centile) are 8.5–10 times more likely than their nonobese peers to develop high blood pressure as young adults (Lauer & Clarke, 1984; Srinivasan et al., 1996). Hyperinsulinaemia plays a key role in the pathogenesis of hypertension. Sympathetic nervous and renin–angiotensin systems activation, decreased renal sodium retention, and a greater sensitivity to sodium intake in obese than in nonobese adolescents, result in enhanced renal absorption of sodium contributing to diastolic and systolic hypertension (Rocchini et al., 1989; Hall 1997).

7.3 Long-term consequences

There is an extensive literature on the short- and mid-term consequences of obesity but few studies have examined the long-term health risks of childhood or adolescent obesity on adult morbidity and mortality. Five major studies with baseline information on obesity before the age of 20 years and adult health outcomes several years later are summarized in Table 7.3. The table is far from complete. Several other prospective and retrospective studies with varying sample sizes and follow-up intervals exist (Paffenbarger & Wing, 1969; Mossberg, 1989; DiPietro et al., 1994; Gunnell et al., 1998). However, the main findings of all studies are similar: adolescent overweight, in men particularly, is associated with an increased morbidity and mortality from CVD, atherosclerosis and colorectal cancer in adult life. All-cause mortality is highest amongst those above the upper quartile for percentage body fat as adolescent men but not for this group as adolescent women. Even after adjustment for adult obesity and for smoking habits, the increased risks remain (Must et al., 1992).

Adolescent overweight is also associated with increased morbidity in adult life from gout in men and arthritis in women (Lake et al., 1997). Men who were obese as children had three times more gout than their peers who were not obese as children.

Women who were overweight in adolescence are twice as likely to report arthritis and eight times more likely to report other limited mobility (Must et al., 1992). Women who were obese in childhood also show increased risk for menstrual problems in early adult life.

Other existing studies of the long-term outcomes for childhood obesity are too preliminary to draw firm conclusions. In the past, few studies have investigated long-term risks using sound objective evidence of child and/or adolescent obesity and of adult adiposity. Even so, there is sufficient evidence to suggest that overweight and obesity in childhood and adolescence influence adult morbidity and mortality. This evidence can only emphasize the importance of primary prevention and early treatment of obesity in children and adolescents. Concern at the increasing numbers of young overweight individuals and the growing evidence of substantial health consequences – short- and long-term, medical, psychosocial – to obesity, underline the importance of further research in this field. There is urgent need for good, objective, studies to clarify this important area of childhood obesity – an area which has so much significance for adult life as well.

Table 7.3. Findings of some long-term follow-up studies of mortality and morbidity risk of overweight and obesity in childhood and adolescence

Author, date, Country	Probands	Study design	Criteria for obesity / Parameters studied	Comments
Abraham et al., 1971, USA	Children: 9–13 years Adults: 42–54 years 86% followed up (1961/1963) after 30–40 years n = 717	Prospective longitudinal study	Overweight: > 120% RBW *Fasting blood glucose, total cholesterol, LDL-cholesterol, blood pressure*	Childhood RBW not significantly related to adult risk parameters. Adult RBW associated with hypertension and cardiovascular disease. Greatest risk for those becoming obese only as adults.
Hoffmans et al., 1988, Netherlands	Adolescents: 18 years Adults: 50 years n = 78 612	Retrospective longitudinal study	BMI classification: < 19; 19–20; 20–25; > 25 *All-cause mortality*	Moderately obese male adolescents had increased mortality risk.
Hoffmans et al., 1989, Netherlands	Adolescents: 18 years Adults: 50 years n = 78 612	Retrospective longitudinal study	BMI classification: < 19; 19–20; 20–25; > 25 *CHD, cancer, especially lung cancer*	Overweight men had increased risk for CHD, but lowest risk for cancer (no information about confounding factors).
Nieto et al., 1992, USA	Children & adolescents 5–18 years Adults followed up 1963, 1975, 1985 n = 13 146	Prospective longitudinal study	Fifths of RBW *All-cause mortality*	Positive association between childhood and adolescent RBW and all-cause mortality at follow up.
Must et al., 1992, USA	Adolescents: 13–18 years Adults: 68–73 years Follow-up after 55 years n = 13 146	Prospective longitudinal study	Overweight: BMI > 75th centile *All-cause mortality, CHD, atherosclerotic cerebrovascular disease, colorectal cancer, breast cancer.*	Increased risk all-cause mortality for men overweight in adolescence but not for women. Increased risk for death from CHD, atherosclerosis, colorectal cancer and gout (men); arthritis (women).
Lake et al., 1997, UK	Children: 7 years Young adults: 23 years n = 5799 women	Prospective longitudinal study	Children: BMI > 20.6 (97th centile at 7 years) Adults: BMI > 28.6 *Menstrual problems, subfertility, hypertension in pregnancy*	Obese: increased menstrual problems at age 23 years; lower rates of conception; increased risk of hypertension in pregnancy.

BMI: body mass index; CHD: coronary heart disease; LDL: low-density-lipoprotein; RBW: relative body weight.

7.4 REFERENCES

Abraham, S., Collins, G. & Nordsieck, M. (1971). Relationship of childhood weight status to morbidity in adults. *Public Health Reports*, **86**, 273–84.

Acalivschi, M.V., Blendea, D., Pascu, M., Georoceanu, A., Bvadea, R.I. & Prelipceanu, M. (1997). Risk of asymptomatic and symtomatic gallstones in moderately obese women: a longitudinal follow-up study. *American Journal of Gastroenterology*, **92**, 127–31.

Bao, W., Srinivasan, S.R., Wattigney, W.A. & Berenson, G.S. (1994). Persistence of multiple cardiovascular risk clustering related to syndrome X from childhood to young adulthood. The Bogalusa Heart Study. *Archives of Internal Medicine*, **154**, 1842–7.

Behrman, R.E. (2000). Torsional and angular deformities. 681.6 Genu varum (bowlegs) 681.7 Genu valgum (knock knees). In eds. R.E. Behrman, R.M. Kliegman & H.B. Jensen, *Nelson's Textbook of Pediatrics*, pp. 2069–71, Philadelphia, PA: W.B. Saunders.

Bennion, L.J., Knowler, W.C., Mott, D.M., Spagnola, A.M. & Bennet, P.H. (1979). Development of lithogenic bile during puberty in Pima Indians. *New England Journal of Medicine*, **300**, 873–9.

Beunen, G.P., Malina, R.M., Lefevre, J.A., Claessens, A.L., Renson, R. & Vanreusel, B. (1994). Adiposity and biological maturity in girls 6–16 years of age. *International Journal of Obesity*, **18**, 542–6.

Burton, B.T., Foster, W.R., Hirsch, J. & Van Itallie, T.B. (1985). Health implications of obesity: an NIH consensus development conference. *International Journal of Obesity*, **9**, 155–69.

Canning, H. & Mayer, J. (1966). Obesity – its possible effect on college acceptance. *New England Journal of Medicine*, **275**, 1172–4.

Canning, H. & Mayer, J. (1967). Obesity: an influence on high school performance? *American Journal of Clinical Nutrition*, **20**, 352–4.

Caprio, S., Bronson, M., Sherwin, R.S., Rife, F. & Tamborlane, W.V. (1996a). Co-existence of severe insulin resistance and hyperinsulinemia in pre-adolescent obese children. *Diabetologica*, **39**, 1489–97.

Caprio, S., Hyman, L.D., McCarthy, S. et al. (1996b). Fat distribution and cardiovascular risk factors in obese adolescent girls: importance of the intra-abdominal fat depot. *American Journal of Clinical Nutrition*, **64**, 12–17.

Caprio, S., Hyman, L.D., Limb, C., McCarthy, S.l., Lange, R., Sherwin, R.S., Shulman, G. & Tamborlane, W.V. (1995). Central obesity and its metabolic correlates in obese adolescent girls. *American Journal of Physiology*, **269**, E118–26.

Charney, E., Goodman, H.C., McBride, M., Lyon, B. & Pratt, R. (1976). Childhood antecedents of adult obesity (Do chubby infants become obese adults?) *New England Journal of Medicine*, **295**, 6–9.

Chay, O.M., Goh, A., Abisheganadeu, J., Tang, J., Lim, W.H., Chan, Y.H. et al. (2000). Obstructive sleep apnoea syndrome in obese Singaporean children. *Pediatric Pulmonology*, **29**, 284–90.

Chehab, F.F., Mounzih, K., Lu, R. & Lim, M.E. (1997). Early onset of reproductive function in normal female mice treated with leptin. *Science*, **275**, 88–90.

Crichlow R.W., Seltzer, M.H. & Jannetta, P.J. (1972). Cholecystitis in adolescents. *American*

Journal of Digestive Diseases, **17**, 68–72.

Dietz, W.H. (1993). Childhood Obesity. In *Textbook of Pediatric Nutrition*, 2nd edn., eds. R.M. Suskind & L. Lewinter-Suskind, pp. 279–84. New York: Raven Press.

Dietz, W.H. (1998). Health consequences of obesity in youth: childhood predictors of adult disease. *Pediatrics*, **101**, 518–25.

Dietz, W.H., Gross, W.L. & Kirkpatrick, J.A. (1982). Blount disease (tibia vara): another skeletal disorder associated with childhood obesity. *Journal of Pediatrics*, **101**, 735–7.

DiPietro, L., Mossberg, H.O. & Stunkard, A.J. (1994). A 40-year history of overweight children in Stockholm: life-time overweight, morbidity and mortality. *International Journal of Obesity*, **18**, 585–90.

Doherty, W. & Harkaway, J. (1990). Obesity and family systems: a family FIRO approach to assessment and treatment planning. *Journal of Marital and Family Therapy*, **16**, 287–98.

Figueroa-Colon, R., Franklin, F.A., Lee, J.Y., Aldridge, R. & Alexander, L. (1997). Prevalence of obesity with increased blood pressure in elementary school-aged children. *Southern Medical Journal*, **90**, 806–13.

Forbes, G.B. (1977). Nutrition and growth. *Journal of Pediatrics*, **91**, 40–2.

Fredrichs, R.R., Webber, L.S., Srinivasan, S.R. & Berenson, G.S. (1978). Relation of serum lipids and lipoproteins to obesity and sexual maturity in white and black children. *American Journal of Epidemiology*, **108**, 486–96.

Freedman, D.S., Shear, C.L., Burke, G.L., Srinivasan, S.R., Webber, L.S., Harsha, D.W. & Berenson, G.S. (1987). Persistence of juvenile-onset obesity over eight years: the Bogalusa Heart Study. *American Journal of Public Health*, **77**, 588–92.

Freedman, D.S., Srinivasan, S.R., Burke, G.L., Shear, C.L., Smoak, C.G., Harsha, D.W., Webber, L.S. & Berenson, G.S. (1989a). Relation of body fat distribution to hyperinsulinemia in children and adolescents: the Bogalusa Heart Study. *American Journal of Clinical Nutrition*, **46**, 403–10.

Freedman, D.S., Srinivasan, Harsha, E.W., Webber, L.S. & Berenson, G.S. (1989b). Relation of body fat patterning to lipid and lipoprotein concentrations in children and adolescents: the Bogalusa Heart Study. *American Journal of Clinical Nutrition*, **50**, 930–9.

Frelut, M.L., Razakarivony, R., Cathelinau, L. & Navarro, J. (1995). Uneven occurrence of fatty liver in morbidly obese children: risk factors and impact of weight loss. *International Journal of Obesity*, **19** Suppl. 2, 122.

Frelut, M.L., Wiling, T.N., Navarro, J. & Debre, R. (1996). Fatty liver and hyperaminotransferasemia (ALT) in obese children: reversibility and correlation with fattening pattern but not overweight degree. *International Journal of Obesity*, **20** Suppl. 4, 147.

Friesen, C.A. & Roberts, C.C. (1989). Cholelithiasis: clinical characteristics in children. *Clinical Pediatrics*, **7**, 294–9.

Fung, K.P., Lau, S.P., Chow, O.K., Lee, J. & Wong, T.W. (1990). Effects of overweight on lung function. *Archives of Disease in Childhood*, **65**, 512–15.

Garn, S.M. (1985). Continuities and changes in fatness from infancy throughout adulthood. *Current Problems in Pediatrics*, **15**, 2–47.

Gennuso, J., Epstein, L.H., Paluch, R.A. & Cerny, F. (1998). The relationship between asthma and obesity in urban minority children and adolescents. *Archives of Paediatric and Adolescent*

Medicine, **152**, 1197–200.

Glueck, C.L., Taylor, H.L., Jacobs, D., Morrison, J.A., Beaglehole, R. & Williams, O.D. (1980). Association with measurements of body mass: the Lipid Research Clinics Program Prevention Study. *Circulation*, **62** Suppl. 4, 62–9.

Goldblatt, P.B., Moore, M.E. & Stunkard, A.J. (1965). Social factors in obesity. *Journal of the American Medical Association*, **192**, 1039–44.

Gortmaker, S.L., Must, A., Perrin, J.M., Sobol, A.M. & Dietz, W.H. (1993). Social and economic consequences of overweight in adolescence and young adulthood. *New England Journal of Medicine*, **329**, 1008–12.

Gunnell, D.J., Frankel, S.J., Nanchahal, K., Peters, T.J. & Smith, G.D. (1998). Childhood obesity and adult cardiovascular mortality: a 57 year follow-up study based on the Boyd Orr cohort. *American Journal of Clinical Nutrition*, **67**, 1111–18.

Guo, S.S., Roche, A.F., Chumlea, W.C., Gardner, J.D. & Siervogel, R.M. (1994). The predictive value of childhood body mass index values for overweight at age 35 y. *American Journal of Clinical Nutrition*, **59**, 810–19.

Halcomb, G.W., O'Neill J.A. & Halcomb, G.W. (1980). Cholecystitis, cholelithiasis and common duct stenosis in children and adolescents. *Annals of Surgery*, **191**, 626–35.

Hall, J.E. (1997). Mechanisms of abnormal renal sodium handling in obesity hypertension. *American Journal of Hypertension*, **10** Suppl., S49–S55.

Hoffmans, M.D.A.F., Kromhout, D. & de Lenzenne Coulander, C. (1988). The impact of body mass index of 78,612 18-year old Dutch men on 32-year mortality from all causes. *Journal of Clinical Epidemiology*, **41**, 749–56.

Hoffmans, M.D.A.F., Kromhout, D. & de Lenzenne Coulander, C. (1989). The impact of body mass index at age of 18 and its effects on 32-year mortality from coronary heart disease and cancer. *Journal of Clinical Epidemiology*, **42**, 513–20.

Honore, L.H. (1980). Cholesterol cholelithiasis in adolescent females. *Archives of Surgery*, **115**, 62–4.

Ingvarrson, T., Hagglund, G., Ramgren, B., Jonsson, K. & Zayer, M. (1997). Long-term results after adolescent Blount's disease. *Journal of Pediatric Orthopedics and Bone Disease*, **6**, 153–6.

Ingvarrson, T., Hagglund, G., Ramgren, B., Jonsson, K. & Zayer, M. (1998). Long-term results after infantile Blount's disease. *Journal of Pediatric Orthopedics and Bone Disease*, **7**, 226–9.

Isnard-Mugnier, P., Vila, G., Nollet-Clemencon, C., Vera, L. & Rault, G. (1993). Etude controllee des conduites alimentaires et des manifestations emotionnelles dans une population d'adolescentes obeses. *Archives Francaises de Pediatrie*, **50**, 479–84.

Johnston F.E. & Mack, R.W. (1980). Obesity, stature and one year relative weight of 15 year old youths. *Human Biology*, **52**, 35–41.

Kaplan, T.A. & Montana, E. (1993). Exercise-induced bronchospasm in non-asthmatic obese children. *Clinical Pediatrics (Philadelphia)*, **32**, 220–5.

Kasapçopur, O., Ozdogan, H. & Yazici, H. (1991). Obesity and erythrocyte sedimentation rate in children. *Journal of Pediatrics*, **119**, 773–5.

Kelsey, J.L., Acheson, J.M. & Keggi, K.J. (1972). The body build of patients with slipped capital epiphysis. *American Journal of Diseases of Children*, **124**, 278–81.

Kimm, S., Sweeney, C. & Janosky, J. (1991). Self-concept measures and childhood obesity: a descriptive analysis. *Journal of Developmental and Behavioural Pediatrics*, **12**, 19–24.

Kinugasa, A., Tsunamoto, K., Furukawa, N., Sawada, T., Kusunoki, T. & Shimada, N. (1984). Fatty liver and its fibrous changes found in simple obesity of children. *Journal of Pediatric Gastroenterology and Nutrition*, **3**, 408–14.

Koffler, M., Raskin, R., Womble, D. & Helderman, J.H. (1991). Immunobiological consequences of regulation of insulin receptor on alloactivated lymphocytes in normal and obese subjects. *Diabetes*, **40**, 364–70.

Kratzsch, J., Dehmel, B., Pulzer, F., Keller, E., Englaro, P., Blum, W.F. & Wabitsch, M. (1997). Increased serum GHBP levels in obese pubertal children and adolescents: relationship to body composition, leptin and indicators of metabolic disturbances. *International Journal of Obesity*, **21**, 1130–6.

Lake, J.K., Power, C. & Cole, T.J. (1997). Women's reproductive health: the role of body mass index in early and adult life. *International Journal of Obesity*, **21**, 432–8.

Lauer, R.M. & Clarke, W.R. (1984). Childhood risk factors for high adult pressure: the Muscatine Study. *Pediatrics*, **84**, 633–41.

Lauer, R.M., Connor, W.E., Leaverton, P.E., Reiter, M.A. & Clarke, W.B. (1975). Coronary heart disease risk factors in school children: the Muscatine Study. *Journal of Pediatrics*, **86**, 697–706.

Lauer, R.M., Lee, J. & Clarke, W.R. (1988). Factors affecting the relationship between childhood and adult cholesterol levels: the Muscatine Study. *Pediatrics*, **82**, 309–18.

Lazar, L., Kauli, R., Bruchis, C., Nordenberg, J., Glaatzer, A. & Perzelean, A. (1995). Early polycystic ovary-like syndrome in girls with central precocious puberty and exaggerated adrenal response. *Journal of Clinical Endocrinology and Metabolism*, **66**, 131–9.

Liddle, R.A., Goldstein, R.B. & Saxton, J. (1989). Gallstone formation during weight reduction dieting. *Archives of Internal Medicine*, **149**, 1750–3.

Loder, R.T., Aronson, D.D. & Greenfield, M.L. (1993). The epidemiology of bilateral slipped capital femoral epiphysis: A study of children in Michigan. *Journal of Bone and Joint Surgery*, **75**, 1141–7.

Lord, G.M., Matarrese, G., Howard, J.K., Baker, R.J., Bloom, S.R. & Lechler, R.I. (1998). Leptin modulates the T-cell immunoresponse and reverses starvation-induced immunosuppression. *Nature*, **394**, 897–902.

Luder, E., Melnik, T.A. & DiMaio, M. (1998). Association of being overweight with greater asthma symptoms in inner city black and Hispanic children. *Journal of Pediatrics*, **132**, 699–703.

Malecka-Tendera, E., Wrzesniewski, N., Kurkowska, M. & Kudla, M. (1998). Overweight in adolescent girls with menstrual irregularities is a risk factor for polycystic ovary syndrome. *International Journal of Obesity*, **22** Suppl. 4, S26.

Mallory, G.B., Fiser, D.H. & Jackson, R. (1989). Sleep-associated breathing disorders in morbidly obese children and adolescents. *Journal of Pediatrics*, **115**, 892–7.

Manolio, T.A., Savage, P.J., Burke, G.L., Liu, K.A., Wagenknecht, L.E., Sidney, S., Jacobs, D.R., Roseman, J.M., Donahue, R.P. & Oberman, A. (1990). Association of fasting insulin with blood pressure and lipids in young adults: the CARDIA Study. *Arteriosclerosis*, **10**, 430–6.

McGill, H.C. Jr., McMahan, C.A., Malcom, G.T., Oalmann, M.C. & Strong, J.P. (1995). Relation of glycohemoglobin and adiposity to atherosclerosis in youth. *Arteriosclerosis, Thrombosis, and Vascular Biology*, **15**, 431–40.

Molnar, D. (1990). Insulin secretion and carbohydrate tolerance in childhood obesity. *Klinische Padiatrie*, **202**, 131–5.

Moran, J.R., Ghishan, F.K., Halter, S.A. & Green, H.L. (1983). Steatohepatitis in obese children: a cause of chronic liver dysfunction. *American Journal of Gastroenterology*, **78**, 374–7.

Mossberg, H.O. (1989). 40-year follow-up of overweight children. *Lancet*, **ii**, 491–3.

Must, A., Jacques, P.F., Dallal, G.E., Bajema, C.J. & Dietz, W.H. (1992). Long-term morbidity and mortality of overweight adolescents: a follow-up of the Harvard Growth Study 1922 to 1935. *New England Journal of Medicine*, **327**, 1350–5.

Nieto, F.J., Szklo, M. & Cornstock, G.W. (1992). Childhood weight and growth rate as predictors of adult mortality. *American Journal of Epidemiology*, **42**, 513–20.

Noguchi, H., Tazawa, Y., Nishinomiya, F. & Takada, G. (1995). The relationship between serum transaminase activities and fatty children with simple obesity. *Acta Paediatrica Japonica*, **37**, 621–5.

Paffenbarger, R.S. & Wing, A.L. (1969). Chronic disease in former college students: the effect of single and multiple characteristics on risk of fatal coronary heart disease. *American Journal of Epidemiology*, **90**, 527–35.

Pinhas-Hamiel, O., Dolan, L.M., Daniels, S.R., Standiford, D., Khoury, P.R. & Zeitler, P. (1996). Increased incidence of non-insulin-dependent diabetes mellitus among adolescents. *Journal of Pediatrics*, **128**, 608–15.

Polito, C., Di Toro, A., Collini, R., Cimmaruta, E., D'Alfonso, C. & Del Giudice, G. (1995). Advanced RUS and normal carpal bone age in childhood obesity. *International Journal of Obesity*, **19**, 506–7.

Power, W., Lake, J.K. & Cole, T.J. (1997). Body mass index and height from childhood to adulthood in the 1958 British birth cohort. *American Journal of Clinical Nutrition*, **66**, 1094–101.

Raitakari, O.T., Porkka, K.V., Rasanden, L., Ronnemaa, T. & Viikari, J.S. (1994). Clustering and six year cluster-tracking of serum total cholesterol, HDL-cholesterol and diastolic blood pressure in children and young adults. The Cardiovascular Risk in Young Finns Study. *Journal of Clinical Epidemiology*, **47**, 1085–93.

Rames, L.K., Clarke, W.R., Connor, W.E., Reiter, M.A. & Lauer, R.M. (1978). Normal blood pressures and the elevation of sustained blood pressure elevation in childhood: the Muscatine Study. *Pediatrics*, **61**, 245–51.

Richards, G.E., Cavalli, A., Meyer, W.J., Prince, M.H., Peters, E.J., Stuart, C.A. & Smith, E.R. (1985). Obesity, acanthosis nigricans, insulin resistance, and hyperandrogenemia: pediatric perspectives and natural history. *Journal of Pediatrics*, **107**, 893–7.

Richardson, S.A., Hastorff, A.H., Goodman, N. & Dornbusch, S.M. (1961). Cultural uniformity in reaction to physical disabilities. *American Sociological Review*, **26**, 241–7.

Riley, D.J., Santiago, T. & Edelman, N.H. (1976). Complications of obesity-hypoventilation syndrome in childhood. *American Journal of Diseases of Children*, **130**, 671–4.

Rocchini, A.P., Key, J., Bondie, D., Chico, R., Moorhead, D., Katch, V. & Martin, M. (1989). The effect of weight loss on the sensitivity of blood pressure to sodium in obese adolescents. *New England Journal of Medicine*, **321**, 580–5.

Sampliner, R.E., Bennet, P.H., Comess, L.J., Rose, F.A. & Burch, T.A. (1970). Gallbladder disease in Pima Indians: demonstration of high prevalence and early onset by cholecystography. *New England Journal of Medicine*, **283**, 1358–64.

Sargent, J.D. & Blanchflower, D.G. (1994). Obesity and stature in adolescence and earnings in young adulthood. *Archives of Pediatrics and Adolescent Medicine*, **148**, 681–7.

Shaffer, E.A. & Small, D.M. (1977). Biliary lipid secretion in cholesterol gallstone disease: the effect of cholecystectomy and obesity. *Journal of Clinical Investigation*, **59**, 828–40.

Silvesti, J.M., Weese-Mayer, D.E., Bass, M.T., Kenny, A.S., Hauptmann, S.A. & Pearsall, S.M. (1993). Polysomnography in obese children with a history of sleep-associated breathing disorders. *Pediatric Pulmonology*, **16**, 124–9.

Sørensen, K.H. (1968). Slipped upper femoral epiphysis. Clinical study on aetiology. *Acta Orthopaedica Scandinavica*, **39**, 499–517.

Srinivasan, S.R., Bao, W., Wattigney, W.A. & Berenson, G.S. (1996). Adolescent overweight is associated with adult overweight and related multiple cardiovascular risk factors: the Bogalusa Heart Study. *Metabolism*, **45**, 235–40.

Styne, D.M. (1996). The testes: disorders of sexual differentiation and puberty. In *Pediatric Endocrinology*, ed. M.A. Sperling, pp. 467. Philadelphia: W.B.Saunders Company.

Sugerman, H.J., Felton, W.L. & Sismani, A. (1999). Gastric surgery for pseudotumor cerebri associated with severe obesity. *Annals of Surgery*, **229**, 634–40.

Thompson, G.H. & Carter, J.R. (1990). Late onset tibia vara (Blount's disease). Current concepts. *Clinical Orthopedics*, **255**, 24–35.

Tracy, V.V., De N.C. & Harper, J.R. (1971). Obesity and respiratory infection in infants and young children. *British Medical Journal*, **1**, 16–18.

Vajro, P., Fontanella, A., Perna, C., Orso, G., Tedesco, M. & De Vicenzo, A. (1994). Persistent hyperaminotransferasemia resolving after weight reduction in obese children. *Journal of Pediatrics*, **125**, 239–41.

Wabitsch, M., Hauner, H., Böckmann, A., Parthon, W., Mayer, H. & Teller, W. (1992). The relationship between body fat distribution and weight loss in obese adolescent girls. *International Journal of Obesity*, **16**, 905–11.

Wabitsch, M., Hauner, H., Heinze, E., Muche, R., Böckmann, A., Parthon, W., Mayer, H. & Teller, W. (1994). Body fat distribution and changes in the atherogenic risk factor profile in obese adolescent girls during weight reduction. *American Journal of Clinical Nutrition*, **60**, 54–60.

Wabitsch, M., Hauner, H., Heinze, E., Muche, R., Böckmann, A., Benz, R., Mayer, H. & Teller, W. (1995). Body fat distribution and steroid hormone concentrations in obese adolescent girls before and after weight reduction. *Journal of Clinical Endocrinology and Metabolism*, **80**, 3469–75.

Wabitsch, M., Braun, S., Hauner, H., Heinze, E., Ilondo, M.M., Shymko, R., De Meyts, P.l. & Teller, W.M. (1996). Mitogenic and antiadipogenic properties of human growth hormone in human adipocyte precursor cells in primary culture. *Pediatric Research*, **40**, 450–6.

Wardle, J., Volz, C. & Golding, C. (1995). Social variation in attitudes to obesity in children. *International Journal of Obesity*, **19**, 562–9.

Weisberg, L.A. & Chutorian, A.M. (1977). Pseudotumor cerebri of childhood. *American Journal of Diseases in Children*, **131**, 1243–8.

Wilcox, P.G., Weiner, D.S. & Leighley, B. (1988). Maturation factors in slipped capital femoral epiphyses. *Journal of Pediatric Orthopedics*, **8**, 196–200.

Whitaker, R.C., Wright, J.A., Pepe, M.S., Seidel, K.D. & Dietz, W.H. (1997). Predicting obesity in young adulthood from childhood and parental obesity. *New England Journal of Medicine*, **337**, 869–73.

Zwiauer, K.F.M., Howanietz, H., Steger, H. & Widhalm, K (1989). Glukosetoleranztest bei hochgradig ubergewichtigen Kinder und Jugendlichten. *Klinische Padiatrie*, **201**, 118–22.

Zwiauer, K., Widhalm, K. & Kerbl, B. (1990). Relationship between body fat distribution and blood lipids in obese adolescents. *International Journal of Obesity*, **14**, 271–7.

Zwiauer, K., R., Müller, T. & Widhalm K. (1992). Cardiovascular risk factors in obese children in relation to overweight and body fat distribution. *Journal of the American College of Nutrition*, **11**, 41–50.

The obese adolescent

Marie-Laure Frelut[1] and Carl-Erik Flodmark,[2]

[1]Robert Debré University Hospital, Paris. [2]Department of Paediatrics, University Hospital in Malmö

8.1 Biophysical factors

8.1.1 Introduction

Adolescence is a key period in life for major physiological and psychological change. Obesity, perhaps dating from infancy, may peak in severity at adolescence. It is thus highly desirable to intervene with vigorous preventive or curative actions early in life. However, adolescents' aspirations and their developing capacity to control their own lives can act as useful adjuncts to the management of obesity in those for whom earlier interventions have been unsuccessful. From the practical point of view, it is critically important that adolescents understand the biological processes affecting them. Stressing the advantages (e.g. growth spurt, increased fat-free mass (FFM) and, as a consequence, increased energy expenditure and requirements) as well as the disadvantages (e.g. increased fat mass in girls) of the pubertal changes in body composition can help adolescents feel more in control of weight management. The differences that develop between sexes should be discussed so that they are understood, accepted and not just seen as further disadvantages for subjects already suffering low self-esteem.

Adolescents also want better understanding of their own behaviour. A recent study from the United States found 24% of a nationally representative sample of adolescents were overweight, but 45% of the girls and 20% of the boys had been dieting, and 13% and 7% of girls and boys, respectively, reported disordered eating. The risk of disordered eating increased during adolescence and correlated with depressive patterns of behaviour (Kaltzman et al., 2000). The potentially favourable independence and the contrasting vulnerability of adolescents mean that interviews and advice need to be handled cautiously and tactfully.

Obesity is a source of rejection by peers which may contribute to conflicts within the family. Advice to obese adolescents should enable them to look positively on their condition by encouraging independent decision making and healthy lifestyles which are perceived as attainable. This chapter presents guidance on the background to obesity in adolescence with the aim of helping those working with these children to develop realistic, positive and sustainable management programmes.

8.1.2 Puberty

Adolescence is the final critical period for the development of obesity in childhood (Dietz, 1996). Early maturation is associated with a greater risk of obesity in adolescence or later (van Lenthe et al., 1996). The risk of being obese in young adult life is strongly related to the level of obesity during adolescence and to the presence of parental obesity. In a recent study in Washington state, Whitaker et al. (1997) found that after adjustment for parental obesity, the odds ratio for adult obesity being associated with childhood obesity ranged from 1.3 at 1–2 years old to 17.5 at 15–17 years old. However, after adjusting for the child's obesity status, the risks of an obese child with one obese parent remaining obese in adult life diminished with age from an odds ratio of 3.2 for children 1–2 years old to only 2.2 for children 15–17 years old. In other words, obesity in older children and adolescents is a significant precursor of adult obesity irrespective of parental nutrition. In children under 10 years, parental obesity more than doubles the risk of adult obesity amongst both obese and nonobese children.

8.1.3 Body composition and energy expenditure

The pubertal growth spurt is associated with changes in body composition which are significantly different for boys and girls. In girls, there is a physiological increase in percentage body fat up to the age of 17 years. In boys, the percentage body fat decreases after the age of 13 years, reaching a minimum around 15 years. This difference is linked to more rapid and greater lean body mass (LBM) development in boys, which continues up to 19 years. In girls, the growth spurt and development of LBM cease around 15 years (Rolland-Cachera et al., 1991; Guo et al., 1997). In parallel with the changes in LBM, energy expenditures which are much the same in prepubertal boys and girls, increase more in boys than girls at puberty, resulting in the markedly higher energy and protein requirements for boys and adult men (World Health Organization, 1985). Puberty is thus associated with changes in body composition which tend to attenuate the development of obesity in boys whilst tending to exacerbate the condition in girls.

Another relevant finding is a tendency for total energy expenditure in girls to fall before puberty. This is not found in boys to the same extent and may be due either to behavioural changes or to energy conserving mechanisms (Goran et al., 1998).

Epidemiological data support the view that about one-third of female obesity in

UK begins in adolescence (Braddon et al., 1986). Although delayed puberty in boys is also associated with an increased fat mass, the risks of developing persistent fatness may be less in boys. However, the change in body shape, reflected in differences in the most typical patterns of fat distribution in adolescence, is less favourable for boys. The android physique, that is increased abdominal fat mass compared with the increased subcutaneous fat of the gynoid physique, is associated with hyperinsulinaemia and increased cardiovascular risk factors and is more common in males than females from adolescence onwards (Rolland-Cachera, 1995; Caprio et al., 1996).

8.1.4 Leptin and puberty

The biological background behind the observed differences in leptin between the sexes is still unclear. Pubic hair development seems to be related to leptin levels during puberty in both sexes, but independently (Wabitsch et al., 1996). Leptin concentrations in girls are 50% higher than in boys at Tanner stage V pubic hair development even for the same fat mass, although only moderate differences were detectable at the onset of puberty. Adolescent girls and women continue to have higher circulating leptin levels than predicted from their higher fat mass, and independent of the degree of obesity (Oslund et al., 1996; Wabitsch et al., 1997). Recent data, linking leptin synthesis in adipose tissue with secondary sexual development and the onset of menarche, support the view that a critical minimum fat mass is necessary to support pregnancy in girls and women (Auwerx & Staels, 1998). By contrast, leptin levels change little in obese boys at puberty (Lahlou et al., 1997). In vitro studies suggest that oestrogen moderately increases, whilst testosterone and dihydrotestosterone significantly decrease, plasma leptin concentrations by decreasing adipocyte mRNA production of leptin (Wabitsch et al., 1996). In adolescent girls, dehydroepiandrosterone (DHEA) has a weakly negative influence on serum leptin whilst testosterone does not reach a level sufficient to affect leptin.

8.1.5 Genetic background and critical periods

Studies of obesity confirm that the heritability of the various obesity phenotypes ranges from 10% to 50% (Pérusse et al., 1998). Further studies are likely to show how different genotypes can lead to the expression of different obese subphenotypes during critical periods for obesity development (Comuzzie & Allison, 1998). Recognition that recessive mutations in the leptin gene and in the leptin receptor (ObR) impair pubertal development and lead to very severe obesity provides a link between nutritional status, as reflected in fat mass, and pubertal achievement.

8.1.6 Cardiovascular risk factors

Obesity in adolescence is an independent risk factor for, and strongly associated with, other cardiovascular risk factors. Increased body mass indexes (BMI) correlate with blood pressure and are predictive of the risk of hypertension by the age of 30 years (Berkey et al., 1998). Waist measurements correlate with increased atherogenic lipoprotein profile and with increased diastolic blood pressure in obese adolescents (Flodmark et al., 1994). The Bogalusa Heart Study showed that the relationship between blood pressure and peripheral body fat weakens during adolescence whilst it remains statistically significant with central body fat, thus contributing to the increased risk profile of the adult with android obesity (Shear et al., 1987). Tell et al. (1985) found an accelerated rate of rise in blood pressure at puberty whilst high-density-lipoprotein (HDL)-cholesterol levels decreased and triglycerides began to rise. Boys exhibited greater negative change in plasma lipids with increasing obesity and this was exacerbated by deleterious behaviours, such as smoking and decreased physical activity.

Cohorts of obese children reviewed in the US after 55 years (Must et al., 1992), and in Sweden after 40 years (Mossberg, 1989), showed that obesity during adolescence was linked with increased mortality in early adult life not only from cerebrovascular accidents but also from breast cancer in women and colon cancer in men. Post-mortem examination of children and young adults involved in the Bogalusa Heart Study demonstrated atherosclerotic lesions of the aorta and coronary arteries in children as young as 2 years of age. Fatty streaks in the coronary arteries increased from 50% at 2–15 years, to 85% at 21–39 years, whilst fibrous-plaque lesions followed the same trend in the aorta. The area of the vessel lining involved was highly correlated with BMI (Berenson et al., 1998). Overweight, together with smoking, despite short exposure to the latter, act synergistically to increase morbidity and mortality. Non-insulin-dependent diabetes mellitus (NIDDM) seems exceptional in obese adolescents although hyperinsulinaemia is by far the most common abnormal biochemical finding revealing the underlying insulin resistance, which precedes pancreatic insufficiency. Only 2% of obese adolescents are diabetic but 85% of young, NIDDM sufferers are obese (Bougnères, 2000). The ten-fold increase in NIDDM amongst morbidly obese adolescents in Cincinnati since 1982 suggests puberty is a critical period for the onset of NIDDM. The mean BMI of the newly diagnosed patients was $37\,kg/m^2$ (Pinhas-Hamiel et al., 1996). Increased visceral fat is likely to be a major contributor to the onset of this complication (Caprio et al., 1996). Some Afro-American populations seem to have a particularly high risk of developing NIDDM.

A study by Strauss et al. (2000) reported fatty liver, assessed by ultrasonography or hyperaminotransferasaemia, in 30–55% of severely obese children and adolescents. Sixty per cent of adolescents with elevated levels of liver aminotransferase were obese. The presence of fatty liver appears to correlate with plasma insulin levels and disappears with weight loss suggesting little underlying structural damage to the liver (Frelut et al., 1995).

8.1.7 Other endocrinological disorders and contraception

Polycystic ovary syndrome (PCOS: Stein–Leventhal syndrome) is defined as the presence of enlarged ovaries with multiple small cysts and thickened white capsule (although this last feature is not essential for diagnosis). Ultrasound appearances are only diagnostic if accompanied by menstrual disorders. Hyperandrogenism, hypothalamo-pituitary abnormalities, insulin resistance, obesity and the presence of other cardiovascular risk factors are associated features of the syndrome. Body weight affects the proportion of androstenedione which converts to oestrone, the major serum oestrogen, and this may explain the propensity of PCOS to develop in association with obesity in adolescence. Obesity is also associated with decreased circulating sex-hormone-binding globulin and this allows higher free testosterone levels which may be another contributing factor. Before the diagnosis of PCOS can be made, it is important to rule out adrenal hyperplasia and ovarian and adrenal tumours (Gordon, 1999).

The contraceptive needs of adolescents must be considered in association with the risk factors linked with obesity and with the psychological backgrounds of obese adolescents requesting contraception. We know of no study which compares the sexual behaviour of obese and nonobese adolescents. We must assume that the obese and nonobese behave similarly.

Obese adolescent girls ask for contraceptive pills more frequently than they ask for any other contraceptive device. The cardiovascular risks associated with contraceptive pills make it advisable to give these girls careful clinical examination, including examination of peripheral veins because of the (very unlikely) risk of deep vein thrombosis. Biochemical checks should include fasting blood glucose, plasma cholesterol, HDL-cholesterol and plasma triglycerides, before recommending oral contraception. Liver aminotransferases should also be measured in morbidly obese children. Irregular menses should raise the possibility of primary or secondary hormonal abnormalities – requiring further investigation – although pregnancy must also be excluded.

The more severe the obesity, the greater is the risk of complications from oral contraception. Nonandrogenic progestogens, derived from 17OH progesterone (chlormadione acetate 5 mg or cyproterone acetate 50 mg) in association with natural 17-β-oestradiols are thus often preferred. The pills are usually prescribed from the 5th to the 25th days of the menstrual cycle.

When discussing sexual activity with adolescents, as with all sexually active individuals, advice on the prevention of sexually transmitted disease is vitally importance. Advice on the use of condoms for example should be offered to both sexes (Atha, 1992; Brown & Cromer, 1997).

8.1.8 Vitamin and mineral status

Adolescence is also characterized by increases in bone mass and mineral density. Peak bone mass is achieved in nonobese subjects around the end of puberty (Martin et al., 1997). Little is known about the development of peak bone mass in obese adolescents (McCormick et al., 1991). Likewise, little is known about Vitamin D status in obese adolescents although alterations in the vitamin D endocrine system have been reported in obese adults (Bell et al., 1985; Norman et al., 1985). Some recent data suggest contradictory results in obese children and adolescents. Manzoni et al. (1996) showed increased total bone mineral content measured by dual X-ray absorptiometry (DEXA) in this population. Total bone mass correlated best with the increase in lean mass. De Schepper et al. (1995) did not find such differences.

In France, where vitamin D supplementation is not provided during adolescence and where dairy products are not supplemented other than when intended for infants, seasonally low levels of 25OH vitamin D occur in 24.5% of nonobese adolescents and, in particular, 38% of adolescents at Tanner pubertal stages 4 and 5 (Zeghoud et al., 1995). In a group of markedly obese adolescents, 13% of boys and 14% of girls of the Paris area were found to have biochemical 25OH vitamin D deficiency during summertime. This was rarely associated with secondary hyperparathyroidism (Frelut et al., 1998). Zamboni et al. (1988) also reported low bone mineral content and plasma 25OH vitamin D_3 in obese adolescents. Such controversial findings may relate to local nutrition as well as to regional differences in exposure to sunshine. The possibility of an impaired social life in adolescent obesity has also to be considered as a risk factor. Clearly, weight loss through dieting requires careful consideration with regard to management of vitamin D status. Obesity cannot necessarily be considered as evidence of adequacy in all nutrients.

We have no other data on vitamin and mineral status in adolescent obesity. However, our personal observation would be that iron deficiency is at least as common as in the general population and is particularly common in pubertal girls.

8.1.9 Complications

The orthopaedic complications of obesity follow different patterns at adolescence. Bone maturation (corresponding to menarche in girls and pubic hair Tanner stage 4 in boys) is linked with a sharp decline in the risk of slipped capital femoral epiphyses which tends to occur more commonly and earlier in obese children (Loder 1996) (Chapter 7). Other problems, such as osteoarthritic changes in the knees, slowly evolve through adolescence into the classical forms of adult obesity related disability.

Other complications usually exist only as mild, reversible forms during adolescence, suggesting a continuum with the more severe and persistent changes in adult obesity. For example, several studies show that morbidly obese adolescents commonly suffer hypopnoea during sleep but life-threatening apnoea is much less frequent. Hypopnoea is often associated with mild daytime sleepiness but is reversible with weight loss. As in adults, mean oxygen saturation (SaO_2) correlates negatively with neck circumference. Obese adolescents, complaining of daytime fatigue, should be assessed for sleep apnoea before their sleepiness is attributed to psychological disturbance (Lecendreux et al., 1998).

Pulmonary hypertension is exceptional in adolescence. Its presence should, in our opinion, indicate the need for cardiovascular investigation to exclude previously undiagnosed cardiovascular malformation. By contrast, in our series of 200 morbidly obese adolescents investigated by ultrasonography before and after weight reduction, minor cardiac abnormalities were extremely common and at least partly reversible (unpublished data). Common findings were mild left atrial enlargement and septal hypertrophy. In morbidly obese adults, such abnormalities indicate marked cardiac dysfunction and associated increased anaesthetic risk (Vaughan, 1992).

8.2 Psychological aspects

Relations with the social environment change dramatically at adolescence. Early in childhood, the family of origin is most important in children's lifestyles and environment. Parents control their children's environment by deciding the foods that are brought home and are thus available. They decide when children should eat and do their best to give their children healthy eating patterns. They guide children by including exercise as a natural part of life, for example by encouraging cycling to school instead of going by bus or car. Parents also have control over the amount of money available to their young children thus influencing how much extra food children can buy at school or with friends.

It is also parents' role to teach their children to take responsibility, adjusting to children's growing capabilities by, for example, increasing pocket money with increasing age and teaching children that older brothers and sisters have different roles. Older children stay up later at night but have more responsibilities helping with family chores.

These examples serve to illustrate the power of the family in preventing the development of severe obesity in young children. We have shown family therapy can be effective in treating obesity when commenced around the age of 10–11 years, that is in the preadolescent period (Flodmark et al., 1993). This should not be a surprise, as the family is regarded as basic to the child's psychological development and the major factor influencing the child's quality of life. Even so, other people, who may be less immediate within the family, such as grandparents, step-parents and adults close to the family, can also be important influences in children's lives.

Children's friends at home or at school are also important to them. They gradually become a significant frame of reference outside the family. In due time, adolescents will leave their family of origin and, after some chaotic years trying to find someone with whom to share their lives, may finally create families of their own. This process of liberation from family influences takes place when obese children are likely to be at their most obese, in the middle of puberty. Family therapy can thus be useful, helping the growth of independence in obese children to proceed without obesity becoming an overwhelming issue for the child or damage to the family.

Families need guidance on how to give children gradually increasing responsibility for their weight regulation. Giving children more and more obligations balanced by more and more freedom accomplishes this. However, it may be only around the age of 15–16 years that obese adolescents really begin to take adult-like responsibilities for their own weight control.

8.2.1 The adolescent psyche

Early adolescence (11–14 years of age) is characterized by the beginning of separation from parents and the increased influence of the peer group. Activities are performed with same-sex peers and the future orientation in thinking is limited. Abstract (formal operational) thinking is developing. The new mental skills of adolescents make them aware of other people's needs but unable to differentiate what is of interest to themselves and of interest to others, often leading to egocentrism. The focus at this stage is largely on body changes: 'Am I normal?' (Joffe, 1994).

Mid-adolescence (14–17 years) usually sees the peak of conflicts and limit testing with parents. Peer influences and conformity with peers are at their most dominant. Sexual behaviour and risk-taking behaviours increase due to a sense of invulnerability. Autonomy is a chief concern. More future-oriented thinking and abstract thinking are established. However, these are not constant and thinking may revert to earlier patterns under stress. Bodily changes have been accepted. The focus is on personal and sexual identity: 'Who am I?'

Late adolescence and young adult life (17–21 years) see the establishment of close friendships and intimate relations with both sexes. Rapprochement with parents takes place and career goals are usually defined. Abstract thinking is well established and future-oriented goals are realistic. Focus is on identity in relation to society: 'What is my role in relation to society?'

8.2.2 What is important for the obese adolescent?

Adolescents need to be accepted and supported by peer groups, usually very close in age. It is important to share common 'identifiers of group' symbols. Clothes become important. This creates problems for obese adolescents. It is difficult for obese adolescents of both sexes to find nice-looking clothes. One of the major benefits of losing weight is the relative ease of finding acceptable clothes. This is a comment made by almost every slimmed child.

Another important issue is acceptability for group activities. Obese adolescents can easily adopt sedentary lifestyles if they are not readily accepted as coparticipants when their group is involved in sport. All kinds of group activities which involve physical exercise – not just formal sporting activities – are significant in this respect. Thus, making it easier for obese adolescents to meet friends at sport clubs, summer camps and so on is an important role for parents. They cannot *make* things happen, but they can provide adolescents with the *means* to make things happen.

8.2.3 How to approach the obese adolescent

Obese adolescents need respect. It is natural for them to try to liberate themselves not only from their parents but also from their weight problems. Similar behavioural mechanisms occur with other chronic diseases such as asthma and diabetes. Family therapy has been effective in these diseases also (Lask, 1987; Dare, 1992).

What is the best approach to obese adolescents for those who are not trained therapists? One basic strategy is to pose questions rather than present answers. This gives the obese adolescent more open space for initiatives of his or her own, but it is important to use the right type of questions.

Linear questions are often used when interviewing parents. For example:

'When did your child develop obesity? When did you move close to school?'

Or:

'When did your child develop obesity? When did you lose your job? Was it after this that you could not afford to buy your child a new bike?'

The questions may seem harmless but, put into the context of the parents of an obese child, they could give parents feelings of guilt. Sometimes we rephrase the question because we realize this danger in advance – and sometimes we do not.

There are other types of questions which are more constructive. One type is the circular question. Circular questions are used to investigate what happens and how a sequence of events takes place. The focus is the interaction between people.

'Who will be the first to notice that XX is increasing weight? What do you do when you notice this? Who will notice this next? What will happen then?'

Curiosity is important in emphasizing the positive chain of events that led to weight control in earlier attempts at losing weight. The questions are thus useful in discussing how to prevent relapses.

Another type of question is the reflexive question. This usually starts with 'If'. One simple example would be questioning a child who seems reluctant to do anything about a weight problem.

Doctor: 'Do you want to lose weight?'
Child: 'No'.

Doctor: 'If it were easy to lose weight, wouldn't you like to start doing something about it?'

So far no-one has responded with a 'no' to the last question.

This classification of questions is particularly useful in the medical setting (Tomm, 1987a,b, 1988). For more examples see Chapter 16.

8.2.4 The severely obese adolescent with problems

Family support cannot guarantee a successful outcome. Difficulties often arise when there are strong genetic influences combined with difficult social situations, for example with some Prader–Willi children. These children with extreme obesity and impaired cognitive function still become adolescents. They want to be responsible adults (as do all adolescents), usually before they are able. They want to live alone but cannot cope with money, since it usually all goes on food. Giving money in small amounts to the adolescent's home assistant can solve this problem but the assistants still need to do the shopping. These children often have reading difficulties so it is important to explain everything carefully so as to avoid misunderstanding. Some young adult Prader–Willi subjects can cope with regular employment and it is then important to find them jobs which give them daily exercise.

Many young adults with impaired intelligence but good family support eventually find partners. Their partners may also be handicapped in some way. Nevertheless, it is very important to include partners in treatment programmes, explaining why energy restriction is so important for Prader–Willi and other handicapped obese subjects. Sometimes it can be helpful to give obese adolescents frozen foods which they can warm up in a microwave oven so they have their own food supply.

Yet, management is not always difficult. Adolescents with impaired cognitive functions are often happy to follow instructions provided they understand the reasons for the instructions! Thorough explanation, at a level which the individual can understand, is worth all the effort this may take!

Prader–Willi adolescents are examples of problem cases where the genetic influences are strong. Social influences can also be very important in management. Children with genetic susceptibilities for obesity living in difficult social situations, such as with drug-addicted parents, usually get little help at home with weight control. These children may be sent to foster homes because of the combination of severe obesity and difficult social circumstances. Then the foster homes need a lot of support so as to keep contact with the biological parents. If done successfully and if the biological parents are allowed to parent whenever possible, then the children have the best chances of controlling weight and developing healthy satisfying lifestyles.

Adolescents with autism and obesity are difficult to treat. The difficulties in communicating with the children and their behavioural problems necessitate specialized treatment which combines the skills of the autism support teams with suitable teaching methods. So far as eating is concerned, it is important to identify children's favourite dishes (which may be few in number) and to offer these in energy-reduced form.

One important, but very, very rare, differential diagnosis in obese adolescents with uncontrollable appetite and social problems is insulinoma (nesidioblastosis). Over-production of insulin leaves these children constantly hungry and, as they grow older, they learn to eat large quantities in order to stave off hunger. Some then become obese, often in combination with delinquency and other behavioural problems. Investigation should include fasting blood glucose, insulin and C-peptide.

8.2.5 Day-care programmes

Adolescents with strong genetic propensities for obesity or from severely disadvantaged social backgrounds may need more support than it is possible to give. It is important to keep them in their own social context, such as their family homes, foster homes or their own apartments. Perhaps they are unable to work or participate in programmes of general education, in which case specialized day-care services should be available. Such obese adolescents could spend the day in home-like environments being trained in group interaction and in learning to take responsibility for themselves. They could be taught how to cook meals of reduced energy content which they can then bring home to eat.

This sort of environmental therapy is also useful in managing adolescents with eating disorders such as bulimia nervosa or binging. Treatment should be combined with other support from child/adolescent guidance clinics. Often, treatment is initiated for problems other than the eating disorder. Most cases of obesity are not due to eating disorders but, when they are, intense treatment is usually necessary.

8.2.6 Eating disorders and obesity

Obesity has not been defined as consistently associated with any psychological or behavioural syndrome (American Psychiatric Association, 1994). However, diagnosis of an eating disorder in association with obesity should be viewed seriously. Eating disorders are divided into bulimia nervosa (BN), anorexia nervosa, binge-eating disorder (BED) and eating disorder not otherwise specified (EDNOS), according to *DSM-IV (Diagnostic and Statistical Manual of Mental Disorders)* (American Psychiatric Association, 1994; Hay & Fairburn, 1998). The *DSM* does not define diseases where there is a common understanding of the pathophysiology. Usually the mechanism is not known and diagnoses are dependent on symptom lists as in medical syndromes. Binge-eating disorder has still to be recognized as a disease in *DSM-IV*, although the criteria for further research have been suggested (American Psychiatric Association, 1994).

Bulimic eating disorders exist on a continuum of clinical severity, from bulimia nervosa purging type (most severe), through bulimia nervosa nonpurging type (intermediate severity), to binge-eating disorder (least severe). There are differences between the conditions in the psychological disturbances and the drop-out rates. Obese nonbinge eaters have least psychopathology, followed by obese binge eaters and then obese bulimia nervosa cases (de Zwaan et al., 1994). The long-term prognosis (6 years) for bulimia nervosa purging type is more favourable than for anorexia nervosa, with a good outcome in 60% of cases (Fichter & Quadflieg, 1997). In one study, 8% of the individuals were obese at the beginning of therapy and at 6-year follow-up this figure was still only 6%. However, bulimic symptoms can remain stable for 10 years (Joiner et al., 1997), indicating that long-term follow-up is necessary. Binge-eating disorder is treated with cognitive therapy or with interpersonal therapy which aims to improve personal relationships (the equivalent of family therapy in adults) (Rissanen, 1998).

Bulimia nervosa is rare or nonexistent before late adolescence, that is age 15 years onwards. Bulimia nervosa could be regarded as a way of compensating for binge eating by vomiting and purging to attempt perceived normal weight.

Stunkard (1990) first described BED in obese adults but the syndrome has been found in people of normal weight. Approximately 29% of subjects in weight-control programmes met the criteria for BED (Stunkard, 1990; Spitzer et al., 1993). The prevalence of eating disorders in obesity was previously thought to be as high as 20–50% among adults seeking help for obesity. It has now been shown that only 7% of adolescents enrolled in an obesity programme have evidence of eating disorders (Decaluwé et al., 2000). The reason for this difference seems to be that diagnostic interviews do not confirm earlier findings developed from the answers to questionnaires (Stunkard et al., 1996; Ricca et al., 2000). Among the obese in the general population and not seeking help for their obesity, the prevalence of eating disorders is likely to be even lower.

Thus, whilst individual psychodynamic psychotherapy may be useful in some cases of eating disorders, it is not useful in cases with obesity. There is no scientific support of its value in obesity without eating disorders (Flodmark, 1997).

8.2.7 Conclusions

Clinically, adolescence is one of the most critical periods for preventing and treating obesity. Most of the risk factors associated with obesity increase and the probability of being an obese adult increases greatly. Nevertheless, the pubertal growth spurt and the psychological and behavioural changes of adolescence can create new positive attitudes which will benefit the adolescent's nutrition.

Psychologically, obese adolescents are in many ways no different from other adolescents with severe chronic diseases. Psychological management should take into account the conflict between the needs for increasing liberation from the family, peer-group acceptability and independence, and the contrasting need for *someone* to be responsible for the adolescent's weight through dietary control and exercise. Guiding the family through this potential battlefield can be particularly helpful. Developing the ideal programme of weight control remains a combined challenge for adolescent, family and professional helper.

8.3 REFERENCES

American Psychiatric Association (1994). *DSM-IV. Diagnostic and Statistical Manual of Mental Disorders.* Fourth Edition. Washington DC: American Psychiatric Association.

Atha, N. (1992). Les adolescentes et la contraception. In *Gynecologie medico chirugicale de l'enfant et de l'adolescente*, eds. Salomon Y., Thibaud E. & Rappaport R. pp. 179–203, Paris: Douin.

Auwerx, J. & Staels, B. (1998). Leptin. *Lancet*, **351**, 737–42.

Bell, N., Epstein, S., Greene, A., Shary, J., Oexmann, M.J. & Shaw, S. (1985). Evidence for alteration of the vitamin D endocrine system in obese subjects. *Journal of Clinical Investigation*, **76**, 370–3.

Berenson, G.S., Srinavasan, S.R., Bao, W. et al. (1998). Association between multiple cardiovascular risk factors and atherosclerosis in children and young adults. The Bogalusa Heart Study. *New England Journal of Medicine*, **338**, 1650–6.

Berkey, C.S., Gardner, J. & Colditz, G.A. (1998). Blood pressure in adolescence and early adulthood related to obesity and birth size. *Obesity Research*, **6**, 187–95.

Bougnères, P.F. (2000). Genèse du risque de diabète chez l'enfant obèse in dépistage et prévention de l'obésité de l'enfant et de l'adolescent, pp. 117–30. Paris: INSERM.

Braddon, F.E.M., Rodgers, B., Wadworth, M.E.J. et al. (1986). Onset of obesity in a 36 years birth cohort. *British Medical Journal*, **293**, 299–303.

Brown, R.T. & Cromer, B.A. (1997). The pediatrician and the sexually active adolescent. *Pediatric Clinics of North America*, **44**, 1379–90.

Caprio, S., Hyman, L.D., McCarthy, S. et al. (1996). Fat distribution and cardiovascular risk factors in obese adolescent girls: importance of the intra-abdominal fat depots. *American Journal of Clinical Nutrition*, **64**, 12–17.

Comuzzie, A.G. & Allison, B. (1998). The search for human obesity genes. *Science*, **280**, 1374–7.

Dare, C. (1992). Change the family, change the child? *Archives of Disease in Childhood*, **67**, 643–8.

Decaluwé, V., Braet, C. & Fairburn, C. (2000). Binge eating in obese children and adolescents. *International Journal of Obesity*, **24** (suppl. 1), S162.

De Schepper, J., Van den Broeck, M. & Jonckheer, M.H. (1995). Study of lumbar spine bone mineral density in obese children. *Acta Paediatrica*, **84**, 313–15.

de Zwaan, M., Mitchell, J.E., Raymond, N.C. & Spitzer, R.L. (1994). Binge eating disorder: clinical features and treatment of a new diagnosis. *Harvard Review of Psychiatry*, **1**, 310–25.

Dietz, W.H. (1996). Prevention of childhood obesity. In *Progress in Obesity Research 7*, eds. A. Angel, H. Anderson, C. Bouchard et al., pp. 223–6. London: John Libbey Company.

Fichter, M.M. & Quadflieg, N. (1997). Six-year course of bulimia nervosa. *International Journal of Eating Disorders*, **22**, 361–84.

Flodmark, C.E. (1997). Childhood obesity. *Clinical Child Psychology and Psychiatry*, **2**, 283–95.

Flodmark, C.E., Ohlsson, T., Ryden, O. & Sveger, T. (1993). Prevention of progression to severe obesity in a group of obese schoolchildren treated with family therapy. *Pediatrics*, **91**, 880–4.

Flodmark, C.E., Sveger, T. & Nilsson-Ehle, P. (1994). Waist measurements correlate to a potentially atherogenic lipoprotein profile in obese 12–14-year-old children. *Acta Paediatrica*, **83**, 941–5.

Frelut, M.L., Rasakarivony, R., Cathelineau, L. & Navarro, J. (1995). Uneven occurence of fatty liver in morbidly obese children. Impact of weight loss. *International Journal of Obesity*, **19** (suppl. 2), 43.

Frelut, M.L., Guibourdenche J., Oberlin F. et al. (1998). Changes in bone mineral density and vitamin D status in obese adolescents during weight loss. *International Journal of Obesity*, **22** (suppl. 4), 33.

Goran, M.I., Gower, B.A., Nagy, T.R. et al. (1998). Developmental changes in energy expenditure and physical activity in children: evidence for a decline in physical activity in girls before puberty. *Pediatrics*, **101**, 887–91.

Gordon, C.M. (1999). Menstrual disorders in adolescence. Excess androgens and polycystic ovary syndrome. *Pediatric Clinics of North America*, **46**, 519–43.

Guo, S.S., Chumlea, W.C., Roche, A.F. & Siervogel, R.M. (1997). Age-and maturity-related changes in body composition during adolescence into adulthood: the FELS Longitudinal Study. *International Journal of Obesity*, **21**, 1167–75.

Hay, P. & Fairburn, C. (1998). The validity of the *DSM-IV* scheme for classifying bulimic eating disorders. *International Journal of Eating Disorders*, **23**, 7–15.

Joffe, A. (1994). Adolescent medicine. In: *Principles and Practice of Paediatrics*. 2nd. edn., ed. F. Oski. Philadelphia: J.B. Lippincott Company.

Joiner, T.E., Jr., Heatherton, T.F. & Keel P.K. (1997). Ten-year stability and predictive validity of five bulimia-related indicators. *American Journal of Psychiatry*, **154**, 1133–8.

Kaltzman, D.K., Golden, N.H., Neumark-Sztainer, D., Yager, J. & Strober, M. (2000). From prevention to progress: clinical research update on adolescent eating disorders. *Pediatric Research*, **47**, 709–12.

Lahlou, N., Landais, P., De Borissieu, D. & Bougneres, P.F. (1997). Circulating leptin in normal children and during the dynamic phase of juvenile obesity: relation to body fatness, energy metabolism, calorie intake and sexual dimorphism. *Diabetes*, **46**, 989–93.

Lask, B. (1987). Family therapy. *British Medical Journal*, **294**, 203–4.

Lecendreux, M., Frelut, M.L., Quera-Salva, M.A. et al. (1998). Weight loss reduces sleep associated breathing disorders in obese children. *Journal of Sleep Research*, **7** (suppl. 2), 152.

Loder, R.T. (1996). The demographics of slipped capital femoral epiphysis. An international multicentered study. *Clinical Orthopaedic Related Research*, **322**, 8–27.

Manzoni, P., Brambilla, P., Pietrobelli, A. et al. (1996). Influence of body composition on bone mineral content in children and adolescents. *American Journal of Clinical Nutrition*, **64**, 603–7.

Martin, A.D., Bailey, D. McKay, H.A. & Whiting, S. (1997). Bone mineral and calcium accretion during puberty. *American Journal of Clinical Nutrition*, **66**, 611–15.

McCormick, D.P., Ponder, S.W., Fawcett, H.D. & Palmer, J.L. (1991). Spinal bone mineral density in 335 normal and obese children and adolescents: evidence for ethnic and sex differences. *Journal of Bone and Mineral Research*, **6**, 507–13.

Mossberg, H.O. (1989). 40-year follow-up of overweight children. *Lancet*, **2**, 491–3.

Must, A., Jacques, P.F., Dallal, G.E. et al. (1992). Long-term morbidity and mortality of overweight adolescents: a follow-up of the Harvard Growth Study of 1922 to 1935. *New England Journal of Medicine*, **327**, 1350–5.

Norman, H., Epstein, S., Grenn, A. et al. (1985). Evidence for alteration of the vitamin D endocrine system in obese subjects. *Journal of Clinical Investigations*, **76**, 370–3.

Oslund, R.E., Yang, J.W., Klein, S. et al. (1996). Relation between plasma leptin concentration and body fat, gender, age, diet and metabolic covariates. *Journal of Clinical Investigations*, **81**, 3909–13.

Pérusse, L., Chagnon, Y.C., Rice, T. et al. (1998). L'épidémiologie génétique et la génétique moléculaire de l'obésité: les enseignements de l'étude des familles du Québec. *Médecine/ Sciences*, **8–9** (24), 914–24.

Pinhas-Hamiel, O., Dolan, L.M., Daniels, S.R. et al. (1996). Increased incidence of non-insulin-dependent diabetes mellitus among adolescents. *Journal of Pediatrics*, **128**, 608–15.

Ricca, V., Mannucci, E., Moretti, S., Di Bernardo, M., Zucchi, T., Cabras, P.L. et al. (2000). Screening for binge eating disorder in obese outpatients. *Comparative Psychiatry*, **41**, 111–15.

Rissanen, A. (1998). Psychological aspects on obesity and eating disorders. In: *Fetma/Fedme (Obesity)*. T. Andersen, A. Rissanen & S. Rössner eds. Lund: Studentlitteratur.

Rolland-Cachera, M.F. (1995). Prediction of adult body composition from infants and child measurements. In *Body Composition Techniques in Health and Disease*, eds. P.S.W. Davies & T.J. Cole. Cambridge: Cambridge University Press.

Rolland-Cachera, M.F., Cole, T.J., Sempé, M. et al. (1991). Body Mass Index variations: centiles fom birth to 87 years. *European Journal of Clinical Nutrition*, **45**, 13–21.

Shear, C.L., Freedman, D., Burke, G. et al. (1987). Body fat patterning and blood pressure in children and young adults. *Hypertension* **9**, 236–84.

Spitzer, R.L., Yanovski, S., Wadden, T., Wing, R., Marcus, M.D., Stunkard, A. et al. (1993). Binge eating disorder: its further validation in a multisite study. *International Journal of Eating Disorders*, **13**, 137–53.

Strauss, R.S., Barlow, S.E. & Dietz, W.H. (2000). Prevalence of abnormal serum aminotransferase values in overweight and obese adolescents. *Journal of Pediatrics*, **136**, 727–33.

Stunkard, A. (1990). A description of eating disorders in 1932. *American Journal of Psychiatry*, **147**, 263–8.

Stunkard, A., Berkowitz, R., Wadden, T., Tanrikut, C., Reiss, E. & Young, L. (1996). Binge eating disorder and the night-eating syndrome. *International Journal of Obesity*, **20**, 1–6.

Tell, G.S., Tuomilheto, J., Epstein, F.H. et al. (1985). Study of atherosclerosis determinants and precursors during childhood and adolescence. *Bulletin of the World Health Organization*, **64**, 595–605.

Tomm, K. (1987a). Interventive interviewing: Part I. Strategizing as a fourth guideline for the therapist. *Family Process*, **26**, 3–13.

Tomm, K. (1987b). Interventive interviewing: Part II. Reflexive questioning as a means to enable self-healing. *Family Process*, **26**, 167–83.

Tomm, K. (1988). Interventive interviewing: Part III. Intending to ask linear, circular, strategic, or reflexive questions? *Family Process*, **27**, 1–15.

Van Lenthe, F.J., Kemper, H.C.G. & Van Melchem, W. (1996). Rapid maturation in adolescence results in greater obesity in adulthood: the Amsterdam Growth and Health Study. *American Journal of Clinical Nutrition*, **64**, 18–24.

Vaughan, R.W. (1992). Anaesthesia and morbid obesity in Obesity, 1st edition, eds. P. Bjorntrop & B.N. Brodoff, pp. 720–30. Philadelphia: J.B. Lippincott Company.

Wabitsch, M., Jensen, P.B., Blum, W.F., Christofferson, C.T. & England, P. (1996). Insulin and cortisol promote leptin production in cultured human fat cells. *Diabetes*, **45**, 1435–8.

Wabitsch, M., Blum, M.F., Muche, R. et al. (1997). Contribution of androgens to the gender difference in leptin production in obese children and adolescents. *Journal of Clinical Investigation*, **100**, 808–13.

Whitaker, R.C., Wright, J.A., Pepe, M.S., Seidel, K.D. & Dietz, W.H. (1997). Predicting obesity in young adults from childhood and parental obesity. *New England Journal of Medicine*, **337**, 869–73.

World Health Organization (1985). *Energy and Protein Requirements*. Technical Report Series 724, Geneva: WH'''O.

Zamboni, G., Soffiati, M., Giovarina, D. et al. (1988). Mineral metabolism in obese children. *Acta Paediatrica Scandinavica*, **77**, 741–6.

Zeghoud, F., Delaveyne, R., Rehel, P. et al. (1995). Vitamine D et maturation pubertaire. Interêt et tolérance d'une supplémentation vitaminique D en période hivernale. *Archives de Pédiatrie*, **2**, 221–6.

Prader–Willi and other syndromes

Giuseppe Chiumello[1] and Elizabeth M.E. Poskitt[2]

[1]Clinica Paediatrica III, Universita degli Studi di Milano. [2]International Nutrition Group, London School of Hygiene and Tropical Medicine

9.1 Introduction

Most children with obesity are basically normal healthy children with simple, primary or exogenous obesity. Some have psychological problems or orthopaedic complaints and simple obesity is also more common in children with mild nonspecific mental retardation. Over time, children with simple obesity also develop the health consequences of severe obesity, but their lack of problems in early childhood is often remarkable. By contrast, children with 'pathological', secondary or endogenous obesity have obesity in association with a wide variety of other problems. Obesity is rarely their presenting problem. True secondary obesity currently accounts for only a small proportion ($<5\%$) of cases of obesity. However developments in understanding of the genetics of obesity may change this in the future as specific diagnoses become possible for increasing numbers of previously 'simple' obesity cases (Farooqi & O'Rahilly, 2000).

Secondary obesity occurs in association with two main types of condition: endocrine disorders and genetic/chromosomal abnormalities (Table 9.1). Clinical features which suggest that obesity may be part of a wider paediatric problem are listed in Table 9.2. Underlying conditions are of two general kinds: acquired endocrine conditions and syndromes which are usually congenital, although obesity may not be apparent in very early life.

9.2 Endocrine problems

9.2.1 Hypothyroidism

Typically hypothyroidism is associated with fat gain and in adult life this may be a major feature. In childhood, however, slowed linear growth is usually the feature which causes most concern. Obesity is rarely more than moderate. Children present with short stature or slowed growth, change of appearance with

Table 9.1. Main clinical obesity-associated syndromes

Chromosomal
   Prader–Willi syndrome
   Down's syndrome

Genetic
   Autosomal dominant
     Biemond syndrome (some cases)
   Autosomal recessive
     Alstrom syndrome
     Bardet–Biedl syndrome
     Biemond syndrome (some cases)
     Carpenter syndrome
     Cohen syndrome
   X-linked inheritance
     Borjeson–Forssman–Lehmann syndrome
   Single gene lesions affecting leptin metabolism
     Congenital leptin deficiency
       truncated leptin protein
       missense mutation in leptin
     Leptin receptor mutation
     Prohormone convertase 1 mutation
     Melanocortin 4 receptor mutation

Endocrine
   Hypothyroidism
   Cushing's disease: hyperadrenocorticism
   Growth hormone deficiency
   Hypothalamic damage secondary to craniopharyngioma, meningitis etc.
   Stein–Leventhal syndrome

myxoedematous skin presenting as pallid face with pink cheeks – the 'peaches and cream' complexion. There may be some hoarsening of the voice and hair loss. Children may feel the cold readily, develop constipation and sleepiness. Provided hypothyroidism has developed post infancy, lowered intelligence is not a problem although there may be slowing of reactions. Typically these children's slow reaction to the usual distractions of childhood make them progress well at school. Treatment may be associated with temporary deterioration in school work as children become more normally restless and inattentive in class (LaFranchi, 2000).

Diagnosis is usually straightforward from measurement of thyroid hormones and thyroid-stimulating hormone (TSH). Treatment with thyroid hormone in

Table 9.2. Clinical features suggesting obesity may be secondary to another condition or syndrome

---

Severe unremitting obesity

Abnormal facies

Disorders of the eyes

   colobomata

   retinal problems, especially retinitis pigmentosa

   narrow palpebral fissures

   abnormally positioned palpebral fissures

   severe squint

Skeletal abnormalities

   polydactyly

   syndactyly

   kyphoscoliosis

Sensorineural deafness

Microcephaly and/or abnormally shaped skull

Mental retardation

Hypotonia

Hypogonadism

   cryptorchidism

   micropenis

   delayed puberty

Renal abnormalities

Cardiac abnormalities

---

replacement doses will be lifelong.

Children with Down's syndrome (Trisomy 21) are, along with many children with some degree of mental retardation, more prone to obesity than normal children. However they are also more prone to hypothyroidism, usually secondary to autoimmune thyroiditis. The Down's syndrome child who develops sudden exacerbation of obesity should be investigated for hypothyroidism.

9.2.2 Cushing's syndrome and hyperadrenocorticism

Cushing's syndrome is not always easy to distinguish clinically from simple obesity in adolescent children who have more or less ceased growing. In younger children hypercortisolism is almost always associated with short stature, in contrast to simple obesity. The moon face, red cheeks and hirsutes typical of Cushing's syndrome can be confused with the plump face of simple obesity as can also the 'buffalo hump' over the upper spine. In simple obesity, plasma cortisol may be elevated but shows normal diurnal variation and should suppress with low dose dexamethasone – unlike Cushing's syndrome and other hypercortisolism. Cushing's syndrome shows raised urinary free cortisol, loss of normal diurnal variation of serum cortisol, and loss of suppressibility of cortisol secretion by low-dose dexamethasone (Weber et al., 1995; Robyn et al., 1997).

9.2.3 Growth hormone deficiency

Here again, short stature usually dominates the clinical features much more than any obesity. Young children with growth hormone (GH) deficiency may be quite thin, with poor appetites, but older children develop some truncal obesity in association with short stature, delayed bone age, immature facies and small hands and feet (Parks, 2000).

Children with craniopharyngioma may have obesity because of GH and/or thyroid hormone deficiency. Treatment may cause further obesity secondary to progressive hypothalamic damage. Poor vision and family indulgence because of the child's sad state may also contribute to obesity through inactivity and overeating.

9.3 Prader–Willi syndrome (PWS)

9.3.1 Description

Prader–Willi–Labhart syndrome is the commonest specific syndrome associated with obesity. It was first described in 1956 (Prader et al., 1956), although specific diagnostic criteria were not established until 1993 (Holm et al., 1993). Estimates of the prevalence of PWS vary from one per 10 000 to one per 15 000 subjects. PWS occurs in both sexes and has been described world-wide (Cassidy, 1997). The syndrome appears to be due to a deletion of the q11–q13 fragment of the paternal chromosome 15, or to the presence of a uniparental disomy (UPD; two complete chromosomes 15, but both maternal in origin) (Ledbetter et al., 1981; Robinson et al., 1991). A third type of genetic alteration, involving the imprinting centre (Horsthemke, unpublished data) is also possible and might explain cases where neither of the other two chromosomal abnormalities are present. Table 9.3 lists features associated with PWS.

Perinatal features

Mothers often report reduced fetal movement. Infants are frequently either pre- or post-term and small for dates. Abnormalities of the fetal hypothalamus may contribute to incorrect timing of the onset of labour (Swaab 1997). In labour, poor fetal tone with neonatal asphyxia is reportedly eight times more common than in the general population (Wharton & Bresman, 1989; Donaldson et al., 1994).

At birth, the main clinical characteristic of the PWS neonate is profound hypotonia. This can also give an impression of perinatal asphyxia even though the

Table 9.3. Clinical features associated with Prader–Willi syndrome

Perinatal
    poor fetal movement
    low birth weight
    neonatal hypotonia
    feeding/sucking difficulties in neonatal period
Facies
    narrow forehead
    antimongoloid slant to eyes
    low-set ears
    anteverted nostrils
    carp-like mouth
    high-arched palate
Skeletal
    small hands and feet
    acromicria: tapering fingers
    small finger nails
    kyphoscoliosis
Short stature
Hypogonadism
    cryptorchidism
    micropenis
    hypoplasia clitoris and labia minora
    primary or secondary amenorrhoea
    poor pubertal development
Mental retardation
Speech disorders
Hyperphagia
Behavioural problems
    temper tantrums
    self harm: skin picking
    stealing, especially food
    manipulative
    emotional vulnerability
Progressive gross obesity from early childhood

abnormal neurology antedates the onset of labour. Muscle tone tends to improve over months or years but never resolves completely. The muscular hypotonia is central and neurological in origin although associated conditions, particularly multiple hormone deficiencies which affect muscle tone, can coexist. The most important consequence of hypotonia during the neonatal period is failure to thrive, due to the feeble sucking reflex and consequent low energy intake. Infants may need tube feeding.

These hypotonic new-borns rarely present with respiratory problems, a feature distinguishing them from many other neonatal hypotonia syndromes. The typical high-pitched weak cry can be a suggestive diagnostic feature (Dubowitz, unpublished data). In males, bilateral cryptorchidism associated with profound hypotonia may draw attention to the diagnosis. Hypoplasia of the external genitalia (labia minora and clitoris) also occurs in girls but is difficult to recognize and, in girls, the diagnosis of PWS is commonly made late.

The facies of the new-born are less specific than later, although dolicocephalic heads, hypomimic facies, micro- or retrognathia and thin upper lips are described. Hands are described as 'delicate', with puffy appearances. Limited hip and knee extension are other features which may be recognized during routine examination of the new-born for congenital dislocation of the hip (Roche et al., unpublished data).

Neonates and infants with PWS show thermoregulatory disturbances. Repeated febrile episodes, without evidence of infection, occur and their significance should be discussed with families and carers so the children are not subjected to unnecessary courses of antibiotics. Febrile episodes should only be treated when there is good evidence of bacterial infection.

Childhood

As the children grow, their facies assume the more typical appearance (Table 9.3) although nonobese PWS children are thought to have less typical facial features than those with obesity. Other clinical features also become more obvious. Orthopaedic problems are common, both as consequences of the syndrome itself and as consequences of the gross obesity. Scoliosis can develop quickly and is often severe. It not only exacerbates the short stature but contributes to deteriorating cardiorespiratory function with age.

Gastrointestinal problems, such as vomiting and rectal bleeding, are not unusual. However, the most notable gastrointestinal feature of PWS is hyperphagia, a continuous hunger, apparently without the normal sensations of satiety, which presents early in childhood and deteriorates in adolescence. Unless appropriately controlled it results in gross obesity. Recently, the insatiable hunger has been attributed to anomalies in the development of the paraventricular nucleus of the hypothalamus. Damage to the oxytocin neurones of this nucleus inhibits food intake in experimental animals. In PWS patients, there is a 40% reduction in cell number (particularly for the putative satiety cells or oxytocin producing neurones) in the paraventricular nucleus, when compared with findings in normal control subjects (Swaab et al., 1995).

Excessive appetite is the major cause of the obesity. Hyperphagia is commonly associated with aggressive (temper tantrums) and self-abusive (skin picking) behaviour, theft of food and pica, as well as poor social relationships and psychotic tendencies (5–10%) in late adolescence and adulthood. Emotional vulnerability, controlling and manipulative behaviours, obsessive–compulsive characteristics and difficulties coping with changes in the daily routine have been reported (Donaldson et al., 1994; Dykens et al., 1996; Cassidy, 1997; Bregani, unpublished data).

Some degree of mental retardation is described in almost all patients, although the degree of developmental and mental delay varies widely. Mean intelligence quotients (IQs) are reported as around 65, whilst the proportion of children with reportedly normal IQ varies between 3% and 12%, and those with borderline IQ between 29% and 63%, depending on the report (Holm, 1981; Greenswag, 1987; Akefeldt et al., 1991). Speech development is commonly delayed with difficulties in articulation, phonation and fluency as the most common reasons for referral. Language problems include defects in grammar and vocabulary. Individualized and relevant treatment programmes are needed to meet each child's particular problems (Defloor et al., unpublished data; Lewis & Freebairn, unpublished data).

Obesity is the major factor contributing to morbidity and mortality in PWS. Life span is probably near normal if severe obesity is avoided. However, with obesity come disadvantageous metabolic alterations (impaired glucose tolerance, Type II diabetes mellitus, hypertension) and circulatory problems such as thrombophlebitis, chronic leg oedema and severely compromised cardiorespiratory function (Cassidy, 1997).

Prader–Willi syndrome has been associated with a propensity for early development of non-insulin-dependent diabetes mellitus (NIDDM). PWS subjects show reduced β-cell response to glucose stimulation and dissociation between obesity and insulin resistance suggesting glucoregulatory mechanisms differ between obese and nonobese PWS subjects (Schuster et al., 1996).

Diabetes mellitus has always been regarded as a common association of PWS. A recent survey of 72 Italian PWS subjects (mean age, 16.3 years; standard error, 0.7 years) showed increased prevalence of altered glucose metabolism with impaired glucose tolerance in 14% of patients and overt NIDDM in 10%. Positive correlations were found between alterations in glucose metabolism and BMI and/or positive familial history for diabetes (Beccaria et al., unpublished data).

The progressive deterioration of cardiac and pulmonary function leading to the Pickwick syndrome, apnoea–hypopnoea syndrome and cardiac failure, frequently leads to severe disability in the early twenties and to early death. The respiratory complications are known to be related mainly to visceral fat deposition in the chest and neck. However there also seems to be a primary disturbance of central respiratory control in PWS patients, detectable in the preobese state, and worsening with the development of obesity (Horner et al., 1989; Shelton et al., 1993; Schuelter et al., 1997; Hertz et al., unpublished data; Wise et al., unpublished data).

PWS children are overweight, not only because of excessive caloric intake, but also because of reduced energy expenditure. Recent studies regarding body composition in PWS patients have shown that, whilst percentage fat mass is higher with respect to other obese subjects of comparable BMI, the lean mass compartment is less. This peculiar body compartment distribution implies a smaller amount of muscle mass, that is, a lesser amount of metabolically active tissue with overall reduced energy expenditure. This observation can also explain the poor muscular performances of PWS subjects and, perhaps, the persistent hypotonia (Davies et al., 1991; Davies & Joughin, 1992; Brambilla et al., 1997).

Nowadays, many PWS patients reach adulthood but burdened with the clinical problems of obesity, hypertension, diabetes, oedema of legs and feet, osteopenia, kyphosis, scoliosis, respiratory problems, cor pulmonale, chronic heart failure, sleep disturbance and digestive problems. Behavioural problems persist with food stealing, stubbornness and psychiatric disturbances (delusion, schizophrenia, obsessive–compulsive behaviour, depression) predominating.

9.3.2 Diagnosis

Prader–Willi syndrome is caused by the absence of normally active paternally inherited genes on chromosome 15 (q11–q13). In approximately 75% of patients with clinically typical PWS, there is a deletion at the 15q11–q13 level of the paternal chromosome. Most of the remaining patients have maternal UPD of chromosome 15.

Karyotyping alone is usually insufficient for definitive diagnosis, except for the rare cases with chromosomal translocations. The two most common techniques for chromosomal diagnosis are, currently, the DNA methylation test, which is able to indicate the presence or absence of the paternal methylated component of chromosome 15 but cannot distinguish between deletion, UPD and imprinting centre mutations, and FISH (fluorescent in situ hybridization), which can identify deletions. In general, a karyotype and a methylation test are sufficient for diagnosis, but further genetic investigations are required if, once diagnosis has been established, further information about the recurrence risk is needed (Brondum-Nielsen, 1997). Clinically however, the Holm & Cassidy criteria remain the first line for diagnosis. A provisional clinical diagnosis of PWS on these criteria is an indication for offering genetic testing.

9.3.3 Endocrinological anomalies

Thyroid function and adrenal function appear substantially normal in most PWS children and do not require routine investigation (Ritzén et al., 1991; Muller, 1997).

However, hyperphagia, obesity, short stature, hypogonadism, disturbances of thermoregulation and aggressive behaviour all suggest a complex defect in hypothalamic and/or hypophyseal function (Miller et al., 1996; Swaab, 1997). Many authors report deficient growth hormone secretion in some PWS children (Lee et al., 1987; Costeff et al., 1990; Angulo et al., 1991, 1996; Blichfeld et al., 1991; Ritzén et al., 1991). The main clinical signs attributable to GH deficit are slow height velocity, short stature, reduced bone mineral content, obesity with central fat distribution, poor lean mass, increased fat mass with visceral fat redistribution, reduced resting metabolic rate, hypotonia and reduced muscle strength (Davies et al., 1991; Klish et al., 1991; Davis & Joughin, 1992; Gertner, 1992). Some behavioural peculiarities have also been attributed to GH deficiency, namely, hyperphagia, feelings of distress, depression and reduced vitality.

Hypogonadism is evident at birth as hypoplasia of the genitalia. Characteristics are: cryptorchidism, scrotal hypoplasia, small penis or hypoplasia of the labia minora and clitoris. Later in life, hypogonadism is shown in partial failure of pubertal development. Pubic and axillary hair may develop early or late but body hair is rarely more than sparse. The degree of development of breast tissue in girls is often obscured by the gross obesity. Although primary amenorrhoea is the rule, menarche can occur spontaneously (up to 28% in a recent epidemiological survey), but secondary amenorrhoea invariably follows (100% in the same survey). Precocious puberty has also been described.

In both males and females, sexual activity is rare and infertility is usual (Cassidy 1997; Crinò et al., unpublished data). Abnormal hypothalamic luteinizing hormone releasing hormone (LHRH) neuronal function seems to account for the decreased levels of sex hormones in PWS children (Swaab, 1997).

Recent data on leptin metabolism in PWS populations seem to indicate that high leptin levels are a reflection of the high fat mass. There is no evidence that the relationship between fat mass and leptin concentration is altered in PWS (Weigle et al., 1997; Butler et al., 1998).

9.3.4 Management

PWS subjects suffer from many, particularly metabolic and cardiorespiratory, complications which contribute to the significant morbidity and frequently lead to early death. Current obesity management has not been very effective with these children. Therapeutic programmes based on diet and physical exercise are still the main approach, but the characteristic behaviour of PWS children creates major obstacles to successful dietary management. Prevention of obesity in PWS is primarily through controlling access to food. Nutritional approaches should be strictly individualized and should take into consideration all aspects of life and the impact of age, physical activity, work, family and social environments and psychological situation in order to achieve compliance. Psychological support is essential for children and their families.

It has been reported that growth hormone treatment in PWS not only improves height prognosis, but also favours major changes in body composition, leading to increments in lean body mass (LBM) and decreased fat mass. Current doses range from a total weekly dose of $15\,U/m^2$ to $20\,U/m^2$ in children and adolescents (Tonini et al., 1993; Donaldson et al., 1994; Angulo et al., 1996; Eiholzer et al., 1997; Hauffa, 1997; Lindgren et al., 1997; Trygstad & Veimo, unpublished data). The positive impact of this therapy seems to be to induce mood and behavioural changes, leading to improvements in the quality of everyday life. Thus GH therapy could improve life expectancy in these subjects. One of the latest reports proposed a higher total weekly dose of $24\,U/m^2$ and the authors concluded that the therapy induced dramatic changes after 1 year. An increase in height velocity was observed in all patients. This, together with an increase in muscle mass, was associated with improved physical performance, decreased fat mass and decreased weight-for-height ratio in obese subjects (Eiholzer et al., 1998).

Cryptorchidism requires early intervention. If human chorionic gonadotropin (HCG) treatment has no effect on testicular descent, orchidopexy is probably indicated. Some PWS subjects present with a hypergonadotrophic hypogonadism as a consequence of failed treatment for cryptorchidism.

PWS adolescents rarely complete puberty spontaneously. Hormone replacement therapy, using the usual protocols for treatment of hypogonadotrophic hypogonadism, can improve the development of secondary sexual characteristics and has beneficial effects on body composition and bone density in older adolescents and adults. Nevertheless, the overwhelming impression of PWS is of children and adults in whom obesity is the major and intractable problem, only made worse by the difficult behaviour and the associated complications of these sad individuals.

9.4 Other obesity syndromes

There are a number of syndromes other than PWS where obesity is only one of many clinical abnormalities. Clinical features seem variable, perhaps due to these syndromes, which are in most cases inherited, reflecting variable genetic expression or even due to failure to distinguish two different conditions. The current separation of Bardet–Biedl and Laurence–Moon syndromes, when they were often

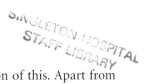

described as one condition in the past, may be an indication of this. Apart from obesity, which is often severe, abnormal facies, visual and auditory degeneration, skeletal abnormalities particularly of the hands and feet, short stature, hypogonadism and mental retardation are frequent associations of these obesity syndromes (Smith & Jones, 1988; McKusick, 1990).

9.4.1 Bardet–Biedl syndrome (BBS)

Bardet–Biedl syndrome, so called by the authors who reported this condition for the first time in 1920 (Bardet) and in 1922 (Biedl), is an autosomal recessively inherited condition. Attempts to locate the BBS gene indicate that the phenotype is probably genetically heterogeneous, resulting from mutations at several different loci including a locus on chromosome 11q (Beales et al., 1997). Modern estimates of prevalence are about 1/17 500 births (Crinò et al., 1994), ten times more frequent than the 1/160 000 reported from Switzerland (Klein & Ammann 1969). The syndrome is characterized by obesity, retinal dystrophy, polydactyly, hypogonadism, mental retardation and, in the vast majority of cases, renal anomalies.

Obesity with a characteristic central distribution develops in a high proportion of cases, usually in association with polyphagia. Reduced glucose tolerance and the development of NIDDM can result from the obese state (Bardet, 1920; Biedl, 1922; Klein & Ammann, 1969). Linear growth is usually within the normal range for age in childhood, although short stature is quite common. Hypogonadism has been detected in nearly half the patients. Micro-orchia, cryptorchidism, and micropenis are the commonest findings. Hypogonadism can lead to poor pubertal growth and more obvious short stature in adolescence. Different genes responsible for the features of BBS may account for variations in characteristics such as height (Beales et al., 1997).

Other dysmorphic features include polydactyly. This is postaxial and affects hands and/or feet. Syndactyly and brachydactyly are also common.

The diagnosis of retinitis pigmentosa is usually made in childhood or adolescence after complaints of hemeralopia (day blindness), blurred vision and/or dyschromatopsia. There is progressive loss of vision with blindness in late childhood or adolescence. Hypoacusia also occurs in a small proportion of patients.

Renal anomalies are common, particularly polycystic kidneys, which may lead to polyuria and renal hypoplasia. Cardiac involvement (left ventricular hypertrophy, aortic stenosis) is usually described as a rare association, although congenital heart disease and/or hypertrophy of the intraventricular septum and dilated cardiomyopathy have been described in 50% of Bedouin subjects with BBS (Elbedour et al., 1994). IQ varies. Mental retardation may be present and severe, although, in some subjects, IQ lies just below normal range.

9.4.2 Laurence–Moon syndrome

Laurence–Moon syndrome, although often linked with Bardet–Biedl syndrome, should be distinguished from the Bardet–Biedl syndrome since it is less common, is characterized by severe neurological extrapyramidal deficit (ataxia and spastic paraparesis) *without obesity* and without finger abnormalities.

9.4.3 Biemond syndrome

Biemond syndrome (Verloes et al., 1997) also resembles BBS. Whilst it appears to be inherited, the form of inheritance has not been fully resolved, perhaps because the syndrome as described reflects several syndromes, at least one of which has autosomal dominant, and one which has autosomal recessive, inheritance. Iris colobomata, mental retardation, obesity, hypogenitalism and postaxial polydactyly have been reported. Coloboma of the iris is the essential clinical feature differentiating the syndrome from the Bardet–Biedl syndrome.

9.4.4 Alstrom syndrome

In Alstrom syndrome, which again resembles BBS, there is no mental retardation, polydactyly nor hypogonadism but retinitis pigmentosa with cone–rod dystrophy, neurosensory deafness, obesity and NIDDM are described (Alstrom et al., 1959).

In contrast to other pigmentary retinopathies in which there is a loss of peripheral vision first, the atypical retinal lesion in Alstrom syndrome causes nystagmus and early loss of central vision. Glaucoma has been described. Neurogenic deafness is progressive.

Reported associated findings are several metabolic abnormalities including hyperuricaemia, elevated serum triglyceride and pre-β-lipoprotein, and acanthosis nigricans (Weinstein & Kliman, 1969). Progressive chronic nephropathy and dilated cardiomyopathy have also been reported.

Alstrom syndrome seems to follow an autosomal recessive pattern of inheritance. Recently, a location for Alstrom syndrome at chromosome 2p12–13 has been reported in a large population of affected French Acadians (Macari et al., 1998).

9.4.5 Borjeson–Forssman–Lehmann syndrome (BFLS)

The diagnostic criteria for BFLS are a characteristic facies with prominent supraorbital ridges, deep-set eyes, ptosis, large ears and round puffy looking face, severe mental retardation, epilepsy, hypotonia, hypogonadism and marked obesity.

An X-linked pattern of inheritance has been suggested (Borjeson et al., 1962; Mathews et al., 1989b; Mulley et al., 1989) possibly with a locus on Xq (Mathews et al., 1989a).

9.4.6 Carpenter syndrome

The diagnostic features of Carpenter syndrome (or acrocephalo-polysyndactyly type II) include: acrocephaly with variable synostosis of sutures, peculiar facies (shallow supraorbital ridges, lateral displacement of the inner canthi with or without inner canthal folds, low-set ears, preauricular pits), short fingers, soft tissue syndactyly in the hands with preaxial polydactyly and syndactyly of the toes (Carpenter, 1909). Obesity, mental retardation and hypogonadism are described in older children (Temtamy, 1966).

Less common features are congenital heart defects, metatarsus varus, coxa valga, genu valgum, accessory spleen, umbilical hernia, short stature and renal abnormalities. Mental retardation is not universal but, in one study, three-quarters of affected individuals had some degree of intellectual impairment (Taravath & Tonsgard, 1993). Carpenter syndrome follows an autosomal recessive pattern of inheritance.

9.4.7 Cohen syndrome (or Pepper syndrome)

The Cohen (or Pepper) syndrome comprises a variable pattern of abnormalities. Short stature, unusual facies, ocular problems, skeletal problems, microcephaly, persistent hypotonia and mental retardation are usual (Cohen et al., 1973; Carey and Hall, 1978). The ocular problems include reduced visual acuity, strabismus, nystagmus and mild to severe optic atrophy, although without severe pigmentary change to the retina (Kitivitie-Kallio et al., 1999). These lead to decreased visual acuity, defective vision in bright light and constricted visual fields.

The facial feature most noticeable in later childhood is the prominence of the maxillary incisors but prominent nasal bridge, short philtrum, mild micrognathia, large ears and mild downslant to the palpebral fissures are also common (Lapeteria et al., 1988). Skeletal abnormalities include narrow hands and feet with short metacarpals and metatarsals and slim fingers, hyperextensible joints, genu and cubitus valgus and lumbar lordosis with mild scoliosis.

Neutropenia associated with increased neutrophil adhesive capacity but more or less normal bone marrow is described in association with Cohen syndrome (Kitivitie-Kallio et al., 1997; Olivieri et al., 1998).

Whilst the obesity, mental retardation, hypotonia and some of the facial features might suggest PWS, children with Cohen syndrome are described as cheerful and of positive social disposition with good scores for responsibility and socialization (Kitivitie-Kallio et al., 1999). These characteristics are in marked contrast to the rather negative behaviour of the typical PWS child.

Transmission is by autosomal recessive inheritance (Friedman & Sack, 1982).

9.4.8 Single-gene defects affecting leptin synthesis and metabolism

Recent developments in molecular genetics have defined several conditions where the synthesis or the metabolism of leptin have been affected by single-gene abnormalities leading to early-onset gross obesity and, in several cases, short stature and hypogonadism as well (Farooqi & O'Rahilly 2000). It seems likely that many more similar abnormalities await to be discovered (Table 9.1). All the conditions so far defined are very rare (Chapter 3).

9.5 REFERENCES

Akefeldt, A., Gillberg, C. & Larsson, C. (1991). Prader–Willi Syndrome in a Swedish rural county: epidemiological aspects. *Developmental Medicine and Child Neurology*, **33**, 715–21.

Alstrom, C.H., Hallgren, B., Nilsson, L.B. & Asander, H. (1959). Retinal degeneration combined with obesity, diabetes mellitus and neurogenous deafness. A specific syndrome (not hitherto described) distinct from Laurence–Moon–Biedl syndrome. A clinical endocrinological and genetic examination based on a large pedigree. *Acta Psychiatrica et Neurologica Scandinavica*, **34** (suppl. 129), 1.

Angulo, M., Castro-Magana, M., Uy, J. & Rosenfeld, W. (1991). Growth hormone evaluation and treatment in Prader–Willi Syndrome. In *Prader–Willi Syndrome and Other Chromosome 15q Deletion Disorders*, ed. S.B. Cassidy, pp. 171–5. NATO ASI Series, 61. Heidelberg: Springer Verlag.

Angulo, M., Castro-Magana, M., Mazur, B., Canas, J.A., Vitollo, P.M. & Serrantonio, M. (1996). Growth hormone secretion and effects of growth hormone therapy on growth velocity and weight gain in children with Prader–Willi syndrome. *Journal of Pediatric Endocrinology and Metabolism*, **9**, 393–400.

Bardet, G. (1920). Sur un syndrome d'obésité congenitale avec polydactylie et retinite pigmentare (contribution à l'etude des formes cliniques de l'obésité hypophysaire), Faculté de Medicine de Paris, Thesis, 470: 107.

Beales, P.L., Warner, A.M., Hitman, G.A., Thakker, R. & Flinter, F.A. (1997). Bardet–Biedl syndrome: a molecular and phenotypic study of 18 families. *Journal of Medical Genetics*, **34**, 92–8.

Biedl, A. (1922). Ein geschwisterpaar mit adiposo-genitaler dystrophie. *Deutsche Medizinische Wochenschrift*, **48**, 1630.

Blichfeld, S., Main, K., Ritzén, M. & Skakkebaek, N.E. (1991). Diminished 24 hour urinary growth hormone excretion in patients with Prader–Willi Syndrome. In *Prader–Willi Syndrome and Other Chromosome 15q Deletion Disorders*, ed. S.B. Cassidy, pp. 175–80. NATO ASI Series, 61. Heidelberg: Springer Verlag.

Borjeson, M., Forssman, H. & Lehmann, O. (1962). An X-linked, recessively inherited syndrome characterized by grave mental deficiency, epilepsy, and endocrine disorder. *Acta Medica Scandinavica*, **171**, 13–21.

Brambilla, P., Bosio, L., Manzoni, P., Pietrobelli, A., Beccaria, L. & Chiumello, G. (1997). Peculiar body composition in patients with Prader Labhart Willi syndrome. *American Journal of Clinical Nutrition,* **65**, 1369–74.

Brondum-Nielsen, K. (1997). The genetic basis for Prader–Willi syndrome: the importance of imprinted genes. *Acta Paediatrica,* **Suppl. 423**, 55–7.

Butler, M.G., Moore, J., Morawiecki, A. & Nicholson, M. (1998). Comparison of leptin protein levels in Prader–Willi syndrome and control individuals. *American Journal of Medical Genetics,* **75**, 7–12.

Carey, J.C. & Hall B.D. (1978). Confirmation of the Cohen syndrome. *Journal of Pediatrics,* **93**, 239–44.

Carpenter, G. (1909). Case of acrocephaly with other congenital malformations, *Proceedings of the Royal Society of Medicine,* **2**, 45–53, 199–201.

Cassidy, S.B. (1997). Prader Willi Syndrome. *Journal of Medical Genetics,* **34**, 917–23.

Cohen, M.M., Hall, B.D., Smith, D.W., Graham, C.B. & Lampert K.J. (1973). A new syndrome with hypotonia, obesity, mental deficiency and facial, oral, ocular and limb anomalies. *Journal of Pediatrics,* **83**, 280–4.

Costeff, H., Holm, V.A., Ruvalcaba, R. & Shaver J. (1990). Growth hormone secretion in Prader–Willi syndrome. *Acta Paediatrica Scandinavica,* **79**, 1059–62.

Crinò, A., Tonini, G., Vido, L., Balsamo, A., De Simone, M., De Toni, T., Bosio, L., Lughetti, L., Livieri, C., Pasquino, A.M., Caruso, M., Ciampalini, P., Digilio, M.C., Antonello, I., Vignutelli, L., Sarni, P., Bernasconi, S., Fazzi, E., Pomella, S., Lo Presti, D., Bosco, D. & Chiumello, G. (1994). Bardet–Biedl syndrome: Italian multicentre study. *Italian Journal of Pediatrics,* **20**, 530–6 (English abstract).

Davies, P.S.W. & Joughin, C. (1992). Assessment of body composition in the Prader–Willi syndrome: implications for management. Prader–Willi Scientific Symposium. (Salt Lake City, Utah. July 18, 1990). *American Journal of Medical Genetics,* **41**, 524–30.

Davies, P.S.W., Joughin, C., Livingstone, M.B.E. & Barnes, N.D. (1991). Energy expenditure in the Prader–Willi Syndrome. In *Prader Willi Syndrome and Other Chromosome 15q Deletion Disorders.* ed. S.B. Cassidy, pp. 181–8. NATO ASI Series, 61. Heidelberg: Springer Verlag.

Donaldson, M.D.C., Chu, C.E., Cooke, A., Wilson, A., Greene, S.A. & Stephenson, J.B.P. (1994). The Prader Willi syndrome. *Archives of Disease in Childhood,* **70**, 58–63.

Dykens, E.M., Leckman, J.F. & Cassidy, S.B. (1996). Obsessions and compulsions in Prader–Willi syndrome. *Journal of Child Psychology and Psychiatry and Allied Disciplines,* **37**, 995–1002.

Eiholzer, U., Weber, R., Stutz, K. & Steinert, H. (1997). Effect of 6 months of growth hormone treatment in young children with Prader–Willi syndrome. *Acta Paediatrica,* **Suppl. 423**, 66–8.

Eiholzer, U., Gisin, R., Weinmann, C., Kriemler, S., Steinert, H., Torresani, T., Zachmann M. & Prader, A. (1998). Treatment with human growth hormone in patients with Prader–Labhart–Willi syndrome reduces body fat and increases muscle mass and physical performance, *European Journal of Pediatrics,* **157**, 368–77.

Elbedour, K., Zucker, N., Zalztein, E., Barki, Y. & Carmi, R. (1994). Cardiac abnormalities in the Bardet–Biedl syndrome: echocardiographic studies of 22 patients. *American Journal of Medical Genetics,* **52**, 164–7.

Farooqi, I.S. & O'Rahilly, S. (2000). Recent advances in the genetics of severe childhood obesity. *Archives of Disease in Childhood,* **83**, 31–4.

Friedman, E. & Sack, J. (1982). The Cohen syndrome: report of five new cases and a review of the literature. *Journal of Craniofacial Genetics and Developmental Biology*, **2**, 193–200.

Gertner, J.M. (1992). Growth hormone actions on fat distribution and metabolism. *Hormone Research*, **38** (Suppl. 2), 41–3.

Greenswag, L.R. (1987). Adults with Prader Willi syndrome: a survey of 232 cases. *Developmental Medicine and Child Neurology*, **29**, 145–52.

Gunay-Aygun, M., Cassidy, S.B. & Nicholls, R.D. (1997). Prader–Willi and other syndromes associated with obesity and mental retardation. *Behavioral Genetics*, **27**, 307–24.

Hauffa, B.P. (1997). One-year results of growth hormone treatment of short stature in Prader–Willi syndrome. *Acta Paediatrica*, **Suppl. 423**, 63–5.

Holm, V.A. (1981). The diagnosis of Prader–Willi syndrome. In *Prader Willi Syndrome*, eds. V.A. Holm, S.J. Schulzbacher & P.L. Pipes. Baltimore: University Park Press.

Holm, V.A., Cassidy, S.B., Butler, M.G., Hanchett, J.M., Greenswag, L.R., Whitman, B.Y. & Greenberg, F. (1993). Prader–Willi syndrome: consensus diagnostic criteria. *Pediatrics*, **91**, 398–402.

Horner, R.L., Mohiaddin, R.H. & Lowell, D.G. (1989). Sites and sizes of fat deposits around the pharynx in obese patients with obstructive spell apnoea and weight matched controls. *European Respiratory Journal*, **2**, 613–22.

Kitivitie-Kallio, S., Rajantie, J., Juvonen, E. & Norio, R. (1997). Granulocytopenia in Cohen syndrome. *British Journal of Haematology*, **98**, 308–11.

Kitivitie-Kallio, S., Larsen, A., Kajasto, K. & Norio, R. (1999). Neurological and psychological findings in patients with Cohen syndrome: a study of 18 patients aged 11 months to 57 years. *Neuropediatrics*, **30**, 181–9.

Klein, D. & Ammann, F. (1969). The syndrome of Laurence–Moon–Bardet–Biedl and allied diseases in Switzerland: clinical, genetic and epidemiological studies. *Journal of Neurological Sciences*, **9**, 479.

Klish, W., Brown, B., Lin, T., Lee, P. & Greenberg, F. (1991). Studies of body composition in patients with Prader–Willi syndrome: implication for management. In Prader–Willi Scientific Symposium. (Salt Lake City, Utah. July 18, 1990), *American Journal of Medical Genetics*, **41**, 524–30.

LaFranchi, S. (2000). Hypothyroidism. In *Nelson Textbook of Pediatrics*, eds. R.E. Behrman, R.M. Kliegman & H.B. Jenson, pp. 1698–704. Philadelphia: W.B. Saunders.

Lapeteria, F., Piantoni, G., Canino, R., Teza, F. & Ferrarini, D. (1988). La sindrome di Cohen. Contributo alla sua delineazione clinica. *Pediatrica Medicina Chirugia*, **10**, 217–21.

Ledbetter, D.H., Riccardi, V.M., Airhart, S.D., Strobel, R.J., Keenan, B.S. & Crawford, J.D. (1981). Deletion of chromosome 15 as a cause of the Prader–Willi syndrome. *New England Journal of Medicine*, **304**, 325–9.

Lee, P.D.K., Wilson, D.N. & Rountree, L. (1987). Linear growth factor to exogenous growth hormone in Prader–Willi syndrome. *American Journal of Medical Genetics*, **28**, 865–71.

Lindgren, A.C., Hagenas, L., Mueller, J., Blichfeld, S., Rosenborg, M., Brismar, T. & Ritzén, E.M., in collaboration with the Swedish National Growth Hormone Advisory Group (1997). Effects of growth hormone treatment on growth and body composition in Prader Willi Syndrome. *Acta Paediatrica*, **Suppl. 423**, 60–2.

Macari, F., Lautier, C., Giradet, A., Dadoun, F., Darmon, P., Dutour, A., et al. (1998). Refinement of genetic localisation of the Alstrom syndrome on chromosome 2p12–13 by linkage analysis in a North African family. *Human Genetics*, **103**, 658–61.

Mathews, K.D., Ardinger, H.H., Nishimura, D.Y., Buetow, K.H., Murray, J.C. & Bartley, J.A. (1989a). Linkage localization for Borjeson–Forssman–Lehmann syndrome. *American Journal of Medical Genetics*, **34**, 470–4.

Mathews, K.D., Buetow, K., Turner, G. & Mulley, J. (1989b). Borjeson–Forssman–Lehmann syndrome localization. *American Journal of Medical Genetics*, **34**, 475.

McKusick, V.A. (1990). *Mendelian Inheritance in Man. Catalogs of Autosomal Dominant, Autosomal Recessive, and X-Linked Phenotypes*, 9th edn. Baltimore: Johns Hopkins University Press.

Miller, L., Angulo, M., Price, D. & Taneja, S. (1996). MR of the pituitary in patients with Prader–Willi syndrome: size determination and imaging findings. *Pediatric Radiology*, **26**, 43–7.

Muller, J. (1997). Hypogonadism and endocrine metabolic disorders in Prader–Willi syndrome. *Acta Paediatrica*, **Suppl. 423**, 58–9.

Mulley, J.C., Turner, G., Gedeon, A., Sutherland, G.R., Rae, J., Power, K. & Arthur, I. (1989). Borjeson–Forssman–Lehmann syndrome: clinical manifestations and gene localization to Xq26–27, *Cytogenetics and Cell Genetics*, **51**, 1049.

Olivieri, O., Lombardi, S., Russo, C. & Corrocher, R. (1998). Increased neutrophil adhesive capability in Cohen syndrome, an autosomal recessive disorder associated with granulocytopenia. *Haematologica*, **83**, 778–82.

Parks, J.S. (2000). Hypopituitarism. In *Nelson Textbook of Pediatrics*, eds. R.E. Behrman, R.M. Kliegman & H.B. Jenson, pp. 1675–80. Philadelphia: W.B. Saunders.

Prader, A., Labhart, A. & Willi, H. (1956). Ein Syndrom von Adipositas, Kleinwuchs, Kryptorchismus and Oligophrenie nach myatonieartigem Zustand im Neugeborenenalter. *Schweizerische Medizinische Wochenschrift*, **86**, 1260–1.

Ritzén, E.M., Bolme, P. & Hall, K. (1991). Endocrine physiology and therapy in Prader–Willi syndrome. In *Prader Willi Syndrome and Other Chromosome 15q Deletion Disorders*, ed. S.B. Cassidy, pp. 153–70. NATO ASI Series, 61. Heidelberg: Springer Verlag.

Robinson, W.P., Bottani, A., Yagang, X., Balakrishnan, J., Binkert, F., Machler, M., Prader, A. & Schinzel, A. (1991). Clinical, molecular and cytogenetic survey of potential Prader–Willi syndrome patients. In *Prader Willi Syndrome and Other Chromosome 15q Deletion Disorders*, ed. S.B. Cassidy, pp. 53–8. NATO ASI Series, 61, Heidelberg: Springer Verlag.

Robyn, J.A., Koch, C.A., Montalto, J., Yong, A., Warne, G.L. & Batch, J.A. (1997). Cushing's syndrome in childhood and adolescence. *Journal of Paediatrics and Child Health*, **33**, 522–7.

Schuelter, B., Buschatz, D., Trowitzsch, E., Asku, F. & Andler, W. (1997). Respiratory control in children with Prader Willi syndrome. *European Journal of Pediatrics*, **156**, 65–8.

Schuster, D.P., Osei, K. & Zipf, W.B. (1996). Characterization of alterations in glucose and insulin metabolism in Prader–Willi subjects. *Metabolism*, **45**, 1514–20.

Shelton, K.E., Woodson, H. & Spencer, G. (1993). Pharyngeal fat in obstructive sleep apnoea. *American Review of Respiratory Disease*, **18**, 462–6.

Smith, D.W. & Jones, K.L. (1988). *Smith's Recognizable Patterns of Human Malformation.*

Philadelphia: W.B. Saunders Co.

Swaab, D.F. (1997). Prader–Willi syndrome and the hypothalamus. *Acta Paediatrica*, **Suppl. 423**, 50–4.

Swaab, D.F., Purba, J.S. & Hofman, M.A. (1995). Alterations in the hypothalamic paraventricular nucleus and its oxytocin neurons (putative satiety cells) in Prader–Willi syndrome: a study of five cases. *Journal of Clinical Endocrinology and Metabolism*, **80**, 573–9.

Taravath, S. & Tonsgard, J.H. (1993). Cerebral malformations in Carpenter syndrome. *Pediatric Neurology*, **9**, 230–4.

Temtamy, S.A. (1966). Carpenter syndrome: acrocephalopoly-syndactyly: an autosomal recessive syndrome. *Journal of Pediatrics*, **69**, 111.

Tonini, G., Bruno, E., Marinoni, S. & Gigio, L. (1993). Growth hormone therapy in syndromes with short stature. *Acta Paediatrica Scandinavica*, **Suppl. 379**.

Verloes, A., Temple, I.K., Bonnet, S. & Bottani, A (1997). Coloboma, mental retardation, hypogonadism, and obesity: critical review of so-called Biemond syndrome type 2, updated nosology, and delineation of three 'new' syndromes. *American Journal of Medical Genetics*, **69**, 370–9.

Weber, A., Trainer, P.J., Grossman, A.B. et al. (1995). Investigation, management and therapeutic outcome in 12 cases of childhood and adolescent Cushing's syndrome. *Clinical Endocrinology*, **43**, 19–28.

Weigle, D.S., Ganter, S.L., Kuijper, J.L., Leonetti, D.L., Boyko, E.J. & Fujimoto, W.Y. (1997). Effect of regional fat distribution in Prader–Willi syndrome on plasma leptin levels. *Journal of Clinical Endocrinology and Metabolism*, **82**, 566–70.

Weinstein, R.L. & Kliman, B. (1969). Familial syndrome of primary testicular insufficiency with normal virilization, blindness, deafness and metabolic abnormalities. *New England Journal of Medicine*, **281**, 967.

Wharton, R.H. & Bresman, M.J. (1989). Neonatal respiratory depression and delay in diagnosis in Prader–Willi syndrome. *Developmental Medicine and Child Neurology*, **31**, 231–6.

10

Hormonal and metabolic changes

Ewa Malecka-Tendera[1] and Dénes Molnár[2]

[1]Department of Pathophysiology, Silesian School of Medicine, Katowice. [2]Department of Paediatrics, University of Pécs

The majority of children who are obese have no underlying medical problems which are recognized as contributing to their obesity. Less than 1% of childhood obesity is caused by endocrine disease. In spite of this, in a hospital-based obesity clinic the referral diagnosis of Cushing syndrome in relatively short children with simple obesity, particularly when they develop pale pink striae of rapid fat accretion, is not uncommon. The contrast between the large body size and the small genitalia hidden in the abdominal fat can be very disturbing for obese boys and their parents consequently seek medical advice because of suspected hypogonadism. In most of the cases, after a careful physical examination, we can reassure the patient, the family and the doctor referring the child to our clinics that no hormonal abnormalities are present. Normal or tall stature, normal intelligence, normal blood pressure, normal or slightly advanced bone age and the absence of dysmorphic features more or less exclude the possibility of pathologic obesity, although the recently described single obesity gene mutations in humans have to be kept in mind. Endocrine abnormalities secondary to increased fat mass are common in simple obesity (Table 10.1), but most abnormalities disappear with successful weight reduction. Hormonal evaluation is seldom indicated unless the diagnosis of simple obesity is uncertain.

The present chapter discusses hormonal changes associated with obesity which are not necessarily abnormal or even dysfunctional. Many of them are compensatory and physiological. For example, the hyperinsulinaemia of obesity compensates for insulin resistance, thereby maintaining euglycaemia. Likewise, the decrease in total serum testosterone observed in moderately obese males, caused by decreased sex-hormone binding globulin, is compensated by an increase in the percentage of free testosterone. This response permits the maintenance of normal androgenic activity. However, some of the hormonal changes in obesity that have a primary compensatory function may also have undesirable secondary effects. For example, hyperinsulinaemia may enhance renal sodium retention and stimu-

Table 10.1. Endocrine abnormalities in obesity

System	Abnormality
Hypothalamic–pituitary–adrenal axis	Increased cortisol turnover
	Increased cortisol in central obesity
	Increased cortisol response to stress
Thyroid	Possible relationship between T3 and RMR
Gonadal	Decreased SHBG
Male	Increased aromatization of adrenal androgens into oestrogens
	Decreased free testosterone
	Hypogonadotrophic hypogonadism in severe obesity
Female	Increased aromatisation of adrenal androgens into oestrogens
	Decreased progesterone
	Increased ovarian androgen production
	Increased free testosterone
GH–IGF	Decreased GH secretion
	Increased GHBP
	Increased IGF-1 (free or total)
Endocrine pancreas	Increased basal and reactive insulin
	Peripheral insulin resistance
Adipose tissue	Raised leptin

T3: triiodothyronine; RMR: resting metabolic rate; SHBG: sex hormone binding globulin; GH: growth hormone; GHBP: growth hormone binding protein; IGF-1: insulin-like growth factor 1.

late ovarian androgen production and thus cause hypertension and hyper-androgenism.

10.1 Pituitary–adrenal axis

Glucocorticoid treatment of laboratory animals results in the development of obesity. Indeed, animal models of obesity invariably have increased levels of corticosterone (York & Bray, 1972). Adrenalectomy results in the reversal or prevention of obesity. This action is most likely mediated via type II glucocorticoid receptors (Thomas et al., 1994). The role of glucocorticoids in human obesity is less clear (Chalew et al., 1995). The secretion rate of cortisol is increased in obese children (Genazzani et al., 1978), reflecting increased lean body mass (LBM), an enlarged intra-adipocyte space for steroid storage, and changes in adrenal steroid metabolism. Plasma cortisol (free and bound), circadian rhythms of cortisol secretion, and urinary free cortisol are all normal in obese subjects, while there is a slight increase in 24-hour integrated serum adrenocorticotrophic hormone (ACTH) concentration (Kobberling & Von zur Muhlen, 1974; Slavnov & Epstein, 1977; Genazzani et al., 1978). The urinary excretion of 17-hydroxy-steroids, which are glucocorticoid metabolites, is normal when corrected for the increased LBM that accompanies obesity (Streeten et al., 1969). The increase in the net excretion of urinary glucocorticoid metabolites, in the context of normal serum cortisol concentrations, suggests that cortisol turnover is increased. The cortisol response to insulin in obese patients was also found slightly higher as compared to lean subjects (Cacciari et al., 1975). The most compelling data for the association between human obesity and cortisol comes from studies that classify obese women into central and peripheral types of obesity. Urinary and serum cortisol increased in parallel with the increase of waist/hip ratio and the sagittal diameter of the abdomen (Marin et al., 1992a). Serum cortisol responses to stress were greater in women with high waist/hip ratio (Marin et al., 1992a; Pasquali et al., 1993), suggesting a role of cortisol response to environmental stressors as a potential factor in abdominal obesity (Björntorp, 1995).

In addition to stimulating cortisol release, the increased ACTH release enhances sex steroid production by the adrenal zona reticularis. Sex steroid production appears to be increased to a greater extent than sex steroid clearance. Serum concentrations of adrenal androgens are higher in obese children than age-matched controls or Tanner-stage-matched lean peers (Genazzani et al., 1978). This phenomenon may explain the earlier adrenarche and the advanced bone age often seen in obese children. By 7 to 9 years of age, obese girls may have circulating adrenal androgen concentrations similar to those of normal adults. Prepubertal obese boys also demonstrate an increase in adrenal androgen production, reaching a plateau in early adolescence (Cacciari et al., 1977).

Dehydroepiandrosterone (DHEA) is an adrenal steroid that serves as a precursor of adrenal sex steroids. DHEA metabolism in obese subjects is of special interest because administration of exogenous DHEA to animals is accompanied by a marked diminution in rates of fat accretion (Cleary et al., 1984). Obese human subjects have elevated serum concentrations of DHEA. These could reflect changes in DHEA synthesis, storage or clearance. Studies in obese humans suggest that there is an increased uptake of DHEA by adipose tissue and a decrease in peripheral conversion of DHEA to its sulphated metabolite (Bird et al., 1972; Fehér & Halmy, 1975). The mechanisms underlying the antiobesity effects of DHEA remain unclear.

10.2 Pituitary–gonadal axis

10.2.1 Ovary

Obesity influences reproductive function early in life. Obese girls have early onset of puberty (Crawford & Osler, 1975). The initiation of menstruation seems to require the attainment of a certain amount of body fat (Frisch, 1987). Certainly the age of menarche tends to be lower in obese girls than in normal-weight individuals.

Obesity is associated with an increased risk of hyperandrogenism, anovulatory cycles and menstruation disorders. Girls that were obese at 7 years of age were found to have an increased risk of menstrual disorders as adult women (Lake et al., 1997). Women that are hyperandrogenic can be divided into two groups. The first group is obese, has evidence for hyperinsulinaemia and normal luteinizing hormone/follicle-stimulating hormone (LH/FSH) ratio. The second group has normal body weight and insulin concentration, but abnormal LH/FSH secretory pattern (Dale et al., 1992). Increased androgenic activity often accompanied by hirsutism and menstrual abnormalities is more frequent in women with abdominal than gluteal–femoral type of obesity (Kirschner et al., 1990). The relationship between hyperandrogenism and abdominal obesity is already present in adolescent girls (Wabitsch et al., 1995b).

The mechanism between obesity and hyperandrogenism is not clear, but certainly there are numerous possible adiposity-related changes in the production of adrenal and gonadal sex steroids, that may account for these menstrual irregularities (Fig. 10.1). Despite insulin resistance in adipose tissue and skeletal muscle, the ovary remains relatively insulin sensitive. In vitro studies on ovarian stroma demonstrated that high ambient concentrations of insulin and insulin-like growth factor 1 (IGF-1) have stimulatory effects on thecal androgen production (Bergh et al., 1993). Hyperinsulinaemia in combination with an elevated luteinizing hormone concentration leads to thecal hyperplasia, increased androgen secretion, arrest of follicular development and, therefore, anovulation with menstrual disturbances. Insulin also acts on the liver. Hyperinsulinaemia inhibits the production of sex-hormone binding globulin and insulin-like growth factor binding protein (IGFBP) (Plymate et al., 1988). Thus, insulin resistance not only increases the secretion of ovarian androgens but also promotes the increase of free active hormones. The inhibition of the production of IGFBP results in an increased concentration of the free form of this hormone, further stimulating ovarian androgen production (Cataldo, 1997). The relationship between hyperinsulinaemia and increased adrenal androgen production is not well established yet (Gonzalez, 1997). There are reports that successful weight reduction and decrease of plasma insulin concentration result in the resumption of normal cyclic menses in obese amenorrhoeic women (Bates & Whitworth, 1982).

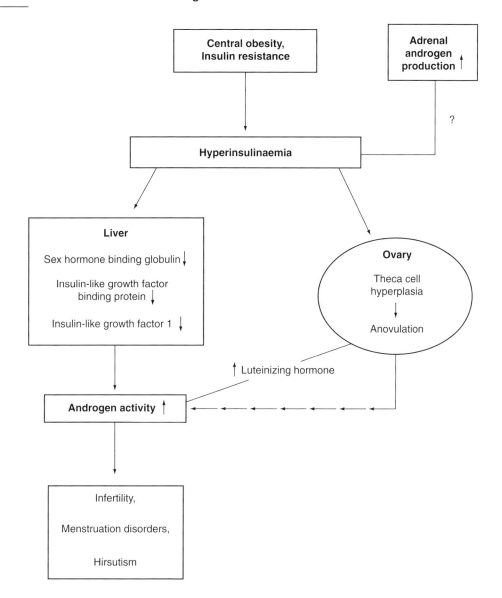

Figure 10.1   Obesity-associated hormonal changes leading to menstruation disorders.

A relatively common reproductive disturbance causing infertility and recurrent abortion in obese women is luteal phase deficiency (Soules et al., 1989). The primary hormonal derangement is inadequate secretion of progesterone by the corpus luteum, resulting in insufficient preparation of the endometrium for implantation of the embryo. The low circulating level of progesterone in luteal insufficiency associated with obesity could be the result of the uptake of progesterone from the circulation into the enlarged fat mass (Evans et al., 1983). Adipose tissue is a reservoir for androgens, oestrogens and progesterone, but not for cortisol (Azziz, 1989). The increased production of oestrogens in obese women is due to the peripheral aromatization of circulating androgens to oestrogens by the stromal vascular cells of adipose tissue. Weight reduction decreases oestrogen concentrations in women (Zumoff & Strain, 1994).

In summary, obese females may have abnormal ovarian function causing oligo-ovulation, amenorrhoea or dysfunctional uterine bleeding. The most common cause of this scenario is polycystic ovarian syndrome. A subset of this disorder is due to hyperinsulinaemia. Obesity may also cause infertility due to luteal phase insufficiency.

10.2.2 Testis

Most obese men have normal reproductive function despite a decrease in serum total testosterone level (Barrett-Connor & Khaw, 1988). Pubertal development in obese children and the libido and potency in obese men are normal. The external genitalia are normal, although the size of the penis may appear small as it recedes into the enlarged fat pad. The decreased total testosterone level is due to an equivalent decrease in sex-hormone binding globulin both in adults (Glass et al., 1977) and in children (Ilyés & Kirilina, 1992). However, the free or unbound testosterone is increased, thus compensating for the decreased total level. Thus, there is no objective evidence of hypogonadism from either the clinical or laboratory standpoint in most obese men.

Some massively obese men (relative body weight $> 200\%$ or body mass index (BMI) > 40) have a decrease in the free as well as total testosterone, which is associated with hypogonadotrophic hypogonadism. This decrement in free and total testosterone may be due to the peripheral conversion of testosterone to oestradiol, which is directly related to the degree of obesity (Pasquali et al., 1988).

Several investigations suggested that testosterone plays an important role in the regulation of visceral fat mass and insulin sensitivity of the skeletal muscle (Marin et al., 1992b, 1995). It has been shown that androgen treatment decreases abdominal adipose tissue (Lovejoy et al., 1995). In the only prospective study to date (Khaw & Barrett-Connor, 1992), an association was observed between low testosterone levels and the presence of increased waist to hip ratio 12 years later.

10.3 Pituitary–thyroid axis

The pituitary–thyroid axis in simple obesity is undisturbed. Plasma thyrotropin (TSH) levels are usually normal in obese subjects and unaffected by fasting. Thyroxin (T4) concentrations are also normal and uninfluenced by overfeeding or fasting. In contrast, triiodotyronine (T3) plays an important role in regulating body weight. Obese children and adults have mildly elevated levels of T3, probably reflecting increased peripheral conversion of T4 to T3. Short-term consumption of a low-energy diet is associated with a significant decrease in plasma T3 concentration (Wadden et al., 1990). This reduction is associated with a decrease in basal metabolic rate suggesting that a fall in T3 is an adaptive mechanism to conserve energy. Decreased peripheral conversion of T4 to T3 probably also plays an important role in preserving lean body mass during underfeeding (Yang & Van Itallie, 1984).

Changes in the pituitary–thyroid axis are generally not causal agents of simple obesity. Secondary obesity that develops in hypothyroidism is associated with impaired somatic growth while the children with simple obesity are usually of average or above average height.

10.4 Growth hormone and insulin-like growth factors

Growth hormone (GH) secretion and dynamics in childhood obesity are of special interest because obese children usually have accelerated growth and in the pre-pubertal and early pubertal period show advanced height and bone age (Minuto et al., 1988; Vignolo et al., 1988). However the pubertal growth spurt is less pronounced and a reduction of the centile for height parallels progression in maturation, so that the final height of obese children is usually not different from that of their lean peers.

A number of abnormalities in GH release as well as in insulin-like growth factors (IGFs) and their binding proteins (IGFBPs) have been described in obese individuals. Basal GH concentrations and GH response to provocative stimulation and GH-releasing hormone (GHRH) are reduced in obese children and adults (Molnár et al., 1981; Ghigo et al., 1992; Slowinska-Srzednicka et al., 1992; Rasmussen et al., 1995). Decreased spontaneous 24-hour GH secretion and pulsatility and accelerated clearance have also been reported (Veldhuis et al., 1991; Chalew et al., 1992). The pulsatile area under the curve and integrated concentration of GH in prepubertal obese children were significantly lower than in lean age-matched controls (Argente et al., 1997). However, when obese children decreased their weight by at least 25% of their initial BMI standard deviation (SD) score, both parameters returned to normal after 1 year, and in all subjects GH secretory pattern was no longer distinguishable from that of the lean controls. After short-term (5–8 weeks) of a low energy diet, integrated concentrations of GH were not restored to normal despite a significant weight reduction (Chalew et al., 1992). Apparently, a longer period of sustained weight loss is needed for GH secretory pattern restoration.

GH binds in plasma with a specific protein – GH-binding protein (GHBP).

GHBP is believed to be derived from the proteolytic cleavage of the extracellular domain of the GH receptor and its concentration in blood corresponds to GH receptor status (Leung et al., 1987). As the liver seems to be a main source of GHBP, serum level of this protein may reflect hepatic growth-hormone receptor (GHR) density. Insulin apparently increases the density of hepatic GHR as GHBP levels are reduced in insulin-dependent diabetes mellitus (IDDM) (Mercado et al., 1992) and increased in obesity (Rasmussen et al., 1996) in which hyperinsulinaemia is a common feature.

In obese subjects, elevated GHBP and positive correlation of GHBP level with BMI have been reported (Hochberg et al., 1992). Increased serum GHBP levels in obese pubertal children decreased significantly after diet-induced weight loss and were paralleled by the decrease of leptin levels (Kratzsch et al., 1997). Authors speculate that leptin may be acting as a link between adipocytes and GHR releasing GHBP. This finding was confirmed in adults with different nutritional status in whom a strong correlation between GHBP and SD score of leptin serum concentration has been reported (Llopis et al., 1998).

The role of elevated GHBP level in obese children is unclear. It may reflect decreased GH clearance, increased density of GHR and perhaps increased GH sensitivity (Hochberg et al., 1992). This phenomenon may be responsible for normal or accelerated growth velocity in spite of the reduced GH secretion in obese children although some other abnormalities in the peripheral GH–insulin-like growth factors (IGFs) system are probably also involved.

Growth-promoting activity of GH is mediated by two insulin-like growth factors – IGF-1 and IGF-2. IGF-2 is the most important growth factor in fetal life, while IGF-1 physiological action is much more pronounced in the postnatal period. Serum concentration of IGF-1 usually reflects 24-hour mean serum concentration of GH and there is a negative feed-back mechanism between IGF-1 and GH secretion by the pituitary. IGFs are synthesized primarily by the liver and they are bound with high-affinity specific proteins – IGF binding proteins (IGFBP). Less than 1% of IGF-1 is circulating in a free form (Blum, 1996). On the basis of their structure at least six classes of IGFBP can be distinguished, of which IGFBP-1, IGFBP-2 and IGFBP-3 are best characterized.

More than 95% of the IGF-1 and IGF-2 in the serum is bound to IGFBP-3. This protein is the main carrier of IGF-1 and because of the short metabolic half-life of free IGF-1 its serum concentration is usually determined on the basis of IGFBP-3 level. IGFBP-3 concentration is regulated mainly by GH. IGFBP-1 is GH independent and primarily influenced by insulin. Increased insulin concentration inhibits its hepatic production (Blum, 1996).

Obesity is usually characterized by normal (Chalew et al., 1992; Slowinska-Srzednicka et al., 1992; Argente et al., 1997) or high IGF-1 levels (Hochberg et al.,

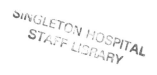

1992). Some authors (Wabitsch et al., 1996b) found increased IGF-1 in younger obese girls, while in subjects older than 14.8 years IGF-1 level was not different from normal. This finding could be attributed to the earlier maturation of obese girls, as IGF-1 is associated with pubertal development and is significantly higher in more mature children (Wilson et al., 1991). The authors speculated that the advanced maturation seen in overnutrition might be due to increased IGF-1 secretion. However, in a study performed in a large group of normal-weight girls (Wilson et al., 1991) serum IGF-1 was not related to BMI, triceps skinfold thickness, waist/hip ratio, height and weight. Normal total but elevated free IGF-1 concentrations have also been reported in obese children (Argente et al., 1997; Attia et al., 1998).

Dynamic studies on IGF and IGFBP levels in obese children before and after weight reduction were conducted independently by two groups of investigators (Wabitsch et al., 1996b; Argente et al., 1997). In a large group of obese pubertal girls, Wabitsch et al. (1996b) reported a decrease in total IGF-1 serum concentration and decreased IGF-1/IGFBP-3 ratio (which represents free IGF-1) after 6 weeks of successful dietary treatment. Obese children in the study of Argente et al. (1997) were prepubertal and they were re-examined after a much longer period of dietary treatment (approximately 1 year). Total IGF concentration remained constant throughout the period, while free IGF increased and reached a level significantly higher than in the lean controls. Serum IGFBP-3 was increased at baseline and returned to normal after weight reduction.

The discrepancies in the results of these studies are probably mostly due to the different follow-up times. The other factor could have been the more restrictive diet in the study by Wabitsch et al. (1996b) The decrease in IGF-1/IGFBP-3 ratio in this study, that could negatively influence growth velocity of obese children during a hypocaloric diet, was not demonstrated by Argente et al. (1997) after 12 months of the isocaloric dietary treatment. Moreover, the latter authors reported a significant increase in free IGF-1 concentration together with the restoration to normal of the initially suppressed GH secretion.

The mechanisms underlying GH–IGF axis abnormalities in obesity remain speculative and the data on IGF and IGFBP levels in obese children are not consistent. This may be due to the dynamic changes of the measured parameters which are dependent on many factors. Since serum IGF-1 level reflects nutritional status, overnutrition possibly leads to increased IGF-1 concentration that, in turn, may be responsible for earlier maturation of obese children. Most changes in IGF and IGFBP concentrations seem to be independent of altered GH secretion and not all of them return to normal after weight reduction. It is likely that the normalization of the whole axis requires a more extended period of time. It would be of special interest to study the GH–IGF axis in postobese children who managed to remain lean for several years. Nevertheless, these abnormalities do not seem to result in impairment of the final height in obese children. Although hypocaloric diets may decrease growth velocity in the short term (Brook et al., 1974), longitudinal clinical studies demonstrate (Epstein et al., 1990) that well balanced diets have no negative effects on the height of the obese children submitted to weight-control treatment.

In addition to its growth promoting activity, growth hormone is known to exert a strong anabolic and lipolytic action. GH-deficient children are generally moderately obese. Their adipose tissue cellularity is different from that of normal-weight and obese children (Wabitsch et al., 1995a). Their fat cell size is larger than normal but the fat cell number is decreased. Treatment with growth hormone shifts the cell number towards normal. Also, treatment with IGF-1 in children with Laron's syndrome decreases the subcutaneous fat. These clinical observations indicate that GH and IGF-1 influence growth of the adipose tissue. GH decreases body fat mass by reducing the volume of mature adipocytes, although it is also capable of differentiating the adipocyte precursors into mature adipocytes. IGF-1 stimulates the differentiation process. Human adipose tissue therefore seems to be a target tissue for GH action. However, administration of leptin antiserum to normally fed rats led to a decrease in plasma GH levels, suggesting that leptin secreted by the adipose tissue may be a metabolic signal regulating GH secretion (Caro et al., 1997). Presence of such regulation could explain low GH levels in obese children and adults with hyperleptinaemia.

Both GH and IGF-1 also have several metabolic effects, mainly on glucose and lipid metabolism. Patients with long-standing GH deficiency show increased mortality from cardiovascular disease and they tend to have increased total cholesterol level and decreased high-density-lipoprotein (HDL)-cholesterol concentration (Carroll et al., 1998). They were also found to be hyperinsulinaemic and insulin resistant. In obese children, increased GHBP level, which may inhibit GH binding to the tissue receptors, correlated positively with total cholesterol, low-density-lipoprotein (LDL)-cholesterol and triglycerides levels (Kratzsch et al., 1997). It is not known whether these metabolic changes may be causally related to the development of dyslipidaemia in future life.

10.5 Hyperinsulinaemia and insulin resistance

Hyperinsulinism is a common feature in obesity. It is at least partially a compensatory response to insulin resistance, a metabolic state in which physiological concentrations of insulin result in a diminished metabolic response. Insulin resistance results in decreased glucose uptake in peripheral tissues and increased glucose release from the liver. These defects are partially compensated by increased insulin secretion. Obese individuals demonstrate an increase in the fasting insulin-to-glucose ratio and in the total amount of insulin required to maintain normal glucose levels during oral glucose tolerance test (OGTT) (Molnár & Soltesz, 1982; Bonora et al., 1984).

The processes that trigger hyperinsulinaemia in human obesity and the cellular mechanism of insulin resistance are not fully identified. In most tissues, insulin is involved in the metabolism of carbohydrates, lipids and amino acids. At the cellular membrane it increases the transport of glucose and other substances. The first step in the interaction of insulin with target cells is binding with the specific protein receptor – a glycoprotein consisting of two α and two β subunits. The α subunit acts as a binding site while the β subunit possesses tyrosine kinase activity for endogenous and exogenous substrates. Experimental studies on human adiposity (Caro et al., 1989) have demonstrated that, although the number of insulin receptors in the adipose tissue was either slightly decreased or normal, it was significantly decreased in the liver and skeletal muscle. Moreover, in skeletal muscle receptors the activity of insulin-sensitive tyrosine kinase was impaired. It indicates that skeletal muscles are more resistant to insulin than adipose tissue. Results of these experiments might explain findings in clinical studies of obese children and adults (Bougneres et al., 1989).

Insulin stimulates glucose transport by initiating redistribution of the glucose transporting protein from the intracellular pool to the plasma membrane. In the adipose and muscle tissue the insulin-responsive glucose transporter is a protein named GLUT-4. This 509 amino acid protein was of special interest because it could be responsible for the insulin resistance in obesity. However, only a modest decrease in its activity was demonstrated (Caro et al., 1989), which could not explain the disturbed glucose transport in human obesity. Hyperinsulinaemia in obese subjects has been primarily attributed to the compensatory hypersecretion of insulin by the pancreatic β cells. However, measurements of C-peptide level in blood of obese adult subjects suggest that, in obesity, fasting hyperinsulinaemia is due to pancreatic hypersecretion, while hyperinsulinaemia after an oral glucose load is a consequence of decreased hepatic metabolism of insulin (Bonora et al., 1984). These findings were confirmed by the Bogalusa Heart Study in obese adolescents (Jiang et al., 1996). White obese individuals had significantly higher values of plasma insulin, C-peptide and insulin-to-glucose ratio. It suggests increased secretion and reduced clearance and sensitivity of insulin in white obese adolescents. Black adolescents had lower insulin secretion and more impaired hepatic insulin clearance than their white peers, despite a lower percentage of body fat. Thus hyperinsulinaemia in black adolescents may be attributed to the decreased insulin clearance and not hypersecretion. This racial difference in insulin sensitivity was confirmed in nonobese children (Arslanian & Suprasongsin,

1996a). At a hyperglycaemic clamp, first- and second-phase insulin levels were respectively 50% and 38% higher in black adolescents compared to their white peers. Black Americans are at increased risk of obesity and non-insulin-dependent diabetes mellitus (NIDDM). It suggests that genetic predisposition may be responsible for at least a part of this metabolic disorder.

Several studies have demonstrated that distribution of body fat is an important factor in determining reduced insulin sensitivity (Despres et al., 1995; Hollmann et al., 1997). High waist-to-hip ratio or even high waist circumference positively correlate with insulin resistance. The mechanism by which visceral fat may influence insulin sensitivity is not clearly defined. It is suggested that increased flow of free fatty acids (FFA) from intra-abdominal fat stores to the liver and systemic circulation promotes the metabolism of fat instead of glucose (Boden et al., 1994). High FFA may also inhibit insulin binding to hepatocytes and therefore reduce its clearance (Bruce et al., 1994). In abdominal obesity, the cluster of metabolic abnormalities known as syndrome X is often present (Fig. 10.2). Its most common manifestations are hyperinsulinaemia, glucose intolerance, increased very-low-density lipoproteins (VLDL) and triglycerides (TG), decreased high-density lipoproteins (HDL) and hypertension. This cluster of metabolic abnormalities is responsible for the increased risk of premature atherosclerosis. The relationship between insulin sensitivity, plasma lipid levels and body composition was examined in prepubertal and pubertal children of normal weight (Arslanian & Suprasongsin, 1996b). A positive correlation between percentage body fat and insulin sensitivity was found in all the subjects examined. In prepubertal children, diastolic blood pressure was negatively correlated with insulin sensitivity and positively with insulin level and in adolescents basal insulin levels correlated positively with VLDL and TG regardless of adiposity. In Finnish children (Ronnemaa et al., 1991), high triglycerides, high systolic blood pressure and low levels of HDL-cholesterol clustered among subjects within the highest insulin quartile. Metabolic syndrome was found in almost 10% of obese Hungarian adolescents and children. Those with longer duration of obesity were at higher risk (Csábi et al., 2000) of multimetabolic syndrome. Longitudinal studies have shown that obese children who became obese adults were at particularly high risk of the metabolic syndrome (Vanhala et al., 1998). The possible mechanism is that a prolonged insulin resistance results in the clustering of hypertension and metabolic abnormalities in the same individual.

Although insulin resistance and hyperinsulinaemia were found already in preadolescent obese children (Molnár et al., 1982; Caprio et al., 1996a), several studies demonstrated that puberty is a critical period for the development of decreased insulin sensitivity (Travers et al., 1995; Arslanian & Suprasongsin, 1996b). Puberty is also associated with increased prevalence of obesity and

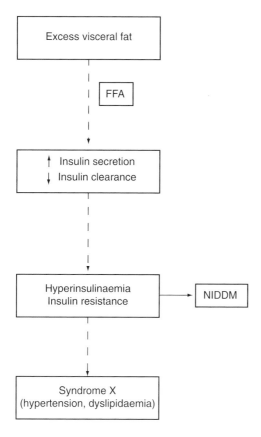

Figure 10.2 Development of insulin resistance in obesity.

adolescent obesity has a high likelihood to persist into adulthood (Power et al., 1997; Whitaker et al., 1997; Roemmich et al., 1998). The percentage of body fat during the consecutive stages of puberty increases in girls and decreases in boys (Guo et al., 1997). In pubertal children (Travers et al., 1995), BMI shows the strongest correlation with insulin sensitivity and boys tend to be more insulin sensitive than girls. Data from the study of Travers et al., as well as the results of the Bogalusa Heart Study (Jiang et al., 1996), show that excess weight gain during adolescence may have long-term adverse health consequence in respect of the impaired insulin secretion and glucose metabolism.

Studies performed in populations with high prevalence of NIDDM have demonstrated that long-lasting hyperinsulinaemia with insulin resistance may precede the decline in pancreatic β-cell function heralding the onset of NIDDM. The majority of members of the Pima Indians population in Arizona is hyperinsulinaemic, insulin resistant and obese. According to the 'thrifty genotype' hypothesis (Neel, 1962), insulin hypersecretion was an advantageous feature during an early stage of evolution because it increased the efficiency of fat tissue storage.

This hypothesis is based on a concept that obesity is a result of insulin resistance and hyperinsulinaemia. However, some observations point to the alternative hypothesis that these metabolic disturbances rather represent physiological adaptation to obesity, limiting further weight gain. In a prospective study of a large group of Pima Indians, a relatively low level of insulin secretion was a strong independent predictor of weight gain in this population (Schwartz et al., 1995). It can be speculated that by increasing central nervous system signalling and suppressing food intake hyperinsulinaemia and insulin resistance may decrease the risk of further weight gain.

Weight loss dramatically improves insulin sensitivity and decreases hyperinsulinaemia in obese adults and children. However, most obese people resist weight reduction. Attempts to lose weight are often not successful or are followed by regaining of the weight lost, so long-term prognosis is usually poor. In hyperinsulinaemic children, treatment was even less effective in terms of weight loss than in normoinsulinaemic peers, but the study was based on a relatively small group of children (Zannolli et al., 1993).

Weight reduction does not seem to restore elevated insulin concentrations to normal in obese children. Prepubertal children remained hyperinsulinaemic after 1 year of a weight loss programme, although they achieved a 50% reduction of their BMI SD score (Argente et al., 1997). Long-term prospective studies of obese children with glucose intolerance revealed that subjects who managed to maintain reduced weight remained hyperinsulinaemic in spite of improved glucose tolerance (Malecka-Tendera et al., 1994). In children who increased their weight over a 6-year period, insulin levels were significantly lower, despite the higher glucose levels on oral glucose tolerance test (OGTT). Results of these clinical studies are in accordance with the hypothesis that insulin resistance may be necessary to prevent additional weight gain (Eckel, 1992). However, long lasting hyperinsulinaemia increases the risk of cardiovascular disease and NIDDM.

NIDDM, once believed to be a disease predominantly of obese adults, is apparently increasing in children. Dramatic increases in NIDDM amongst adolescents in Greater Cincinnati have been documented (Pinhas-Hamiel et al., 1996). Before 1992, children with a diagnosis of NIDDM represented only 2% to 4% of all the newly diagnosed diabetics aged between birth and 19 years, but by 1994 NIDDM accounted for 16% of all the cases in this age-group. Among the children with NIDDM, 92% had BMI over $40\,kg/m^2$. A retrospective analysis of the children with NIDDM, diagnosed in Arkansas, 1988–1995, demonstrated that children with NIDDM were mostly African-Americans characterized by significant obesity (BMI $> 35\,kg/m^2$) and acanthosis nigricans (Scott et al., 1997).

The obese youth with newly diagnosed diabetes mellitus should always raise suspicion of NIDDM, particularly if there is no history of prior weight loss and physical examination reveals acanthosis nigricans and hypertension. Obese adolescents with NIDDM are similar to obese adults, in that they risk complications such as retinopathy, nephropathy and neuropathy. Their severe obesity puts them also at risk of orthopaedic complications as well as hypertension and lipid disturbances promoting premature atherosclerosis. As they grow into adulthood the long duration of their condition may lead to more severe complications. Many of them will probably need lifelong therapy with oral hypoglycaemic drugs and regular metabolic monitoring. It is well established in adults that the risk of developing NIDDM rises exponentially with increasing BMI. With the increasing prevalence of childhood and adolescent obesity and with the growing number of super-obese children NIDDM may soon be a common paediatric problem.

10.6 Leptin

In 1994, the *ob* gene was identified in ob/ob mice and its product, a 167-amino acid peptide was named leptin from the Greek word 'leptos', meaning 'thin'. Since that time over 1500 papers concerning leptin have been published and our knowledge on its biological functions has been constantly expanding. Leptin is encoded by a gene located in human chromosome 7q31.3.

At first, leptin was seen as an adipocyte-derived signalling molecule, limiting food intake and increasing energy expenditure (Zhang et al., 1994), and having plasma levels which correlated positively with fat mass. Now it is recognized that brown adipose tissue (Dessolin et al., 1997), placenta (Hoggard et al., 1997) and several fetal tissues, including heart, bone/cartilage and hair follicles (Hoggard et al., 1998), are also production sites for the hormone. Leptin was also believed to be secreted in the stomach (Bado et al., 1998) but there is a body of evidence which suggests it is locally concentrated and stored, but not produced, in gastric mucosa (Breidert et al., 1999).

Human leptin is secreted in a circadian and pulsatile fashion with a nocturnal rise and an organized pattern of pulsatility, with an average of 32 pulses/day, each pulse lasting 33 min (Prolo et al., 1998). In the plasma, leptin circulates, either free or complexed to a binding protein, and the proportion of bound/free leptin varies with BMI. Free leptin increases in obese individuals (Houseknecht et al., 1996). Plasma leptin half-life is 24.9 ± 4.4 min in humans (Klein et al., 1996) and it is the same in obese and normal-weight individuals. The short half-life of leptin in the circulation is mainly determined by renal clearance, mediated by glomerular filtration (Cumin et al., 1996). The leptin receptor belongs to the class-I cytokine receptor family and one or more of its splice variants are expressed in most, if not all, tissues including choroid plexus, hypothalamus, heart, liver, lung, kidney, skeletal muscle, small intestine, prostate, testis, adipose tissue, adrenal medulla,

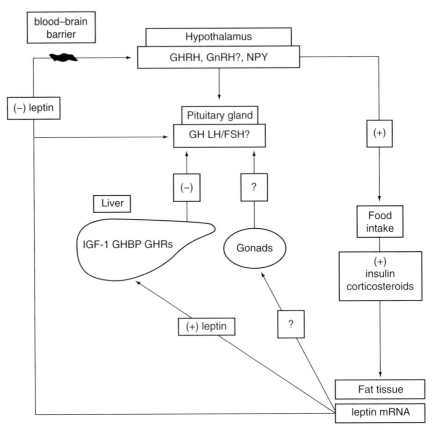

Figure 10.3　Hypothetical leptin action: GHRs: growth-hormone receptors; GHBP: growth-hormone binding proteins; IGF-1: insulin-like growth factor 1; GH: growth hormone; GHRH: growth-hormone releasing hormone; GnRH: gonadotrophin-releasing hormone; NPY: neuropeptide Y; LH: luteinizing hormone; FSH: follicle-stimulating hormone.

β-cells of the pancreas, ovaries, placenta and fetal tissues (Hoggard et al., 1997; Stephens & Caro, 1998; Trayhurn et al., 1999). The extensive distribution of leptin-receptor gene expression is indicative of the hormone having a range of targets and is consistent with the growing evidence of a multiplicity of functions.

10.6.1 Leptin and obesity

The primary physiological role of leptin seems to be to send signals to the brain about the energy stores of the body and so to act as part of a feedback mechanism that can function as a 'lipostat'. A decrease of body weight is associated with dramatic reduction in serum leptin concentration even if the change in body weight is moderate. Weight reductions of about 10% result in falls in leptin levels of obese adults of 34% (Havel et al., 1996) to 53% (Considine et al., 1996). During weight-maintenance periods, leptin levels rise again slightly or remain stable.

Fasting reduces leptin levels acutely by 60–70% (Boden et al., 1996) in obese as well as normal-weight subjects. In contrast, in response to massive overfeeding resulting in 10% weight gain over 5 weeks, leptin levels were more than three-fold higher than would have been expected by the rise in BMI (Kolaczynski et al., 1996).

Treatment with leptin induces weight reduction in morbidly obese ob/ob mice and decreases their plasma glucose and insulin levels. Peripherally injected leptin can alter feeding behaviour in ob/ob mice but its potency is 100 times greater when it is injected directly into the lateral ventricle of the brain (Stephens & Caro, 1998). High-affinity leptin receptors have been discovered in the hypothalamus and chronic leptin treatment decreases both hypothalamic synthesis and release of neuropeptide Y (NPY). This peptide is one of the most powerful food-intake stimulators and most animal models of obesity, such as ob/ob mice with leptin deficiency, are characterized by high hypothalamic NPY expression.

The results of animal and human studies indicate that relative leptin deficiency in the central nervous system might be a mechanism leading to obesity. One possible defect may be impaired transportation through the blood–brain barrier, because plasma leptin levels were about 300% higher in the obese than in the nonobese, whilst cerebrospinal fluid concentrations were only 30% higher (Caro et al., 1996). However, true 'leptin resistance', mediated by receptor or postreceptor defects, similar to the defects in insulin resistance, can also be involved in the development of some human obesity. A good example of the receptor type of leptin resistance is the mutation in a splice donor site of the leptin receptor gene described by Clément et al. (1998). Also, impaired reactions by other molecules, such as NPY, on which leptin acts in the brain may contribute to impaired sensitivity to leptin in obese subjects. However, some obese subjects show lower concentrations of leptin, which may result from an abnormal secretion of leptin from fat stores. This may partially explain the high failure rate of dieting (Friedman, 1997).

Abnormalities in leptin regulation are expressed early in the natural history of human adiposity as hyperleptinaemia was already present in prepubertal obese children (Caprio et al., 1996b). After weight loss, leptin levels decreased markedly. Most values were in the range of normal-weight children, although the subjects were still obese (Wabitsch et al., 1996a). Although marked decrease in circulating leptin levels during weight loss may be one of the reasons for the poor long-term prognosis with hypocaloric diets, few data are available on whether leptin levels predict future weight change. Relatively low plasma leptin levels were found to predict subsequent weight gain in obese Pima Indians (Ravussin et al., 1997) as well as in prepubertal children (Caprio et al., 1998). Thus, it could be speculated that individuals with low leptin concentrations gain more weight because of inadequate satiety signals. However, in Japanese Americans (Chessler et al., 1998) and in a Swedish study of serum stored for 29 years (Lissner et al., 1998), relatively high levels of leptin were found to be risk factors for subsequent weight gain, suggesting the importance of leptin resistance in the pathophysiology of human adiposity.

The final argument supporting a role of leptin in the control of body weight was provided by identification of a frame-shift mutation of the leptin gene involving the deletion of a single guanine nucleotide at codon 133 which resulted in a truncated protein in two severely obese children in the same highly consanguineous pedigree (Montague et al., 1997a). Both of them had normal birth weight but suffered from severe obesity from an early age. They were constantly hungry and demanding food continuously. In one of them, treatment with recombinant human leptin (RmetHuleptin) induced significant weight loss (Farooqi et al., 1998). Subsequently, Strobel and colleagues (1998) described a Turkish family in which three severely obese siblings were found to be leptin deficient due to a missense mutation in the leptin gene.

10.6.2 Leptin and body fat distribution

Although several studies have shown strong positive correlations between percentage body fat and plasma leptin concentration, there is nevertheless significant variation in leptin levels amongst subjects with the same amount of body fat (Ostlund et al., 1996). In obese subjects, leptin concentrations are, on average, significantly higher than in lean subjects, but there is considerable overlap in the values. Leptin levels may relate to body fat distribution also but the interaction of fat distribution and leptin levels is not yet clear. Lönnqvist et al. (1995) found no significant difference in *ob* gene expression between subcutaneous and omental fat, while Montague et al. (1997b) and Lefebvre et al. (1998) demonstrated higher leptin mRNA levels in subcutaneous than in omental adipocytes. These latter data could indicate that leptin plays a role in the control of adipose tissue distribution. Most studies published so far relating leptin to body fat distribution, used anthropometric parameters and came to different conclusions (Dua et al., 1996; Haffner et al., 1996; Weigle et al., 1997; Van Gaal et al., 1999; Sudi et al., 2000). However, the correlations between leptin levels and subcutaneous body fat were stronger than those between leptin and intra-abdominal fat (Caprio et al., 1996b).

10.6.3 Leptin and sexual dimorphism

Women have higher absolute leptin levels than men, regardless of fat mass (Saad et al., 1998). Significantly higher leptin concentrations were also found in obese adolescent girls compared to boys at the same degree of adiposity (Blum et al., 1997; Garcia-Mayor et al., 1997; Wabitsch et al., 1997). At the early stages of puberty, gender differences were less pronounced, but at Tanner stage 5, leptin concentrations in obese girls were over 50% higher than in boys for the same percentage body fat (Blum et al., 1997). Gender difference in serum leptin concentration may be explained by a suppressive effect of androgens on leptin production. Testosterone had a potent negative effect on serum leptin in obese boys (Blum et al., 1997; Wabitsch et al., 1997). These findings were confirmed by in vitro studies of cultured human adipocytes. They revealed that testosterone and dihydrotestosterone are able to reduce leptin secretion into the culture medium (Wabitsch et al., 1997). Recent findings that hypogonadal men with low serum testosterone concentrations have significantly increased serum leptin levels compared to men without any endocrine disorder (Behre et al., 1997) further support the above theory.

10.6.4 Leptin and puberty

Besides its role in signalling energy deficiency, leptin is an important integrator of neuroendocrine function (Fig. 10.3). It has been speculated for more than 20 years that young women need a certain cut-off weight/body fat to attain menarche or to avoid secondary amenorrhoea (de Courten et al., 1997). Chehab et al. (1996) demonstrated that leptin-deficient mice are infertile and that sterility can be corrected by treatment with leptin. Surprisingly enough, normal reproductive function was reported in leptin-deficient patients with lipoatrophic diabetes, suggesting that leptin is not fundamental to the maintenance of normal reproductive function in humans (Andreelli et al., 2000). In rodents, a rapid fall of plasma leptin level in response to energy deprivation results in the activation of the hypothalamic–pituitary–adrenal axis and suppression of the thyroid and reproductive axes. These adaptive changes to starvation promote increased hepatic gluconeogenesis, a fall in metabolic rate and limited reproduction in females. Starvation-induced changes in gonadal, adrenal and thyroid axes can be prevented with administration of exogenous leptin (Lönnqvist & Schalling, 1997). Starvation also results in a suppression of GH and IGF-1 in rodents, while in humans there is an increase of GH and suppression of IGF-1 production. A significant correlation between IGF-1 and leptin concentrations in women with anorexia nervosa was found (Grinspoon et al., 1996) suggesting the existence of a similar adaptive mechanism. Leptin most probably exerts its function through the hypothalamus. Initially, NPY was viewed as a key target. However, the same adaptive changes to starvation were found in mice with destruction of the *NPY* gene.

To clarify its neuroendocrine function in the regulation of puberty in humans, leptin has been studied in healthy children and individuals with precocious puberty (Blum et al., 1997; Garcia-Mayor et al., 1997; Mantzoros et al., 1997; Palmert et al., 1998). In boys, leptin levels rose by 50% just before the onset of puberty and decreased to baseline in the postpubertal period, while, in girls, increase in leptin plasma level paralleled pubertal stage. Leptin level was also found to be inversely related to age of menarche in girls (Matkovic et al., 1997). Patients homozygous for a mutation in the leptin receptor gene were sexually immature (Clement et al., 1998). Taken together, the results of these studies suggest that the onset of puberty is associated with sufficient or threshold serum leptin levels and that leptin may be one of the several signals that regulate the hypothalamic–pituitary–gonadal axis and trigger the initiation of puberty.

Insulin is probably important in long-term regulation of leptin as insulin resistance was found to be associated with elevated leptin concentrations independent of adiposity and fat distribution (Zimmet et al., 1998). This suggests that hyperleptinaemia could be the missing link in the multimetabolic syndrome. Studies in vitro show that insulin provokes a dose-dependent rise in leptin protein (Wabitsch et al., 1996c). However, insulin does not seem to influence leptin secretion acutely, because short-term infusions of insulin do not alter plasma leptin levels in humans (Ryan & Elahi, 1996). In contrast, leptin has a dose-dependent direct inhibitory effect on glucose-induced insulin secretion by islet cells from ob/ob mice (Emilsson et al., 1997), which suggests that leptin overproduction could be involved in the development of the diabetic syndrome in obese subjects with insulin resistance.

Glucocorticoids probably act, at least in part, directly on adipose tissue to stimulate leptin synthesis and secretion in humans (Wabitsch et al., 1996c; Masuzaki et al., 1997). The diurnal rhythm seen in circulating leptin levels is opposite to those of ACTH and cortisol, suggesting the existence of hypothalamic–pituitary–adrenal regulation and a negative feedback (Saad et al., 1998).

According to recent results, sympathetic nervous system activity also plays a dominant role in the regulation of leptin production in white adipose tissue through modulating the transcription of the *ob* gene (Rayner et al., 1998; Sakane et al., 1998).

10.6.5 Other functions of leptin

Serum leptin levels increase during pregnancy (Highman et al., 1998), especially during the first two trimesters (Tamás et al., 1999) as a result of increased fat accretion and of the leptin produced by the placenta. The concentration of the hormone is also high in the cord blood of the neonate (Hassink et al., 1997). Leptin production is detectable in the fetus from 18 to 24 weeks and it increases parallel with the increase of the fat content of the fetus (Jaquet et al., 1998). The exact role of the leptin produced by the placenta and the fetus is not known. One possible explanation is that placental leptin production evolved as a signal to maintain hypothalamic–pituitary, thyroid and reproductive hormones during periods in which adipose tissue leptin production might be reduced by food deprivation. In this way, the placenta could ensure its survival and that of the fetus. A second possibility for placental leptin is that the hormone acts in a paracrine or autocrine manner on the placenta or the fetus, perhaps regulating growth or partitioning of nutrients. Maternal leptin levels show positive correlation with the measures of adiposity of the mother and a negative correlation with placental size at delivery, but do not correlate with the birth weight of the new-born (Schubring et al., 1996; Hassink et al., 1997). Leptin concentrations in the cord blood correlate with adiposity indices of the new-born, indicating the role of leptin in the fetal development (Schubring et al., 1996; Hassink et al., 1997). Leptin concentration decreases rapidly after birth in both mother and new-born due to the abrupt cessation of placental leptin production (Marchini et al., 1998). The decrease in leptin levels is probably an important factor initiating food intake in the new-born after birth. After the first few postnatal days, leptin concentrations start to increase again in parallel with weight gain (Ertl et al., 1999). One additional function of leptin in reproduction can be inferred from the finding of the hormone in breast milk (Casabiell et al., 1997). Leptin in breast milk appears to be derived from the maternal circulation but may also be synthesized by mammary epithelial cells (Casabiell et al., 1997; Smith-Kirwin et al., 1998). The concentration of leptin in the milk does not correlate with percentage milk fat but could be an important growth factor in the neonate or may serve as a coordinating signal for the hypothalamic–pituitary axis. Leptin probably also participates in the regulation of haematopoiesis, cellular growth, angiogenesis, sympathetic activity and the immune system (for review see Considine & Caro, 1999). The detailed discussion of these latter functions is far beyond the scope of this chapter.

10.7 REFERENCES

Andreelli, F., Hanaire-Broutin, H., Laville, M., Tauber, J.P., Riou, J.P. & Thivolet, C. (2000). Normal reproductive function in leptin-deficient patients with lipoatropic diabetes. *Journal of Clinical Endocrinology and Metabolism*, **85**, 715–9.

Argente, J., Caballo, N., Barrios, V., Pozo, J., Munoz, M.T., Chowen, J.A. & Hernandez, H. (1997). Multiple endocrine abnormalities of the growth hormone and insulin-like growth factor axis in prepubertal children with exogenous obesity: effect of short- and long-term weight reduction. *Journal of Clinical Endocrinology and Metabolism*, **82**, 2076–83.

Arslanian, S. & Suprasongsin, C. (1996a). Differences in the in vivo insulin secretion and sensitivity of healthy black versus white adolescents. *The Journal of Pediatrics*, **129**, 440–3.

Arslanian, S. & Suprasongsin, C. (1996b). Insulin sensitivity, lipids and body composition in childhood: is 'syndrome X' present? *Journal of Clinical Endocrinology and Metabolism*, **81**,

1058–62.

Attia, N., Tamborlane, W.V., Heptulla, R., Maggs, D., Grozman, A., Sherwin, R.S. & Caprio, S. (1998). The metabolic syndrome and insulin-like growth factor I regulation in adolescent obesity. *Journal of Clinical Endocrinology and Metabolism*, **83**, 1467–71.

Azziz, R. (1989). Reproductive endocrinologic alterations in female asymptomatic obesity. *Fertility and Sterility*, **52**, 703–25.

Bado, A., Levasseur, S., Attoub, S., Kermorgant, S., Laigneau, J.P., Bortoluzzi, M.N., Moizo, L., Lehy, T., Guerre-Millo, M., LeMarchand-Brustel, Y. & Lewin, M.J. (1998). The stomach is a source of leptin. *Nature*, **394**, 790–3.

Barrett-Connor, E. & Khaw, K.T. (1988). Endogenous sex hormones and cardiovascular disease in men: a prospective population-based study. *Circulation*, **78**, 539–45.

Bates, G.W. & Whitworth, N.S. (1982). Effects of body weight reduction on plasma androgens in obese, infertile women. *Fertility and Sterility*, **38**, 406–9.

Behre, H.M., Simoni, M. & Nieschlag, E. (1997). Strong association between serum levels of leptin and testosterone in men. *Clinical Endocrinology*, **47**, 237–40.

Bergh, C., Carlsson, B., Olsson, J.H., Selleskog, U. & Hillensjo, T. (1993). Regulation of androgen production in cultured human thecal cells by GF-1 and insulin. *Fertility and Sterility*, **59**, 323–31.

Bird, C.E., Murphy, J., Boroomand, K., Finnis, W., Dressel, D. & Clark, A.F. (1972). Dehydroepiandrosterone: kinetics of metabolism in normal women. *Journal of Clinical Endocrinology and Metabolism*, **47**, 818–25.

Björntorp, P. (1995). Insulin resistance: The consequence of a neuroendocrine disturbance? [review]. *International Journal of Obesity*, **19** (Suppl. 1), S6–10.

Blum, W.F. (1996). Insulin-like growth factors and their binding proteins. In *Diagnostics of Endocrine Function in Children and Adolescents*, 2nd edn, ed. M.B. Ranke, pp. 190–3, Heidelberg-Leipzig: Johann Ambrosius Barth Verlag.

Blum, W.F., Englaro, P., Hanitsch, S., Juul, A., Hertel, N.T., Muller, J., Skakkebaek, N.E., Heiman, M.L., Birkett, M., Attanasio, A.M., Kiess, W. & Rascher, W. (1997). Plasma leptin levels in healthy children and adolescents: dependence on body mass index, body fat mass, gender, pubertal stage and testosterone. *Journal of Clinical Endocrinology and Metabolism*, **82**, 2904–10.

Boden, G., Chen, X., Ruiz, J., White, J.V. & Rossetti, L. (1994). Mechanisms of fatty acid-induced inhibition of glucose uptake. *Journal of Clinical Investigation*, **92**, 91–8.

Boden, G., Chen, X., Mozzoli, M. & Ryan, I. (1996). Effect of fasting on serum leptin in normal human subjects. *Journal of Clinical Endocrinology and Metabolism*, **81**, 3419–23.

Bonora, E., Zavaroni, I., Bruschi, F., Alpi, O., Pezzarosa, A., Guerra, L., Dall'Aglio, E., Coscelli, C. & Butturini, U. (1984). Peripheral hyperinsulinemia of simple obesity: pancreatic hypersecretion or impaired insulin metabolism? *Journal of Clinical Enocrinology and Metabolism*, **59**, 1121–7.

Bougneres, P.F., Artavia-Loria, E., Henry, S., Basdevant, A. & Castano, L. (1989). Increased basal glucose production and utilisation in children with recent obesity versus adults with long-standing obesity. *Diabetes*, **38**, 477–83.

Breidert, M., Miehlke, S., Glasow, A., Orban, Z., Stolte, M., Ehniger, G., Bayerdorffer, E.,

Nettesheim, O., Halm, U., Haidan, A. & Bornstein, R. (1999). Leptin and its receptor in normal human gastric mucosa and in *Helicobacter pylori-associated gastritis. Scandinavian Journal of Gastroenterology*, **34**, 954–61.

Brook, C.D.G., Lloyd, J.K. & Wolf, O.H. (1974). Rapid weight loss in children. *British Medical Journal*, **3**, 44–5.

Bruce, R., Godsland, I., Walton, C., Crook, D. & Wynn, V. (1994). Associations between insulin sensitivity, and free fatty acid and triglyceride metabolism independent of uncomplicated obesity. *Metabolism*, **43**, 1275–81.

Cacciari, E., Cicognani, A., Pirazzoli, P., Tassoni, P., Zappulla, F., Salardi, S. & Bernardi, F. (1975). Relationship among the secretion of ACTH, GH, and cortisol during the insulin-induced hypoglycemia test in the normal and obese child. *Journal of Clinical Endocrinology and Metabolism*, **40**, 802–9.

Cacciari, E., Cicognani, A., Pirazzoli, P., Zappulla, F., Tassoni, P., Bernardi, F., Salardi, S. & Mazzanti, L. (1977). Effect of obesity on the hypothalamo-pituitary-gonadal function in childhood. *Acta Paediatrica Scandinavica*, **66**, 345–50.

Caprio, S., Bronson, M., Sherwin, R.S., Rife, F. & Tamborlane, W.V. (1996a). Co-existence of severe insulin resistance and hyperinsulinemia in pre-adolescent obese children. *Diabetologia*, **39**, 1489–97.

Caprio, S., Tamborlane, W.V., Silver, D., Robinson, C., Leibel, R., McCarthy, S., Grozman, A., Belous, A., Maggs, D. & Sherwin, R.S. (1996b). Hyperleptinemia: an early sign of juvenile obesity. Relation to body fat depots and insulin concentrations. *American Journal of Physiology*, **271**, E626–30.

Caprio, S., Savoye, M., DeStefano, R., Bronson, M., Lavietes, S., Silver, D. & Tamborlane, W. (1998). Importance of low plasma leptin levels in predicting weight gain in obese children: 3 year longitudinal study. *International Journal of Obesity*, **22** (S3), 201.

Caro, J.F., Dohm, G.L., Pories, W.J. & Sinha, M.K. (1989). Cellular alteration in liver, skeletal muscle and adipose tissue responsible for insulin resistance in obesity and type II diabetes. *Diabetes and Metabolism Reviews*, **5**, 665–89.

Caro, J.F., Kolaczynski, J.W., Nyce, M.R., Ohannesian, J.P., Opentanova, I., Goldman, W.H., Lynn, R.B., Zhang, P.L., Sinha, M.K. & Considine, R.V. (1996). Decreased cerebrospinal-fluid/serum leptin ratio in obesity: a possible mechanism for leptin resistance. *Lancet*, **348**, 159–61.

Caro, E., Senaris, R., Considine, R.V., Casanueva, F.F. & Dieguez, C. (1997). Regulation of in vivo growth hormone secretion by leptin. *Endocrinology*, **138**, 2203–6.

Carroll, P.V., Christ, E.R., Christiansen, J.S., Clemmons, D., Hintz, R., Ho, K., Laron, Z., Sizonenko, P., Sonksen, P.H., Tanaka, T. & Thorner, M. (1998). Growth hormone deficiency in adulthood and the effects of growth hormone replacement: a review. *Journal of Clinical Endocrinology and Metabolism*, **83**, 382–95.

Casabiell, X., Pineiro, V., Tome, M.A., Peino, R., Dieguez, C. & Casanueva, F.F. (1997). Presence of leptin in colostrum and/or breast milk from lactating mothers: a potential role in the regulation of neonatal food intake. *Journal of Clinical Endocrinology and Metabolism*, **82**, 4270–3.

Cataldo, N.A. (1997). Insulin like growth factor binding proteins: do they play a role in polycystic ovary syndrome? *Endocrinology*, **15**, 123–36.

Chalew, S.A., Lozano, R.A., Armour, K.M. & Kowraski, A.A. (1992). Reduction of plasma insulin levels does not restore integrated concentration of growth hormone to normal in obese children. *International Journal of Obesity*, **16**, 459–63.

Chalew, S., Nagel, H. & Shore, S. (1995). The hypothalamic–pituitary–adrenal axis in obesity [review]. *Obesity Research*, **3**, 371–82.

Chehab, F., Lim, M. & Lu, R. (1996). Correction of sterility defect in homozygous obese female mice treated with human recombinant leptin. *Nature Genetics*, **12**, 318–20.

Chessler, S.D., Fujimoto, W.Y., Shofer, J.B., Boyko, E.J. & Weigle, D.S. (1998). Increased plasma leptin levels are associated with fat accumulation in Japanese Americans. *Diabetes*, **47**, 239–43.

Cleary, M.P., Shepherd, A. & Jenks, B. (1984). Effect of dehydroepiandrosterone on growth in lean and obese Zucker rats. *Journal of Nutrition*, **114**, 1242–51.

Clément, K., Vaisse, Ch., Lahlou, N., Cabrol, S., Pelloux, V., Cassuto, D., Gourmelen, M., Dina, Ch., Chambaz, J., Lacorte, J.-M., Basdevant, A., Bougnieres, P., Lebouc, Y., Froguel, P. & Guy-Grand, B. (1998). A mutation in the human leptin receptor gene causes obesity and pituitary dysfunction. *Nature*, **392**, 398–401.

Considine, R.V. & Caro, J.F. (1999). Pleiotropic cellular effects of leptin. *Current Opinion in Endocrinology and Diabetes*, **6**, 163–9.

Considine, R.V., Sinha, M.K., Heiman, M.L., Kriauciunas, A., Stephens, T.W., Nyce, M.R., Ohannesian, J.P., Marco, Ch.C., McKee, L.J., Bauer, T.L. & Caro, J.F. (1996). Serum immunoreactive-leptin concentrations in normal-weight and obese humans. *New England Journal of Medicine*. **334**, 292–5.

Crawford, J.D. & Osler, D.C. (1975). Body composition at menarche: The Frisch–Ravelle hypothesis revisited. *Pediatrics*, **56**, 449–58.

Csábi, Gy., Török, K., Jeges, S. & Molnár, D. (2000). Presence of metabolic cardiovascular syndrome in obese children. *European Journal of Pediatrics*, **159**, 91–4.

Cumin, F., Baum, H-P. & Levens, N. (1996). Leptin is cleared from the circulation primarily by the kidney. *International Journal of Obesity*, **20**, 1120–6.

Dale, P.O., Tanbo, T., Vaaler, S. & Abyholm, T. (1992). Body weight, hyperinsulinemia, and gonadotropin levels in the polycystic ovarian syndrome: evidence of two distinct populations. *Fertility and Sterility*, **58**, 487–91.

De Courten, M., Zimmet, P., Hidge, A., Collins, V., Nicholson, M., Staten, M., Dowse, G. & Alberti, K.G.M.M. (1997). Hyperleptinaemia: the missing link in the metabolic syndrome? *Diabetic Medicine*, **14**, 200–8.

Despres, J.P., Lemieux, S., Lamarche, B., Prud'homme, B., Moorjani, S., Brun, L.D., Gagne, C. & Lupien, P.J. (1995). The insulin resistance-dyslipidemic syndrome: contribution of visceral obesity and therapeutic implications. *International Journal of Obesity*, **19** (Suppl. 1), S76–S86.

Dessolin, S., Schalling., M., Champigny, O., Lomnqvist, F., Ailhaud, G., Dani, C. & Ricquier, D. (1997). Leptin gene is expressed in rat brown adipose tissue at birth. *FASEB Journal*, **11**, 382–7.

Dua, A., Hennes, M.I., Hoffmann, R.G., Maas, D.L., Krakower, G.R., Sonnenberg, G.E. & Kissebah, A.H. (1996). Leptin: a significant indicator of total body fat but not of visceral fat

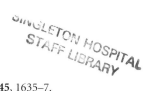

and insulin insensitivity in African-American women. *Diabetes*, **45**, 1635–7.

Eckel, R.H. (1992). Insulin resistance: an adaptation for weight maintenance. *The Lancet*, **340**, 1452–3.

Emilsson, V., Liu, Y.L., Cawthorne, M.A., Morton, N.M. & Davenport, M. (1997). Expression of the functional leptin receptor mRNA in pancreatic islets and direct inhibitory action of leptin on insulin secretion. *Diabetes*, **46**, 313–6.

Epstein, L.H., McCurley, J., Valoski, A. & Wing, R.R. (1990). Growth in obese children treated for obesity. *American Journal of Diseases of Childhood*, **144**, 1360–4.

Ertl, T., Funke, S., Sárkány, I., Szabó, I., Rascher, W., Blum, W.F. & Sulyok, E. (1999). Postnatal changes of leptin levels in full-term and preterm neonates: Their relation to intrauterine growth, gender and testosterone. *Biology of the Neonate*, **75**, 167–76.

Evans, D.J., Hoffmann, R.G., Kalkhoff, R.K. & Kissebah, A.H. (1983). Relationship of androgenic activity to body fat topography, fat cell morphology, and metabolic aberrations in premenopausal women. *Journal of Clinical Endocrinology and Metabolism*, **57**, 304–10.

Farooqi, L.S., Jeeb, S., Cook, G., Cheetham, C.H., Lawrence, E., Prentice, A., Hughes, L.A., McCamish, M. & O'Rahilly, S. (1998). Treatment of congenital leptin deficiency in man, *8th International Congress on Obesity. Paris 1998*, eds. G. Ailhand & B. Guy, International Association for the Study of Obesity. Hot topic lectures. p. 7.

Fehér, T. & Halmy, L. (1975). The production and fate of adrenal DHEA in normal overweight subjects. *Hormone Research*, **6**, 303–4.

Friedman, J.M. (1997). Role of leptin and its receptors in the control of body weight. In *Leptin: The Voice of Adipose Tissue*, eds. W. Blum, W. Kiess & W. Rascher, pp. 3–22. Leipzig: Johann Ambrosius Barth Verlag.

Frisch, R.E. (1987). Body fat, menarche, fitness and fertility. *Human Reproduction*, **2**, 521–33.

Garcia-Mayor, R.V., Andrade, A., Rios, M., Lage, M., Dieguez, C. & Casanueva, F.F. (1997). Serum leptin levels in normal children: relationship to age, gender, body mass index, pituitary-gonadal hormones and pubertal stage. *Journal of Clinical Endocrinology and Metabolism*, **82**, 2849–55.

Genazzani, A.R., Pintor, C. & Corda, R. (1978). Adrenal and gonadal steroids in obese prepubertal girls. *Journal of Clinical Endocrinology and Metabolism*, **47**, 974–9.

Ghigo, E., Procopio, M., Boffano, G.M., Arvat, E., Valente, F., Maccario, M., Mazza, E. & Cammani, F. (1992). Arginine potentiates but does not restore the blunted growth hormone response to growth hormone-releasing hormone in obesity. *Metabolism*, **41**, 560–3.

Glass, A.R., Swerdloff, R.S., Bray, G.A., Dahms, W.T. & Atkinson, R.L. (1977). Low serum testosterone and sex-hormone-binding-globulin in massively obese men. *Journal of Clinical Endocrinology and Metabolism*, **45**, 1211–19.

Gonzalez, F. (1997). Adrenal environment in polycystic ovary syndrome. *Seminars in Reproductive Endocrinology*, **15**, 137–57.

Grinspoon, S., Gulick, T., Askari, H., Landt, M., Lee, K., Anderson, E., Ma, Z., Vignati, L., Bowsher, R., Herzog, D. & Klibanski, A. (1996). Serum leptin levels in women with anorexia nervosa. *Journal of Clinical Endocrinology and Metabolism*, **81**, 3861–3.

Guo, S.S., Chumlea, W.C., Roche, A.F. & Siervogel, R.M. (1997). Age and maturity-related changes in body composition during adolescence into adulthood: the Fels longitudinal study.

International Journal of Obesity, **21**, 1167–75.

Haffner, S.M., Gingerich, R.L., Miettinen, H. & Stern, M.P. (1996). Leptin concentrations in relation to overall adiposity and regional body fat distribution in Mexican Americans. *International Journal of Obesity*, **20**, 904–8.

Hassink, S.G., de Lancey, E., Sheslow, D.V., Smith-Kirwin, S.M., O'Connor, D.M., Considine, R.V., Opentanova, I., Dostal, K., Spear, M.L., Leef, K., Ash, M., Spitzer, A.R. & Funanage, V.L. (1997). Placental leptin: an important new growth factor in intrauterine and neonatal development? *Pediatrics*, **100**, 124 (E1).

Havel, P.J., Kasim-Karakas, S., Mueller, W., Johnson, P.R., Gingerich, R.L. & Stern, J.S. (1996). Relationship of plasma leptin to plasma insulin and adiposity in normal weight and over-weight women: effects of dietary fat content and sustained fat loss. *Journal of Clinical Endocrinology and Metabolism*, **81**, 4406–13.

Highman, T.J., Friedman, J.E., Huston, L.P., Wong, W.W. & Catalano, P.M. (1998). Longitudinal changes in maternal serum leptin concentrations, body composition, and resting metabolic rate in pregnancy. *American Journal of Obstetrics and Gynecology*, **178**, 1010–15.

Hochberg, Z., Hertz, P., Colin, V., Ish-Shalom, S., Yeshurun, D., Youdim, M.B.H., & Amit, T. (1992). The distal axis of growth hormone (GH) in nutritional disorders: GH-binding protein, insulin-like growth factor-I (IGF-I), and IGF-I receptors in obesity and anorexia nervosa. *Metabolism*, **41**, 106–12.

Hoggard, N., Hunter, L., Duncan, J., S., Williams, L., M., Trayhurn, P. & Mercer, J., G. (1997). Leptin and leptin receptor mRNA and protein expression in murine foetus and placenta. *Proceedings of the National Academy of the Sciences of the United States of America*, **94**, 11073–8.

Hoggard, N., Hunter, L., Trayhurn, P., Williams, N.M. & Mercer, S.W. (1998). Leptin and reproduction. *Proceedings of the Nutrition Society (London)*, **57**, 421–7.

Hollman, M., Runnebaum, B. & Gerhard, I. (1997). Impact of waist-hip-ratio and body mass index on hormonal and metabolic parameters in young, obese women. *International Journal of Obesity*, **21**, 476–83.

Houseknecht, K.L., Mantzoros, C.S., Kuliawat, R., Hadro, E., Flier, J.S. & Kahn, B.B. (1996). Evidence for leptin binding to proteins in serum of rodents and humans: modulation with obesity. *Diabetes*, **45**, 1638–43.

Ilyés, I. & Kirilina, Sz. (1992). Sex hormone binding globulin (SHBG) in children with obesity. *Acta Paediatrica Hungarica*, **32**, 149–57.

Jaquet, D., Leger, J., Levy-Marchal, C., Oury, J.F. & Czemechov, P. (1998). Ontogeny of leptin in human fetuses and newborns: effect of intrauterine retardation on serum leptin concentrations. *Journal of Clinical Endocrinology and Metabolism*, **83**, 1243–6.

Jiang, X., Srinivasan, S.R. & Berenson, G.S. (1996). Relation of obesity to insulin secretion and clearance in adolescents: the Bogalusa Heart Study, *International Journal of Obesity*, **20**, 951–6.

Khaw, K.T. & Barrett-Connor, E. (1992). Lower endogenous androgens predict central adiposity in men. *Annals of Epidemiology*, **2**, 675–82.

Kirschner, M.A., Samojlik, E., Drejka, M., Szmal, E., Schneider G. & Ertel, N. (1990). Androgen-estrogen metabolism in women with upper body versus lower body obesity. *Journal of Clinical*

Endocrinology and Metabolism, **70**, 473–9.

Klein, S., Coppack, S.W., Mohamed-Ali, V. & Landt, M. (1996). Adipose tissue leptin production and plasma leptin kinetics in humans. *Diabetes*, **45**, 984–7.

Kobberling, J. & Von zur Muhlen, A. (1974). The circadian rhythm of free cortisol determined by urine sampling at two-hour intervals in normal subjects and in patients with severe obesity or Cushing's syndrome. *Journal of Clinical Endocrinology and Metabolism*, **38**, 313–19.

Kolaczynski, J.W., Ohannesian, J.P., Considine, R.V., Marco, Ch.C. & Caro, J. (1996). Response of leptin to short-term and prolonged overfeeding in humans. *Journal of Clinical Endocrinology and Metabolism*, **81**, 4162–5.

Kratzsch, J., Dehmel, B., Pulzer, F., Keller, E., Englaro, P., Blum, W.F. & Wabitsch, M. (1997). Increased serum GHBP levels in obese pubertal children and adolescents: relationship to body composition, leptin and indicators of metabolic disturbances. *International Journal of Obesity*, **21**, 1130–6.

Lake, J.K., Power, C. & Cole, T.J. (1997). Women's reproductive health: the role of body mass index in early and adult life. *International Journal of Obesity*, **21**, 432–8.

Lefebvre, A.-M., Laville, M., Vega, N., Riou, J.P., Van Gaal, L., Auwerx, J. & Vidal, H. (1998). Depot-specific differences in adipose tissue gene expression in lean and obese subjects. *Diabetes*, **47**, 98–103.

Leung, D.W., Spencer, S.A., Cachianes, G., Hammond, R.G., Collins, C., Henzel, W.J., Bernard, R., Watars, M.J. & Wood, W.I. (1987). Growth hormone receptor and serum binding protein: purification, cloning and expression. *Nature*, **330**, 537–43.

Lissner, L., Karlsson, C., Lindroos, A.K., Sjostrom, L., Carlsson, B., Carlsson, L. & Bengtsson, C. (1998). Relations between leptin and body weight history in Swedish female population, using serum stored 29 years. *International Journal of Obesity*, **22** (S3), 37.

Llopis, M.A., Granada, M.L., Cuatrecasas, G., Formiguera, X., Sanchez-Planell, L., Sanmarti, A., Alastrue, A., Rull, M., Corominas, A. & Foz, M. (1998). Growth hormone-binding protein directly depends on serum leptin levels in adults with different nutritional status. *Journal of Clinical Endocrinology and Metabolism*, **83**, 2006–11.

Lönnqvist, F. & Schalling, M. (1997). Role of leptin and its receptors in human obesity. *Current Opinion in Endocrinology and Diabetes*, **4**, 164–71.

Lönnqvist, F., Arner, P., Nordfors, L. & Schalling, M. (1995). Overexpression of the obese (*ob*) gene in adipose tissue of human obese subjects. *Nature Medicine*, **1**, 950–3.

Lovejoy, J.C., Bray, G.A., Greeson, C.S., Klemperer, M., Morris, J., Partington, C. & Tulley, R. (1995). Oral anabolic steroid treatment, but not parenteral androgen treatment, decreases abdominal fat in obese, older men. *International Journal of Obesity*, **19**, 614–24.

Malecka-Tendera, E., Koehler, B., Wiciak, B. & Ramos, A. (1994). Impaired glucose tolerance in obese children – a long term prospective study. In *Obesity in Europe 1993*. eds. H. Ditschuneit, F.A. Gries, H. Hauner, V. Schusdziarra & J.G. Wechsler. pp. 153–8. London: John Libbey & Company Ltd.

Mantzoros, C.S., Flier, J.S. & Rogol, A.D. (1997). A longitudinal assessment of hormonal and physical alterations during normal puberty in boys. V. Rising leptin levels may signal the onset of puberty. *Journal of Clinical Endocrinology and Metabolism*, **82**, 1066–70.

Marchini, G., Fried, G., Östlund, E. & Hagenas, L. (1998). Plasma leptin in infants: Relationship to birth weight and weight loss. *Pediatrics*, **101**, 429–32.

Marin, P., Darin, N., Amemiya, T., Andersson, B., Jern, S. & Björntorp, P. (1992a). Cortisol secretion in relation to body fat distribution in obese premenopausal women. *Metabolism*, **41**, 882–6.

Marin, P., Holmang, S., Jonsson, L., Sjostrom, L., Kvist, H., Holm, G., Lindstedt, G. & Björntorp, P. (1992b). The effects of testosterone treatment on body composition and metabolism in middle-aged obese men. *International Journal of Obesity*, **16**, 991–7.

Marin, P., Oden, B. & Björntorp, P. (1995). Assimilation and mobilization of triglycerides in subcutaneous abdominal and femoral adipose tissue in vivo in men: Effects of androgens. *Journal of Clinical Endocrinology and Metabolism*, **80**, 239–43.

Masuzaki, H., Ogawa, Y., Hosoda, K., Miyawaki, T., Hanaoka, I., Hiraoka, J., Yasuno, A., Nishimura, H., Yoshimasa, Y., Nishi, S. & Nakao, K. (1997). Glucocorticoid regulation of leptin synthesis and secretion in humans: elevated plasma leptin levels in Cushing's syndrome. *Journal of Clinical Endocrinology and Metabolism*, **82**, 2542–7.

Matkovic, V., Ilich, J.Z., Skugor, M., Badenhop, E., Goel, P., Clairmont, A., Klisovic, D., Nahhas, R.W. & Landoll, J.D. (1997). Leptin is inversely related to menarche in human females. *Journal of Clinical Endocrinology and Metabolism*, **82**, 3239–45.

Mercado, M., Mollitch, M.E. & Bauman, G. (1992). Low plasma growth hormone binding protein in IDDM. *Diabetes*, **41**, 605–9.

Minuto, F., Barecca, A., Del-Monte, P., Fortini, P., Resetini, M., Morabito, F. & Giordano, G. (1988). Spontaneous growth hormone and somatomedin-C/insulin-like growth factor-I secretion in obese subjects during puberty, *Journal of Endocrinological Investigation*, **11**, 489–95.

Molnár, D. & Soltesz, G. (1982). Metabolic and hormonal effects of fasting in obese children. *Acta Paediatrica Hungarica*, **23**, 45–50..

Molnár, D., Kardos, M. & Soltesz, G. (1981). Effect of glucagon infusion on blood glucose, plasma immunoreactive insulin, growth hormone and adenosine 3'5'-monophosphate in obese children. *Acta Paediatrica Hungarica*, **22**, 325–9.

Molnár, D., Kardos, M., Soltesz, G. & Baranyai, S. (1982). Intravenous glucose tolerance test in childhood obesity: metabolite levels and their relation to glucose utilisation rate. *Acta Paediatrica Hungarica*, **23**, 127–35.

Montague, C.T., Farooqi, S., Whitehead, J.P., Soos, M.A., Rau, H., Wareham, N.J., Sewter, C.P., Digby, J.E., Mohammed, S.N., Hurst, J.A., Cheetham, Ch.H, Earley, A.R., Barnett, A.H., Prins, J.B. & O'Rahilly, S. (1997a). Congenital leptin deficiency is associated with severe early-onset obesity in humans. *Nature*, **387**, 903–8.

Montague, C.T., Prins, J.B., Sanders, L., Digby, J.E., O'Rahilly, S. (1997b). Depot- and sex-specific differences in human leptin mRNA expression. Implications for the control of regional fat distribution. *Diabetes*, **46**, 342–7.

Neel, J.V. (1962). Diabetes mellitus: a 'thrifty' genotype rendered detrimental by 'progress?'. *American Journal of Human Genetics*, **14**, 353–62.

Ostlund, R.E., Yang, J.W., Klein, S. & Gingerich, R. (1996). Relation between plasma leptin concentration and body fat, gender, diet, age and metabolic covariates. *Journal of Clinical Endocrinology and Metabolism*, **81**, 3909–13.

Palmert, M.R., Radovick, S. & Boepple, P. (1998). Leptin levels in children with central precocious puberty. *Journal of Clinical Endocrinology and Metabolism*, **83**, 2260–5.

Pasquali, R., Casimirri, F., Melchionda, N., Fabbri, R., Capelli, M., Plate, L., Patrono, D., Balestra, V. & Barbara, L. (1988). Weight loss and sex steroid metabolism in massively obese men. *Journal of Clinical Investigation*, **11**, 205–10.

Pasquali, R., Cantobelli, S., Casimirri, F., Capelli, M., Bortoluzzi, L., Flamia, R., Labate, A.M. & Barbara, L. (1993). The hypothalamic–pituitary–adrenal axis in obese women with different patterns of body fat distribution [see comments]. *Journal of Clinical Endocrinology and Metabolism*, **77**, 341–6.

Pinhas-Hamiel, O., Dolan, L.M., Daniels, S.R., Standiford, D., Khoury, P.R. & Zeitler, P. (1996). Increased incidence of non-insulin-dependent diabetes mellitus among adolescents. *Journal of Pediatrics*, **128**, 698–715.

Plymate, S.R., Matej, L.A., Jones, R.E. & Friedl, K.E. (1988). Inhibition of sex hormone-binding globulin production in the human hepatoma (Hep G2) cell line by insulin and prolactin. *Journal of Clinical Endocrinology and Metabolism*, **67**, 460–4.

Power, C., Lake, J.K. & Cole, T.J. (1997). Measurement and long-term health risks of child and adolescent fatness. *International Journal of Obesity*, **21**, 507–26.

Prolo, P., Wong, M.-L. & Licinio, J. (1998). Molecules in focus. leptin. *International Journal of Biochemistry and Cell Biology*, **30**, 1285–90.

Rasmussen, M.H., Juul, A., Kjems, L.L., Skakkebaek, N.E. & Hilsted, J. (1995). Lack of stimulation of 24-hour growth hormone release by hypocaloric diet in obesity. *Journal of Clinical Endocrinology and Metabolism*, **80**, 796–801.

Rasmussen, M.H., Ho, K.K.Y., Kjems, L. & Hilsted, J. (1996). Serum growth hormone-binding protein in obesity: effect of a short-term, very low calorie diet and diet induced weight loss. *Journal of Clinical Endocrinology and Metabolism*, **81**, 1519–24.

Ravussin, E., Pratley, R.E., Maffei, M., Wang, H., Friedman, J.M., Bennett, P.H. & Bogardus, C. (1997). Relatively low plasma leptin concentrations precede weight gain in Pima Indians. *Nature Medicine*, **3**, 238–40.

Rayner, D.V., Simón, E., Duncan, J.S., Trayhurn, P. (1998). Hyperleptinaemia in mice induced by administration of the tyrosine hydroxylase inhibitor α-methyl-*p*-tyrosine. *FEBS Letters*, **429**, 395–8.

Roemmich, J.N., Clark, P.A., Mai, V., Berr, S.S., Weltman, A., Veldhuis, J.D. & Rogol, A.D. (1998). Alteration in growth and body composition during puberty: III. Influence of maturation, gender, body composition, fat distribution, aerobic fitness, and energy expenditure on nocturnal growth hormone release. *Journal of Clinical Endocrinology and Metabolism*, **83**, 1440–7.

Ronnemaa, T., Knip, M., Lautala, P., Viikari, J., Uhari, M., Leino, A., Kaprio, E.A., Salo, M.K., Dahl, M., Nuutinen, E.M., Pesonen, E., Pietikainen, M. & Akerblom, H.K. (1991). Serum insulin and other cardiovascular risk indicators in children, adolescents and young adults. *Annals of Medicine*, **23**, 67–72.

Ryan, A.S. & Elahi, D. (1996). The effects of acute hyperglycemia and hyperinsulinemia on plasma leptin levels: its relationships with body fat, visceral adiposity and age in women, *Journal of Clinical Endocrinology and Metabolism*, **81**, 4433–8.

Saad, M.F., Riad-Gabrielm, M.G., Khan, A., Sharma, A., Michael, R., Jinagouda, S.D., Boyad-jian, R. & Steil, G.M. (1998). Diurnal and ultradian rhythmicity of plasma leptin: effects of gender and adiposity. *Journal of Clinical Endocrinology and Metabolism*, **83**, 453–9.

Sakane, N., Yoshida, T., Mizutani, T., Nakagawa, Y. (1998). Serum leptin levels in a patient with pheochromocytoma. *Journal of Clinical Endocrinology and Metabolism*, **83**, 1400.

Schubring, C., Kiess, W., Englaro, P., Rascher, W. & Blum, W. (1996). Leptin concentrations in amniotic fluid, venous and arterial cord blood and maternal serum: high leptin synthesis in the foetus and inverse correlation with placental weight. *European Journal of Pediatrics*, **155**, 830.

Schwartz, M.W., Boyko, E.J., Kahn, S.E., Ravussin, E. & Bogardus, C. (1995). Reduced insulin secretion: an independent predictor of body weight gain. *Journal of Clinical Endocrinology and Metabolism*, **80**, 1571–6.

Scott, C.R., Smith, J.M., Cradock, M.M. & Pihoker, C. (1997). Characteristics of youth-onset noninsulin-dependent diabetes mellitus and insulin-dependent diabetes mellitus at diagnosis. *Pediatrics*, **100**, 84–91.

Slavnov, V.N. & Epstein, E.V. (1977). Somatotrophic, tyrotrophic, and adrenocorticotrophic functions of the anterior pituitary in obesity. *Endocrinologie*, **15**, 213–8.

Slowinska-Srzednicka, J., Zgliczynski, W., Makowska, A., Jeske, W., Brzezinska, A., Soszynski, P. & Zgliczynski, S. (1992). An abnormality of the growth hormone/insulin-like growth factor-I axis in women with polycystic ovary syndrome due to coexistent obesity. *Journal of Clinical Endocrinology and Metabolism*, **74**, 1432–5.

Smith-Kirwin, S.M., O'Conner, D.M., Johnston, J., De Lancey, E., Hassink, S.G. & Funanage, V.L. (1998). Leptin expression in human mammary epithelial cells and breast milk. *Journal of Clinical Endocrinology and Metabolism*, **83**, 1810–3.

Soules, M.R., McLachlan, R.I., Ek, M., Dahl, K.D., Cohen, N.L. & Bremner, W.J. (1989). Luteal phase deficiency: characterization of reproductive hormones over the menstrual cycle. *Journal of Clinical Endocrinology and Metabolism*, **69**, 804–12.

Stephens, T.W. & Caro, J.F. (1998). To be lean or not to be lean. Is leptin the answer? *Experimental and Clinical Endocrinology and Diabetes*, **106**, 1–15.

Streeten, D.H.P., Stevenson, G.T. & Dalakos, T.G. (1969). The diagnosis of hypercortisolism: Biochemical criteria differentiating patients from lean and obese normal subjects and from females on oral contraceptives. *Journal of Clinical Endocrinology and Metabolism*, **29**, 1191–211.

Strobel, A., Issad, T., Camoin, L., Ozata, M. & Strossberg, A., D. (1998). A leptin missense mutation associated with hypogonadism and morbid obesity. *Nature Genetics*, **18**, 213–15.

Sudi, K.M., Gallistl, S., Tafeit, E., Moller, R. & Borkenstein, M.H. (2000). The relationship between different subcutaneous adipose tissue layers, fat mass and leptin in obese children and adolescents. *Journal of Pediatric Endocrinology and Metabolism*, **13**, 505–12.

Tamás, P., Sulyok, E., Ertl, T., Szabó, I., Vizer, M., Rascher, W. & Blum, W.F. (1999). Changes of maternal serum leptin levels during pregnancy. *Gynecological and Obstetrical Investigations*, **46**, 169–71.

Thomas, T.L., Devenport, L.D. & Stith, R.D. (1994). Relative contribution of type I and II corticosterone receptors in VMH lesion-induced obesity and hyperinsulinemia. *American*

Journal of Physiology, **266**, R1623–29.

Travers, S.H., Jeffers, B.W., Bloch, C.A., Hill, J.O. & Eckel, H. (1995). Gender and Tanner stage differences in body composition and insulin sensitivity in early pubertal children. *Journal of Clinical Endocrinology and Metabolism*, **80**, 172–8.

Trayhurn, P., Hoggard, N., Mercer, J.G. & Rayner D.V. (1999). Leptin: fundamental aspects. *International Journal of Obesity*, **23** (Suppl. 1), 22–8.

Van Gaal, L.F., Wauters, M.A., Mertens, I.L., Considine, R.V. & De Leeuw, I.H. (1999). Clinical endocrinology of human leptin. *International Journal of Obesity*, **23** (Suppl 1), 29–36.

Vanhala, M., Vanhala, P., Kompusalo, E., Halonen, P. & Takala, J. (1998). Relation between obesity from childhood and the metabolic syndrome: population based study. *British Medical Journal*, **317**, 319–20.

Veldhuis, J.D., Iranmanesh, A., Ho, K.K.Y., Waters, M.J., Johnson, M.L. & Lizarralde, G. (1991). Dual defects in pulsatile growth hormone secretion and clearance subserve the hyposomatotropism of obesity in man. *Journal of Clinical Endocrinology and Metabolism*, **72**, 51–9.

Vignolo, A., Naseli, A., Di Battista, E., Mostart, M. & Aicardi, G. (1988). Growth and development in simple obesity. *The European Journal of Pediatrics*, **147**, 242–4.

Wabitsch, M., Hauner, H., Heinze, E. & Teller, W. (1995a). The role of hormone/insulin-like growth factors in adipocyte differentiation, *Metabolism*, **44**, 45–9.

Wabitsch, M., Hauner, H., Heinze, E., Bockman, A., Benz, R., Mayer, H. & Teller, W. (1995b). Body fat distribution and steroid hormone concentrations in obese adolescent girls before and after weight reduction. *Journal of Clinical Endocrinology and Metabolism*, **80**, 3469–75.

Wabitsch, M., Blum, W., Heinze, E., Mayer, H. & Teller, W. (1996a). Serum concentrations of leptin in obese children and adolescents before and after weight loss. *Hormone Research*, **46** (S2), 2.

Wabitsch, M., Blum, W.F., Muche, R., Heinze, E., Haug, C., Mayer, H. & Teller, W. (1996b). Insulin-like growth factors and their binding proteins before and after weight loss and their associations with hormonal and metabolic parameters in obese adolescent girls. *International Journal of Obesity*, **20**, 1073–80.

Wabitsch, M., Jensen, P.B., Blum, W., Christoffersen, C.T., Englaro, P., Heinze, E., Rascher, W., Teller, W., Tornqvist, H. & Hauner, H. (1996c). Insulin and cortisol promote leptin production in cultured human fat cells. *Diabetes*, **45**, 1435–8.

Wabitsch, M., Blum, W.F., Muche, R., Braun, M., Hube, F., Rascher, W., Heinze, E., Teller, W., & Hauner, H. (1997). Contribution of androgens to the gender difference in leptin production in obese children and adolescents. *Journal of Clinical Investigation*, **100**, 808–13.

Wadden, T.A., Mason, G., Foster, G.D., Stunkard, A.J. & Prange, A.J. (1990). Effects of a very low calorie diet on weight, thyroid hormones and mood. *International Journal of Obesity*, **14**, 249–58.

Weigle, D.S., Ganter, S.L., Kuijper, J.L., Leonetti, D.L., Boyko, E.J. & Fujimoto, W.Y. (1997). Effect of regional fat distribution and Prader–Willi syndrome on plasma leptin levels. *Journal of Clinical Endocrinology and Metabolism*, **82**, 566–70.

Whitaker, R.C., Wright, J.A., Pepe, M.S., Seidel, K.D. & Dietz, W.H. (1997). Predicting obesity in young adulthood from childhood and parental obesity. *New England Journal of Medicine*, **337**, 869–73.

Wilson, D.M., Killen, J.D., Hammer, L.D., Litt, I.F., Vosti, C., Miner, B., Hayward, C. & Taylor, C.B. (1991). Insulin-like growth factor-I as a reflection of body composition, nutrition, and puberty in sixth and seventh grade girls. *Journal of Clinical Endocrinology and Metabolism*, **73**, 907–12.

Yang, M.U. & Van Itallie, T.B. (1984). Variability in body protein loss during protracted, severe caloric restriction: role of triiodothyronine and other possible determinants. *American Journal of Clinical Nutrition*, **40**, 611–22.

York, D. A. & Bray, G. A. (1972). Dependence of hypothalamic obesity on insulin, the pituitary and adrenal gland. *Endocrinology*, **90**, 425–32.

Zannolli, R., Rebeggiani, A., Chiarelli, F. & Morgese, G. (1993). Hyperinsulinism as a marker in obese children. *American Journal of Diseases of Children*, **147**, 837–41.

Zhang, Y., Proenca, R., Maffei, M., Barone, M., Leopold, L. & Friedman, J.M. (1994). Positional cloning of the mouse obese gene and its human homologue. *Nature*, **372**, 425–32.

Zimmet, P.Z., Collins, V.R., de Courten, M.P., Hodge, A.M., Collier, G.R., Dowse, G.K., Alberti, K.G., Tuomilehto, J., Hemraj, F., Gareeboo, H., Chitson, P.& Fareed, D. (1998). Is there a relationship between leptin and insulin sensitivity independent of obesity? A population-based study in the Indian Ocean nation of Mauritius. *International Journal of Obesity*, **22**, 171–7.

Zumoff, B. & Strain, G.W. (1994). A perspective on the hormonal abnormalities of obesity: are they cause or effect? *Obesity Research*, **2**, 56–67.

Risk of cardiovascular complications

David S. Freedman,[1] Sathanur R. Srinivasan[2]
and Gerald S. Berenson[2]

[1]Centers for Disease Control and Prevention, Atlanta. [2]Tulane Center for Cardiovascular Health, Tulane University School of Public Health, New Orleans

11.1 Introduction

The prevalence of obesity among children and adults has increased over the last few decades (Kuczmarski et al., 1994; Troiano et al., 1995; Freedman et al., 1997), and the obese are at increased risk of diabetes, coronary heart disease, hypertension and certain cancers (Kushner, 1993; Hodge & Simmet, 1994; Baumgartner et al., 1995). Because substantial weight loss is difficult to maintain (Dyer, 1994), several studies have focused on the development of overweight and its consequences.

As with adults, numerous studies have found that obese children tend to have adverse levels of lipids, blood pressure, insulin and other risk factors for coronary heart disease (CHD) (Berenson et al., 1993). Furthermore, obesity in early life is associated with the early stages of atherosclerosis, including fatty streaks and raised lesions (Berenson et al., 1998), and coronary calcification (Mahoney et al., 1996). It is also likely that obesity in early life influences the subsequent risk for various diseases in adulthood, and there is some evidence that this association exists independent of adult weight (Must et al., 1992). The secular trend in overweight among youths (Troiano et al., 1995; Freedman et al., 1997) suggests a possible increase in the incidence of CHD and other diseases (Pinhas-Hamiel et al., 1996) among adults.

The current chapter reviews the associations between obesity and CHD risk factors in early life, and the evidence suggesting that child-onset obesity influences subsequent clinical disease. Many of the data presented are from the Bogalusa Heart Study, a long-term study of the early natural history of cardiovascular disease (Berenson, 1986; Freedman et al., 1997; Berenson et al., 1998; Freedman et al., 1999a). Seven cross-sectional studies of children and young adults in this biracial community of approximately 20 000 were conducted between 1973 and 1994.

11.1.1 Classification of overweight

Many issues concerning the measurement of body fat have been addressed in Chapter 1, and will be only briefly discussed here. Overweight among youth has typically been assessed through various power indices, in which weight (W) is divided by height (H) raised to a power (p). The exponent is frequently chosen to maximize the correlation with body fat and to minimize the correlation with height, and several values of p have been proposed that range from 1.5 to 3 (Keys et al., 1972; Cole, 1991). The optimal exponent among adults is near 2 among men, and between 1 and 2 among women. The Quetelet index (W/H^2) is now widely used in clinical and epidemiological studies, and in reference standards. Although W/H^2 is also referred to as BMI or body mass index, it was a 19th-century Belgian mathematician – Adolphe Quetelet – who noted that the weight of adults was proportional to height^2 (Garrow & Webster, 1985).

Although the Quetelet index is also widely used as a measure of relative weight among children, it is moderately correlated ($r = 0.5$–0.6) with height and age. The median value of this index, for example, increases by about 25% between the ages of 5 and 17 years (Najjar & Rowland, 1987; Freedman et al., 1997). It is therefore important to adjust Quetelet index for age, as a girl with a Quetelet index of 17.6 kg/m^2 could be either an overweight (90th centile) 5-year-old, an average 10-year-old, or a thin (10th centile) 15-year-old (Najjar & Rowland, 1987). Comparing the Quetelet indices of similarly aged children of differing heights may also be problematic: taller children will tend to have higher levels of this index.

Because levels of many risk factors increase with age, these intercorrelations may confound the observed associations with Quetelet index. We have found, for example, that age adjustment reduces the correlation between Quetelet index and diastolic blood pressure (DBP) from 0.47 to 0.25. Although other indices, such as W/H^3, have been used as measures of relative weight among children (Berenson, 1986; Resnicow & Morabia, 1990; Freedman et al., 1997), they have not gained widespread acceptance.

Because of the difficulties in using biological endpoints to define overweight/obesity (see Chapter 1), recent recommendations have used the sex- and age-specific 85th centile and 95th centile of body mass index from various studies (Himes & Dietz, 1994) (Table 11.1). It has been suggested that children above the 95th centile be considered overweight[1] and referred for further assessment, while those between the 85th centile and 95th centile would be considered 'at risk for overweight' and would be examined for various risk factors (Himes & Dietz, 1994). A simple approximation to the 95th centile among 10- to 17-year-olds can be obtained by adding 13 (for boys) or 14 (for girls) to years of age.

---

[1] Editors' note: usage in this chapter differs from elsewhere in the book, where a body mass index over the 95th centile is described as obesity, and over the 85th centile is overweight.

Table 11.1. Recommended cut-points for overweight based on levels of body mass index (kg/m²) among children and adolescents (Must et al., 1992)

Age (years)	Centiles				
	Boys		Girls	
	85th	95th	85th	95th
6	16.6	18.0	16.2	17.5
7	17.4	19.2	17.2	18.9
8	18.1	20.3	18.2	20.4
9	18.8	21.5	19.2	21.8
10	19.6	22.6	20.2	23.2
11	20.4	23.7	21.2	24.6
12	21.1	24.9	22.2	26.0
13	21.9	25.9	23.1	27.1
14	22.8	26.9	23.9	28.0
15	23.6	27.8	24.3	28.5
16	24.4	28.5	24.7	29.1
17	25.3	29.3	25.2	29.7

11.2 Secular trends

There has been a substantial increase in the prevalence of overweight among schoolchildren in the US (Troiano et al., 1995), with the proportion of children above the 95th centile increasing two-fold between 1963 and 1991. Furthermore, it appears that most of the increase has occurred since 1980. The secular increase in overweight among adults also appears to have accelerated since the 1980s (Kuczmarski et al., 1994).

These secular trends were further examined in the Bogalusa Heart Study, where levels of several anthropometric variables increased substantially from 1973 to 1994 (Freedman et al., 1997). Among 5- to 14-year-olds during this approximately 20-year period, mean levels of weight ($+3.4$ kg), body mass index ($+1.5$ kg/m²) and skinfold thickness ($+2.2$ mm) all increased; furthermore, adjustment for differences in height, age and other covariates had little influence on the results. Several of the estimates, however, varied across subgroups, with the largest proportional increase in weight (9% of the initial value) seen among 19- to 24-year-olds. Increases in weight and skinfolds tended to be larger during the latter part of the period, but there was little difference across race–sex groups.

The increase in relative weight was particularly striking at the upper end of the weight distribution, as indicated by a comparison of various centiles of the Rohrer

Table 11.2. Prevalence (%) of overweight in the Bogalusa Heart Study based on centiles from the 1973–74 Examinations

	Age group (years)							
	5–14				15–17			
			Skinfolds				Skinfolds	
Year	n	BMI	Triceps	Subscap	n	BMI	Triceps	Subscap
1973–74	3508	15 (5)[a]	15 (5)	—	—	—	—	—
1976–77	3073	20 (7)	27 (11)	—	992	15 (5)	15 (5)	—
1978–79	2908	21 (8)	34 (16)	15 (5)	671	15 (5)	19 (7)	15 (5)
1981–83	2749	22 (9)	37 (19)	20 (8)	554	19 (6)	19 (9)	20 (7)
1983–86	2604	23 (10)	25 (11)	22 (9)	662	23 (10)	20 (9)	33 (14)
1987–91	2688	27 (12)	27 (12)	24 (9)	548	30 (12)	22 (10)	38 (15)
1992–94	2582	32 (11)	37 (22)	31 (17)	534	30 (15)	28 (16)	37 (21)

[a]Values represent percentage of participants above the 85th (95th) centile.
BMI: body mass index.

index (W/H^3). Whereas the median increased by 0.8 kg/m^3 (from 12.3 kg/m^3 to 13.1 kg/m^3) over the study period, the 90th centile increased by 2.4 kg/m^3. Among the 5- to 14-year-olds, 31–37% of those examined in 1992–94 would have been considered overweight or obese based on the 85th centile from 1973–74; corresponding percentages based on the 95th centile ranged from 11% (body mass index) to 22% (triceps skinfold thickness) (Table 11.2). More than four times the expected number of children in 1992 was above the 95th centile of triceps skinfold thickness based on the 1973 levels.

The secular trends in overweight among youths suggest a possible increase in the incidence of CHD and other diseases among adults in the future. For example, it has been reported that the incidence of non-insulin-dependent diabetes among adolescents increased ten-fold between 1982 and 1994 (Pinhas-Hamiel et al., 1996). As the mean body mass index of these newly diagnosed patients was approximately 37 kg/m^2, the observed increases may be related to the substantial increase in the proportion of overweight youths.

11.3 Associations with risk factors

Overweight children and adolescents have adverse levels of lipids, insulin and blood pressure (Laskarzewski et al., 1980; Williams et al., 1992; Berenson et al., 1993; Raitakari et al., 1994; Dwyer & Blizzard, 1996). Furthermore, longitudinal changes in relative weight are associated with changes in these characteristics

Table 11.3. Relation of body mass index to adverse risk factors in 3599
5 to 10-year-olds

	BMI centiles[a]							Correlation with BMI[b]
	< 25	25–49	50–74	75–84	85–94	95–97	> 97	
n	904	817	798	340	384	100	256	
Age (years)	8.2	8.1	8.2	8.5	8.5	9.0	8.7	
TC > 200 mg/dl (%)	9[c]	10	10	13	18	17	23	0.10
TG > 130 mg/dl (%)	2	3	3	6	10	10	21	0.27
LDLC > 130 mg/dl (%)	8	8	9	10	18	12	23	0.12
HDLC < 35 mg/dl (%)	5	5	6	4	8	7	18	−0.14
Insulin > 95th centile	2	2	3	3	4	10	27	0.46
SBP > 95th centile	2	2	4	6	7	12	22	0.34
DBP > 95th centile	2	2	4	9	7	9	14	0.29

[a] Sex- and age-specific centiles based on US national data.

[b] All correlations are significant, $P < 0.001$.

[c] Values represent percentage of subjects with adverse risk factor levels within each body mass index category.

TC: total cholesterol; TG: triglycerides; LDLC: low-density-lipoprotein cholesterol; HDLC: high-density-lipoprotein cholesterol; SBP: systolic blood pressure; DBP: diastolic blood pressure; BMI: body mass index.

(Freedman et al., 1985), and the tracking of multiple risk factors increases with relative weight (Bo et al., 1994). In general, various measures of overweight and obesity have been found to be related weakly to levels of total cholesterol and low-density-lipoprotein (LDL) cholesterol ($r \sim 0.05$–0.15), but more strongly to levels of high-density-lipoprotein (HDL) cholesterol, blood pressure and insulin (Lauer et al., 1975; Laskarzewski et al., 1980; Raitakari et al., 1994; Chu et al., 1998; Freedman et al., 1999b).

Some of these results, however, are difficult to interpret. For example, the nonlinearity of the associations has not always been examined and it is possible that associations may not have been adequately represented in linear or correlation analyses. For example, Resnicow & Morabia (1990) found that total cholesterol levels among schoolchildren appeared to increase exponentially above the 50th centile of relative weight but little association was seen at lower centiles. There is also little information on either (a) the probability that an overweight child will have adverse risk-factor levels (predictive value), or (b) the proportion of children with adverse risk factors that can be detected by examining overweight children (sensitivity).

A recent analysis of data in the Bogalusa Heart Study (Freedman et al., 1999b) also found that the relation of body mass index to adverse risk factor levels tended to be nonlinear. In general, most risk factors varied only slightly below the 75th or 85th centile of body mass index, and particularly among the 5- to 10-year-olds (Table 11.3). The prevalence of a high LDL-cholesterol level, for example, increased from 8% to only 10% between the thinnest (below the 25th centile) children and those with a body mass index between the 75th and 85th centiles. In contrast, the prevalence of various risk factors increased substantially above the 85th centile, and even among overweight (above the 95th centile) schoolchildren, body mass index remained associated with risk factor levels. The secular increase in the proportion of children at the upper end of the relative weight distribution may therefore be particularly relevant. Of the examined risk factors, insulin levels showed the strongest association with body mass index, the prevalence of high levels increasing from 2% to 27%.

Associations with total cholesterol (*a*) and insulin (*b*) are shown in Fig. 11.1 for 5- to 10-year-old white girls. Rohrer index (kg/m^3) was used as a measure of relative weight because it is less strongly correlated with age than is body mass index – in this sample the observed correlation coefficients with age were -0.13 (Rohrer) vs. 0.31 (body mass). Lines were fitted using lowess, a robust method that relies only on the data to determine the functional form of the relationship (Cleveland, 1985). These figures illustrate the large variability in the relation of relative weight to different CHD risk factors. Whereas the association with total cholesterol (TC) largely resembles a 'data cloud', the fitted line is fairly linear with TC levels increasing by about 20 mg/dl over the relative weight range. In contrast, the association with insulin levels is markedly nonlinear, with an inflection point at approximately 15 kg/m^3 (the 80th centile of Rohrer index). These data indicate the difficulties involved in classifying overweight based on associations with risk factors.

The relation of overweight to adverse risk factor levels among schoolchildren is shown in Table 11.4. The sensitivity (23–62%) and positive predictive value (9–24%) of overweight was generally low. For example, only 24% of the 747 children with an elevated TC level were also overweight; furthermore, only 18% of the overweight children had an elevated TC level. Many of the odds ratios (ORs), however, were substantial. As compared with other children, for example, an overweight child was 7.1 times as likely to have a high triglyceride level. The largest ORs were seen with insulin, and 62% of the 273 persons with an insulin level over the 95th centile were also overweight. The magnitudes of the ORs with Rohrer index were comparable to those observed for body mass index, but associations with triceps skinfold thickness were weaker. We also found that the triceps skinfold thickness provided very little additional information on risk factor levels

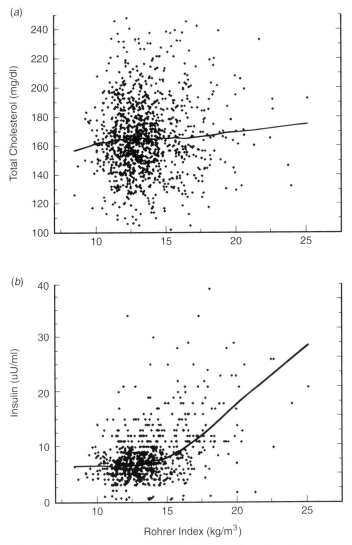

Figure 11.1 Relation of relative weight to total cholesterol (*a*) and insulin (*b*) among 5- to 10-year-old white girls (*n* = 1132 and *n* = 802 respectively), with fitted curves constructed using lowess (Cleveland, 1985).

if weight and height were known. This supports other evidence (Spataro et al., 1996) that weight–height indices predict adverse health outcome as well as the triceps skinfold thickness.

Although overweight does not accurately identify children with adverse levels of individual risk factors, it is better at screening for multiple risk factors (Table 11.5). Among the 5- to 10-year-olds, for example, overweight children represented 7% (sensitivity) of the 1670 children with no risk factors, but 80% [(24 + 8)/

Table 11.4. Associations between overweight (body mass index > 95th centile) and adverse risk factor levels

| Risk factor | n^c | Screening[a] for BMI > 95th centile | | Odds Ratios[b] (BMI > 95th centile vs. < 85th centile) | | |
		Sensitivity (%)	Positive predictive value (%)	Body mass index	Rohrer index	Triceps skinfold
TC > 200 mg/dl	747	24	18	2.4	2.5	2.3
TG > 130 mg/dl	502	47	24	7.1	6.2	5.1
LDLC > 130 mg/dl	653	28	18	3.0	2.9	2.5
HDLC < 35 mg/dl	702	25	17	3.4	3.1	2.6
Insulin > 95th centile	273	62	21	12.6	11.7	8.6
SBP > 95th centile	371	34	13	4.5	4.5	3.4
DBP > 95th centile	395	23	9	2.4	2.9	2.6

[a] Sensitivity is the proportion of children with risk factor who are also overweight. Positive predictive value is the proportion of overweight children who have adverse risk factor level.
[b] ORs are based on the cross-tabulation of overweight and specified risk factors. An OR of 2.4 for TC indicates that the percentage of overweight children with high TC levels is 2.4 times higher than the corresponding percentage of nonoverweight children.
[c] Number of children with risk factor. Of the 9167 children, 1147 were excluded with a Body Mass index between the 85th and 94th centile.
Abbreviations as Table 11.3.

$(32 + 8)]$ of those with three or more risk factors. Compared to nonoverweight children, overweight children were 9.7 times more likely to have two risk factors and over 40 times more likely to have three risk factors. Of the 302 overweight 5- to 10-year-olds, 183 (61%) had at least one risk factor, and the corresponding positive predictive value among 11- to 17-year-olds was 58% (295/511). Of the 80 children with high levels of both insulin and triglycerides, 90% were also overweight.

These findings agree well with other analyses that have examined risk factor clustering. Up to six times as many children and adolescents as expected have high levels of both relative weight and various risk factors (Srinivasan et al., 1996). Furthermore, 55% of overweight girls and 70% of overweight boys have at least one risk factor (Chu et al., 1998). Because of the large increase in fibrous plaques in the coronary arteries of children and young adults who have multiple CHD risk factors (Berenson et al., 1998), the use of overweight as a screening tool may be particularly effective in the early identification of high-risk subjects.

Table 11.5. Relation of overweight to clustering of adverse risk factor levels

Age-Group (years)	Number of risk factors[a]	n	n (%) who are overweight[b]	Female (%)	Black (%)	Adjusted OR
5–10	0	1670	119 (7%)	48	36	1.0 (ref.)
	1	464	103 (22%)	49	39	3.8
	2	118	48 (41%)	53	25	9.7
	3	32	24 (75%)	62	25	43.5
	4 +	8	8 (100%)	50	12	—
	Overall	2292	302			
11–17	0	2214	216 (10%)	48	37	1.0 (ref.)
	1	677	155 (23%)	51	37	2.8
	2	223	90 (40%)	51	24	6.5
	3	58	40 (69%)	48	21	22.6
	4 +	13	10 (77%)	62	8	29.8
	Overall	3185	511			

[a] Number of risk factors is the sum of TG > 130 mg/dl, LDLC > 130 mg/dl, HDLC < 35 mg/dl, insulin > 95th centile, and either SBP > 95th centile or DBP > 95th centile. All analyses are for 5477 schoolchildren examined in the last four examinations.

[b] Values in parentheses represent percentage of subjects in risk factor category who are overweight. Abbreviations as in Table 11.3 and OR: odds ratio.

11.3.1 Overweight and lipid testing

Lipid guidelines for children in the US, which use the presence of parental coronary disease or hypercholesterolaemia as an initial screening tool, would result in a quarter of all children undergoing lipid testing, 80% of them because of parental TC levels (National Cholesterol Education Program, 1991). Overall, the guidelines would identify 40% of all children and adolescents with an LDL-cholesterol level greater than or equal to 130 mg/dl. The use of a parental TC level of 300 mg/dl or more would achieve a sensitivity of 28% by screening 14% of all children, similar to using overweight (above the 95th centile) as an initial screening tool. Screening children with a relative weight above the 85th centile would yield a sensitivity of 43%, similar to that for the current lipid guidelines.

The current lipid guidelines in the US rely on *recorded* parental TC levels, which may often not be available. It has been found that a reported parental TC level of 240 mg/dl would result in 6% of children undergoing lipid screening, with very low values for sensitivity (6%) and positive predictive value (14%) (Resnicow & Cross, 1993).

Compared to the current recommendations concerning the use of parental TC levels, it is likely that overweight (a) would be simpler to use as a screening trigger, and (b) would more accurately identify adverse levels of LDL cholesterol and other risk factors. Because several risk factors are more strongly associated with relative weight than are levels of LDL cholesterol, this approach would probably identify youths with multiple risk factors.

11.4 Body fat patterning

Systematic methods to categorize human body shape were first introduced in the 1930s and the relation of fat patterning to various chronic diseases was recognized by Vague and others in the 1950s (Vague, 1956). Cohort studies have since shown that a preponderance of adult body fat in the abdomen, upper body or trunk is predictive of diabetes mellitus and CHD (Ducimetiere et al., 1986; Seidell, 1992), and is associated with adverse levels of lipoproteins, blood pressure, insulin and other metabolic risk factors (Björntorp, 1990; Haffner et al., 1987). Although associations are often assumed to be independent of the general level of obesity, there is a correlation ($r \sim 0.2$–0.5) (Ducimetiere et al., 1986; Haffner et al., 1987; Freedman et al., 1999a) between relative weight and various fat patterns. The role of intra-abdominal fat in these metabolic and clinical outcomes has been emphasized (Björntorp, 1990), but other fat depots may also be important. For example, there appear to be increased risks associated with chest circumference (Freedman et al., 1989) and subcutaneous adipose tissue (Abate et al., 1996).

The importance of fat distribution among children is less certain. Although associations with various risk factors have been reported (Zwiauer et al., 1992; Brambilla et al., 1994), negative results have also appeared (Mueller & Wohlleb, 1981; Caprio et al., 1996). The contradictory findings are hard to interpret because of differences in the risk factors examined, the age ranges studied, the circumferences or skinfolds measured and the statistical techniques used. The study of fat patterning in early life is made more difficult because (a) there is only a small amount of intra-abdominal fat present before adulthood (Goran et al., 1995), (b) there are marked changes in circumferences and skinfold thicknesses during growth and development (Malina & Bouchard, 1988; Weststrate et al., 1989; Freedman et al., 1999a), and (c) the anthropometric indices typically used in adult studies may not be appropriate in childhood (Sangi & Mueller, 1991).

A recent study (Freedman et al., 1999a) examined the relation of skinfolds (subscapular and triceps) and circumferences (waist and hips) to various risk factors among 5- to 17-year-olds ($n = 2996$). As expected, most anthropometric dimensions were highly intercorrelated, emphasizing the need to adjust for the overall level of relative weight. Both weight–height indices were strongly related to the circumferences ($r \sim 0.9$) and skinfolds ($r \sim 0.8$), and the circumferences and skinfolds were also strongly intercorrelated. In contrast, only a moderate associ-

Table 11.6. Relation of waist, hip and skinfold thickness measures to levels of lipids and insulin

		LDL cholesterol (mmol/l)	Triglycerides (mmol/l)	HDL cholesterol (mmol/l)	Insulin (pmol/l)
Individual measures	Waist	$+0.12^a$	$+0.09$	-0.07	$+7$
	Hip	—	-0.04	$+0.04$	-5
	Subscapular skinfold	$+0.13^b$	$+0.08$	—	—
	Triceps skinfold	—	—	—	—
	F-statistic	(28)	(27)	(22)	(21)
Ratios	Waist/hip	$+0.12$	$+0.08$	-0.08	$+7$
	Subscapular/triceps	—	$+0.07$	-0.05	—
	F-statistic	(19)	(24)	(31)	(31)
Principal components	Generalized obesity	$+0.19$	$+0.08$	—	—
	Central fat patterning^c	$+0.08$	$+0.08$	-0.09	$+6$
	F-Statistic	(28)	(36)	(46)	(31)

[a] Values represent the predicted change in lipid or insulin level associated with a change for each anthropometric dimension between the 10th and 90th centiles, based on stepwise regression and adjusted for race, sex, age, height and weight. Dashes indicate that the variable was not significant, $P > 0.01$.

[b] F-statistic tests that all added anthropometric characteristics have zero coefficients. An F-statistic of ~7 is significant, $P < 0.001$.

[c] The second principal component was a linear contrast of the waist circumference with the hip circumference and triceps skinfold thickness.

LDL: low-density-lipoprotein; HDL: high-density-lipoprotein.

ation was seen between the ratio of waist to hip circumference (WHR) and the ratio of subscapular to triceps skinfold ($r \sim 0.35$), suggesting that each might capture a different aspect of fat distribution (Haffner et al., 1987).

Given the strong intercorrelations, it is not surprising that each characteristic showed fairly similar associations with levels of lipids and insulin. Compared to a child at the 10th centile, for example, the excess LDL-cholesterol level for a child at the 90th centile varied from $+0.30$ mmol/l (weight and hip circumference) to $+0.34$ mmol/l (subscapular skinfold). Predicted differences (90th centile vs. 10th centile) in levels of other risk factors also varied only slightly across the anthropometric characteristics, with insulin levels showing the strongest associations.

Forward stepwise regression was used to identify the circumferences and skinfolds that best predicted the presence of risk factors, after adjusting for weight, height, age, sex and race (Table 11.6). Waist circumference was consistently significant, along with hip circumference (for triglycerides, HDL-cholesterol and insulin) and subscapular skinfold (for LDL-cholesterol and triglycerides). Hip circumference was only significant when waist circumference was present, and triceps skinfold thickness provided no additional information.

Similar analyses were conducted for the ratios and principal components. Ratios were included because they are widely used in studies of body fat distribution, but they have several limitations (Kronmal, 1993). For example, the use of WHR is analogous to modelling an interaction between waist and hip^{-1} in a regression model without including the main effects; and even if the interaction is not present, the importance of each variable cannot be assessed. As an alternative to ratios, principal component analysis has been advocated (Mueller & Wohlleb, 1981; Harrison, 1985). This statistical technique replaces a set of correlated variables (skinfolds and circumferences) with several uncorrelated components:

$$PC_i = \beta_1 l_1 + \beta_2 l_2 + \cdots + \beta_n l_n$$

where PC_i is the ith principal component and the l_is are the skinfolds and circumferences. Regression coefficients β_i are chosen to (a) yield components that are uncorrelated with each other, and (b) maximize the variance of each component. In studies of fat patterning, the first component typically represents the general level of fatness, while the second component generally contrasts adipose tissue at truncal and peripheral sites (Mueller & Wohlleb, 1981). A major advantage of principal component analysis is that the relation of risk factors to the second principal component, which is independent of the first component, can be examined without fear of confounding by the overall level of obesity. In these analyses, the first principal component was positively correlated ($r \sim 0.5$–0.9) with all anthropometric dimensions, while the second was related positively to the waist circumference ($r \sim 0.8$) and negatively ($r \sim -0.35$) to the hip circumference and the triceps skinfold thickness (i.e. a central fat pattern).

The relations of risk factors to the two ratios and two principal components are also shown in Table 11.6. The principal components were, in general, more strongly related to risk factor levels than were the two ratios. The second principal component was associated with adverse levels of all risk factors.

An illustration of the additional information supplied by the waist circumference in predicting risk factor levels is shown in Fig. 11.2. The nine panels summarize the relation of waist circumference to levels of HDL-cholesterol among 675 black girls within categories of Rohrer index. Despite some inconsistencies, an increase in waist circumference from 60 cm to 80 cm was typically associated with a 0.15–0.25 mmol/l decrease in HDL-cholesterol.

These results indicate that a relative excess of adipose tissue in the abdominal or central region is associated with adverse levels of lipids and insulin. The associ-

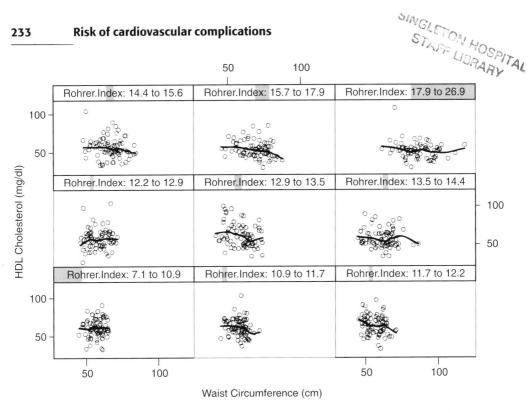

Figure 11.2 Relation of waist circumference to HDL-cholesterol among black females. Each of the nine panels shows this relation, summarized using lowess curves, for a given range of the Rohrer index (kg/m³); each subject is represented by an open circle. Rohrer index increases from left to right, and from bottom to top; the shaded part of the label indicates the position of the specified stratum relative to the overall range.

ations were independent of weight, height, age and other covariates, and were similar in magnitude regardless of whether fat distribution was quantified using waist circumference, WHR or a principal component contrasting waist circumference with the sum of hip circumference and triceps skinfold thickness. Of the individual anthropometric dimensions, waist circumference showed the most consistent, and generally the strongest, associations with adverse risk factor levels.

These findings may reflect the ability of waist circumference to act as an index of both fat distribution and generalized obesity, as well as its relation to other characteristics associated with lipid levels. Waist circumference, for example, is related to both age and body mass index, and mean levels differ substantially between boys and girls. Because the waist circumference is also relatively easy to measure, it may be particularly appropriate for epidemiological and intervention studies, and may help to identify children who have adverse risk factor levels.

11.5 Longitudinal analyses

11.5.1 Tracking of overweight and obesity

Although childhood levels of obesity and overweight are predictive of later levels, a wide range of correlation coefficients ($r = 0$–0.84) has been reported between serial measurements over periods of up to 45 years (Clarke & Lauer, 1993; Serdula et al., 1993; Power et al., 1997). Estimates of the proportion of overweight children who remain overweight as adults are also varied (26–77%), as are the increased risks (1.5–7) for overweight in later life (Johnston, 1985; Dietz, 1998). In general, the estimates depend on the initial age at which measurements are made, and are stronger (a) for weight–height indices than for skinfolds, (b) for shorter time intervals, and (c) if at least one parent is overweight (Whitaker et al., 1997).

Many of these trends are illustrated in an analysis of data from the Fels Longitudinal Study (Siervogel et al., 1991). Although body mass index among 35-year-olds could be predicted fairly well at age 18 ($r \sim 0.60$–0.75), correlations from age 7 years were only 0.3 (boys) and 0.5 (girls). Furthermore, the probability of overweight in adulthood increased with the age at first measurement. For example, a 17-year-old girl with a body mass index at the 85th centile had a 40–80% chance of being overweight at age 35 years, but more extreme overweight (95th centile) at age 8 years was associated with a less than 30% chance of being overweight at follow-up.

11.5.2 Relation of childhood overweight to subsequent disease

Childhood relative weight could act directly to influence the risk of adult disease, or any association could be indirect. For example, a relation could be mediated by the tracking of obesity from childhood through adulthood, with any complications mediated through adult obesity. The scarcity of longitudinal data from early life through adulthood complicates the assessment of these associations. Much of the relevant information has been previously reviewed (Must, 1996; Power et al., 1997).

Several cohort studies have focused on adolescent males. For example, overweight 18-year-old men with a BMI above 31 kg/m^2 (Sørensen & Sonne-Holm, 1977) or above 25 kg/m^2 (Hoffmans et al., 1988) had excess all-cause mortality. Waaler (1984), in a study of the entire population of Norway, found that 15- to 19-year-old males with a BMI above 27 kg/m^2 had an increased overall mortality rate during 10 years of follow-up; no association, however, was seen among women. CHD mortality was also increased among male college alumni over the 75th centile of relative weight, particularly those dying before age 45 years (Paffenbarger & Wing, 1969). An increase in all-cause mortality has also been reported among women who were relatively heavy (over the 80th centile) during adolescence (Nieto et al., 1992).

A large, long-term (55 years) follow-up of men in the Harvard Growth Study indicated that overweight male adolescents (over the 75th centile) had an increase in both total and CHD mortality (Must et al., 1992). The risk associated with overweight in adolescence was stronger than for adult overweight; furthermore, overweight in adolescence remained statistically significant even after accounting for weight at age 50 years. In contrast, women did not show an increased risk associated with adolescent overweight, though, given the relatively small numbers, this sex difference is uncertain. While there appears to be a long-term risk associated with overweight, additional studies are needed to confirm the associations among women, to assess the role of puberty in these associations, and to examine the role of adult weight in mediating any association.

11.6 Conclusions

There are numerous studies that document cross-sectional associations between childhood obesity and CHD risk factors among children, but the specific shape of these relationships has received less attention. The relative importance of moderate vs. severe obesity should be further examined, as well as the magnitude of the associations with various weight–height indices, skinfolds and circumferences. Consideration should be given to the strong association of the anthropometric dimensions with age among children.

It is also important to obtain additional information on the correlations between levels of overweight/obesity and body fat patterning among children and adults. These findings, along with those of studies examining the relation of childhood overweight/obesity levels to disease risk, may allow effective interventions to be targeted better.

11.7 REFERENCES

Abate, N., Garg, A., Peshock, R.M., Stray-Gundersen, J., Adams-Huet, B. & Grundy, S.M. (1996). Relationship of generalised and regional adiposity to insulin sensitivity in men with NIDDM. *Diabetes*, **45**, 1684–93.

Baumgartner, R., Heymsfield, S.B. & Roche, A.F. (1995). Human body composition and the epidemiology of chronic disease. *Obesity Research*, **3**, 73–95.

Berenson, G.S. (ed.) (1986). *Causation Of Cardiovascular Risk Factors in Children. Perspectives on Cardiovascular Risk in Early Life*. New York: Raven Press.

Berenson, G.S., Srinivasan, S.R., Wattigney, W.A. & Harsha, D.W. (1993). Obesity and cardiovascular risk in children. *Annals of the New York Academy of Sciences*, **699**, 93–103.

Berenson, G.S., Srinivasan, S.R., Bao, W., Newman, W.P., Tracy, R.E. & Wattigney, W.A. (1998). Association between multiple cardiovascular risk factors and atherosclerosis in children and young adults. The Bogalusa Heart Study. *New England Journal of Medicine*, **338**,

1650–6.

Björntorp, P. (1990). 'Portal' adipose tissue as a generator of risk factors for cardiovascular disease and diabetes. *Arteriosclerosis*, **10**, 493–6.

Bo, W., Srinivasan, S.R., Wattigney, W.A. & Berenson, G.S. (1994). Persistence of multiple cardiovascular risk clustering related to syndrome X from childhood to young adulthood. The Bogalusa Heart Study. *Archives of Internal Medicine*, **154**, 1842–7.

Brambilla, P., Manzoni, P., Sironi, S., Simone, P., Del Maschio, A., di Natale, B. & Chiumello, G. (1994). Peripheral and abdominal adiposity in childhood obesity. *International Journal of Obesity*, **18**, 795–800.

Caprio, S., Hyman, L.D., McCarthy, S., Lange, R., Bronson, M. & Tamborlane, W.V. (1996). Fat distribution and cardiovascular risk factors in obese adolescent girls: importance of the intraabdominal fat depot. *American Journal of Clinical Nutrition*, **64**, 12–17.

Chu, N.F., Rimm, E.B., Wang, D.J., Liou, H.S. & Shieh, S.M. (1998). Clustering of cardiovascular disease risk factors among obese schoolchildren: the Taipei Children's Heart Study. *American Journal of Clinical Nutrition*, **67**, 1141–6.

Clarke, W.R. & Lauer, R.M. (1993). Does obesity track into adulthood? *Critical Reviews in Food Science and Nutrition*, **33**, 423–30.

Cleveland, W.S. (1985). *The Elements of Graphing Data*, pp. 170–8. Monterey, CA: Wadsworth Advanced Books and Software.

Cole, T.J. (1991). Weight-stature indices to measure underweight, overweight, and obesity. In *Anthropometric Assessment of Nutritional Status*, ed. J.H. Himes, pp. 83–111. New York: Wiley-Liss.

Dietz, W.H. (1998). Health consequences of obesity in youth: childhood predictors of adult disease. *Pediatrics*, **101** (suppl), 518s–25s.

Ducimetiere, P., Richard, J. & Cambien, F. (1986). The pattern of subcutaneous fat distribution in middle-aged men and the risk of coronary heart disease: the Paris Prospective Study. *International Journal of Obesity*, **10**, 229–40.

Dwyer, T. & Blizzard, C.L. (1996). Defining obesity in children by biological endpoint rather than population distribution. *International Journal of Obesity*, **20**, 472–80.

Dyer, R.G. (1994). Traditional treatment of obesity: does it work? *Baillieres Clinical Endocrinology and Metabolism*, **8**, 661–88.

Freedman, D.S. & Rimm, A.A. (1989). The relation of body fat distribution, as assessed by six girth measurements, to diabetes mellitus in women. *American Journal of Public Health*, **79**, 715–20.

Freedman, D.S., Burke, G.L., Harsha, D.W., Srinivasan, S.R., Cresanta, J.L., Webber, L.S. & Berenson, G.S. (1985). Relationship of changes in obesity to serum lipid and lipoprotein changes in childhood and adolescence. *Journal of the American Medical Association*, **254**, 515–20.

Freedman, D.S., Srinivasan, S.R., Valdez, R.A., Williamson, D.F. & Berenson, G.S. (1997). Secular increases in relative weight and adiposity among children over two decades: the Bogalusa Heart Study. *Pediatrics*, **99**, 420–5.

Freedman, D.S., Serdula, M.K., Srinivasan, S.R. & Berenson, G.S. (1999a). The relation of circumferences and skinfolds to levels of lipids and insulin: the Bogalusa Heart Study.

American Journal of Clinical Nutrition, **69**, 308–17.

Freedman, D.S., Dietz, W., Srinivasan, S.R. & Berenson, G.S. (1999b). The relation of overweight to cardiovascular risk factors among children and adolescents: The Bogalusa Heart Study. *Pediatrics*, **103**, 1175–82.

Garrow, J.S. & Webster, J. (1985). Quetelet's index (W/H^2) as a measure of fatness. *International Journal of Obesity*, **9**, 147–53.

Goran, M.I., Kaskoun, M. & Shuman, W.P. (1995). Intra-abdominal adipose tissue in young children. *International Journal of Obesity*, **19**, 279–83.

Haffner, S.M., Stern, M.P., Hazuda, H.P., Pugh, J. & Patterson, J.K. (1987). Do upper-body and centralized adiposity measure different aspects of regional body-fat distribution? Relationship to non-insulin-dependent diabetes mellitus, lipids, and lipoproteins. *Diabetes*, **36**, 43–51.

Harrison, G.G. (1985). Anthropometric differences and their clinical correlates. In *Recent Advances in Obesity Research: IV. Proceedings of the 4th International Congress on Obesity*, eds. J. Hirsch & T.B. Van Itallie, pp. 144–9. London: John Libbey and Company.

Himes, J.H. & Dietz, W.H. (1994). Guidelines for overweight in adolescent preventive services: recommendations from an expert committee. *American Journal of Clinical Nutrition*, **59**, 307–16.

Hodge, A.M. & Simmet, P.Z. (1994). The epidemiology of obesity. *Baillieres Clinical Endocrinology and Metabolism*, **8**, 577–99.

Hoffmans, M.D.A.F., Kromhout, D. & de Lezenne Coulander, C. (1988). The impact of body mass index of 78 612 Dutch men on 32-year mortality. *Journal of Clinical Epidemiology*, **41**, 749–56.

Johnston, F.E. (1985). Health implications of childhood obesity. *Annals of Internal Medicine*, **103** (6, suppl., part 2), 1068–72.

Keys, A., Fidanza, F., Karvonen, M.J., Kimura, N. & Taylor, H.L. (1972). Indices of relative weight and obesity. *Journal of Chronic Diseases*, **25**, 329–43.

Kronmal, R.A. (1993). Spurious correlation and the fallacy of the ratio standard revisited. *Journal of the Royal Statistical Society Series A*, **156**, 379–92.

Kuczmarski, R.J., Flegal, K.M., Campbell, S.M. & Johnson, C.L. (1994). Increasing prevalence of overweight among US adults: the National Health and Nutrition Examination Surveys, 1960 to 1991. *Journal of the American Medical Association*, **272**, 205–11.

Kushner, R. (1993). Body weight and mortality. *Nutrition Reviews*, **51**, 127–36.

Laskarzewski, P., Morrison, J.A., Mellies, M.J., Kelly, K., Gartside, P.S., Khoury, P. & Glueck, C.J. (1980). Relationships of measurements of body mass to plasma lipoprotein in schoolchildren and adults. *American Journal of Epidemiology*, **111**, 395–406.

Lauer, R.M., Connor, W.E., Leaverton, P.E., Reiter, M.A. & Clarke, W.R. (1975). Coronary heart disease risk factors in school children: the Muscatine Study. *Journal of Pediatrics*, **86**, 697–706.

Mahoney, L.T., Burns, T.L., Stanford, W., Thompson, B.H., Witt, J.D., Rost, C.A. & Lauer, R.M. (1996). Coronary risk factors measured in childhood and young adult life are associated with coronary artery calcification in young adults: the Muscatine Study. *Journal of the American College of Cardiology*, **27**, 277–84.

Malina, R.M. & Bouchard, C. (1988). Subcutaneous fat distribution during growth. In *Fat Distribution During Growth and Later Health Outcomes*, eds. C. Bouchard & F.E. Johnston, pp. 63–84. New York: Alan R. Liss.

Mueller, W.H. & Wohlleb, J.C. (1981). Anatomical distribution of subcutaneous fat and its description by multivariate methods: How valid are principal components? *American Journal of Physical Anthropology*, **54**, 25–35.

Must, A. (1996). Morbidity and mortality associated with elevated body weight in children and adolescents. *American Journal of Clinical Nutrition*, **63** (suppl.), 445s–7s.

Must, A., Jacques, P.F., Dallal, G.E., Bajema, C.J. & Dietz, W.H. (1992). Long-term morbidity and mortality of overweight adolescents. A follow-up of the Harvard Growth Study of 1922 to 1935. *New England Journal of Medicine*, **327**, 1350–5.

Najjar, M.F. & Rowland, M. (1987). *Anthropometric Reference Data and Prevalence of Overweight, United States, 1976–80.* Washington (DC): Public Health Service, Vital and Health Statistics, series 11, no. 238. US Department of Health and Human Services Publication No. (PHS) 87-1688.

National Cholesterol Education Program (1991). *Report of the Expert Panel on Blood Cholesterol Levels in Children and Adolescents.* Washington, DC: US Department of Health and Human Services National Institutes of Health Publication No. 91-2732.

Nieto, F.J., Szklo, M. & Comstock, G.W. (1992). Childhood weight and growth rate as predictors of adult mortality. *American Journal of Epidemiology*, **136**, 201–13.

Paffenbarger, R.S. & Wing, A.L. (1969). Chronic disease in former college students: the effects of single and multiple characteristics on risk of fatal coronary heart disease. *American Journal of Epidemiology*, **90**, 527–35.

Pinhas-Hamiel, O., Dolan, L.M., Daniels, S.R., Standiford, D., Khoury, P.R. & Zeitler, P. (1996). Increased incidence of non-insulin-dependent diabetes mellitus among adolescents. *Journal of Pediatrics*, **128**, 608–15.

Power, C., Lake, J.K. & Cole, T.J. (1997). Measurement and long-term health risks of child and adolescent fatness. *International Journal of Obesity*, **21**, 507–26.

Raitakari, O.T., Porkka, K.V.K., Rönnemaa, T. & Åkerblom, H.K. (1994). Clustering of risk factors for coronary heart disease in children and adolescents. The Cardiovascular Risk in Young Finns Study. *Acta Paediatrica*, **83**, 935–40.

Resnicow, K. & Cross, D. (1993). Are parents' self-reported total cholesterol levels useful in identifying children with hyperlipidemia? An examination of current guidelines. *Pediatrics*, **92**, 347–53.

Resnicow, K. & Morabia, A. (1990). The relation between body mass index and plasma total cholesterol in a multiracial sample of US schoolchildren. *American Journal of Epidemiology*, **132**, 1083–9.

Sangi, H. & Mueller, W.H. (1991). Which measure of body fat distribution is best for epidemiologic research among adolescents? *American Journal of Epidemiology*, **133**, 870–83.

Seidell, J.C. (1992). Regional obesity and health. *International Journal of Obesity*, **16** (suppl. 2), S31–4.

Serdula, M.K., Ivery, D., Coates, R.J., Freedman, D.S., Williamson, D.F. & Byers, T. (1993). Do obese children become obese adults? A review of the literature. *Preventive Medicine*, **22**, 167–77.

Siervogel, R.M., Roche, A.F., Guo, S., Mukhergee, D. & Chumlea, W.C. (1991). Patterns of change in weight/stature^2 from 2 to 18 years: Findings from the long-term serial data for children in the Fels Longitudinal Growth Study. *International Journal of Obesity*, **15**, 479–85.

Sørensen, T.I.A. & Sonne-Holm, S. (1977). Mortality in extremely overweight young men. *Journal of Chronic Diseases*, **30**, 359–67.

Spataro, J.A., Dyer, A.R., Stamler, J., Shekelle, R.B., Greenlund, K. & Garside, D. (1996). Measures of adiposity and coronary heart disease mortality in the Chicago Western Electric Company Study. *Journal of Clinical Epidemiology*, **49**, 849–57.

Srinivasan, S.R., Bao, W., Wattigney, W.A. & Berenson, G.S. (1996). Adolescent overweight is associated with adult overweight and related multiple cardiovascular risk factors: the Bogalusa Heart Study. *Journal of Chronic Diseases*, **45**, 235–40.

Troiano, R.P., Flegal, K.M., Kuczmarski, R.J., Campbell, S.M. & Johnson, C.L. (1995). Overweight prevalence and trends for children and adolescents. The National Health and Nutrition Examination Surveys, 1963 to 1991. *Archives of Pediatrics and Adolescent Medicine*, **149**, 1085–91.

Vague, J. (1956). The degree of masculine differentiation of obesities: a factor determining predisposition to diabetes, atherosclerosis, gout, and uric calculous disease. *American Journal of Clinical Nutrition*, **4**, 20–34.

Waaler, H.T. (1984). Height, weight and mortality: the Norwegian experience. *Acta Medica Scandinavica*, **679** (Suppl), 1–56.

Weststrate, J.A., Deurenberg, P. & van Tinteren, H. (1989). Indices of body fat distribution and adiposity in Dutch children from birth to 18 years of age. *International Journal of Obesity*, **13**, 456–77.

Whitaker, R.C., Wright, J.A., Pepe, M.S., Seidel, K.D. & Dietz, W.H. (1997). Predicting obesity in young adulthood from childhood and parental obesity. *New England Journal of Medicine*, **227**, 869–73.

Williams, D.P., Going, S.B., Lohman, T.G., Harsha, D.W., Srinivasan, S.R., Webber, L.S. & Berenson, G.S. (1992). Body fatness and risk for elevated blood pressure, total cholesterol, and serum lipoprotein ratios in children and adolescents. *American Journal of Public Health*, **82**, 358–63.

Zwiauer, K.F.M., Pakosta, R., Mueller, T. & Widhalm, K. (1992). Cardiovascular risk factors in obese children in relation to weight and body fat distribution. *Journal of the American College of Nutrition*, **11**, 41s–50s.

Part III

Prevention and management

12

Prevention

Inge Lissau,[1] Walter Burniat,[2] Elizabeth M.E. Poskitt[3] and Tim Cole[4]

[1]National Institute of Public Health, Copenhagen. [2]University Hospital for Children 'Reine Fabiola', Free University of Brussels. [3]International Nutrition Group, London School of Hygiene and Tropical Medicine. [4]Department of Paediatric Epidemiology and Biostatistics, Institute of Child Health, London

12.1 Prevention before management

It seems almost *de rigueur* to end medical and nutritional texts with a section on prevention of the problem under discussion. Yet is this intelligent planning? The editors had lengthy discussions on the most logical order for the chapters in this book. No current programme for the treatment of obesity is particularly success-ful. Thus, control of the epidemic of obesity sweeping many countries in the developed world, and indeed beginning to affect countries in the developing world, is likely to depend more on effective prevention than on 'cure' of obesity. For this reason, priority in the management of childhood obesity has been given to this chapter on prevention.

12.2 Why prevention?

There are many reasons for promoting obesity prevention in childhood:
1. the prevalence of obesity is rising in industrialized countries (Chapter 2);
2. childhood obesity is likely to lead to obesity in adult life (Chapter 2);
3. it limits physical activity (Chapter 5);
4. it is associated with psychosocial disadvantage (Chapter 6);
5. it is associated with a higher risk of adult conditions such as Type II diabetes mellitus and hypertension (Chapters 7, 8, 10 and 11);
6. it is difficult to treat successfully (Chapters 13–20).

12.2.1 Primary prevention

The focus for preventive health programmes operates at three levels (WHO, 1998):
• primary prevention, aimed at reducing the number of new cases (incidence);

- secondary prevention, aimed at reducing the numbers of established cases (prevalence);
- tertiary prevention, aimed at reducing the degree of disability associated with the condition (treatment).

These definitions generate a paradox: is obesity a disease or a risk factor for disease? The physical, psychosocial and long-term complications of childhood obesity are so pervasive that, for preventive policies at least, obesity should be considered a disease. Thus, the levels of obesity prevention can be defined as follows:

- primary, preventing the development of obesity;
- secondary, controlling or treating existing obesity to reduce its prevalence and/or severity;
- tertiary, reducing the adverse consequences of obesity, which may or may not reduce its prevalence as well.

It might be expected that the rising prevalence of obesity at all ages would make preventive programmes a high priority in obesity research. This does not seem to be the case. A recent Cochrane review found few preventive projects with sufficient power to set clear directions for the prevention of childhood obesity. Most projects have been set up in one country, the USA, and have involved 'middle-aged' children only – those between 7 and 12 years old. The conclusion of this review was that it was impossible to conclude that any one strategy or combination of strategies had greater effect than other strategies. There remains an urgent need for further sound studies in the field of obesity prevention in childhood (Campbell et al., 2001).

This chapter focuses on what is known and what can be recommended as potentially effective in primary prevention. It identifies the key risk factors for later obesity, that is those amenable to change, then discusses which individuals and groups of individuals have responsibility to instigate change in the risk factors, and finally proposes strategies to encourage change within the different groups. The conclusion is that change should be instigated at all levels of society, and that an integrated approach is the only realistic way forward.

12.2.2 The target population

Should a programme to prevent child obesity target the whole population (population strategy), or alternatively should it focus only on those children particularly at risk (risk-group strategy)? Power et al. (1997) have argued strongly for a population-based strategy, on the grounds that most children at risk of adult obesity cannot be identified with any confidence in childhood – most obese adults become obese only in late adolescence or early adulthood. Any attempt to target at-risk groups in childhood is likely to be ineffective. A population-based ap-

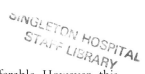

proach to the prevention of childhood obesity seems preferable. However, this does not rule out the possibility of testing particular intervention strategies on at-risk groups, in order to monitor their effectiveness.

12.2.3 Risk factors

A recent systematic review identified several proven risk factors for obesity: parental fatness, social factors, birth weight, timing or rate of maturation, physical activity, dietary factors, and other behavioural and psychological factors (Parsons et al., 1999). Several social factors are also relevant for future obesity: poverty, psychosocial deprivation and membership of certain ethnic groups. What is not understood is what it is about these factors that makes them relevant to the development of childhood obesity, since the same factors are also associated with children at increased risk of failure to thrive – within the same society. Other clearly identifiable minority groups with increased risk of obesity are children with special educational needs, those with a handicap that restricts physical exercise, and those with certain obesity-related syndromes such as Down's syndrome or Prader–Willi syndrome (Chapter 9).

Though the list of risk factors is long, most of them can be disregarded immediately in the context of prevention as they are not amenable to change. Parental fatness, birth weight and maturation, for example, are all determined by the time a child is born, and so are irrelevant for later prevention. Perhaps, all that can be said about them is that children should choose their parents carefully...!

The two risk factors that are clearly amenable to change are physical activity and diet, and it is on these two factors that any obesity prevention strategy should hang.

12.3 Prevention strategy

The thermodynamic basis for obesity is positive energy balance. If energy consumed in the diet exceeds energy expended through exercise, then surplus energy is stored as fat. So the way to prevent obesity is (in theory) very simple – ensure negative energy balance. This encourages the conversion of stored fat into energy, with resulting loss in weight.

Consequently, obesity should be preventable through:
• increasing energy output (physical activity);
• reducing energy intake (diet).

The aim for individuals and populations should be to keep energy output greater than energy intake. The rising tide of obesity indicates that, at the population level, this aim is not being achieved. The reasons for this are not hard to find. Over the last 20–30 years, levels of activity, whether at school, work or home, have fallen dramatically. Though dietary intakes in many westernized countries have also fallen, they have failed to fall as fast as activity. Indeed the Bogalusa Heart Study showed no change in the energy intakes of 10-year-olds from 1973 to 1998 (Nicklas et al., 1993).

12.3.1 Increase energy expenditure

Though emphasis is often on increasing physical activity, reducing sedentary activity is probably more important for the prevention of obesity. Time spent exercising has always been only a small fraction of the day, so the level of activity when not exercising may be the sphere of activity which has changed most since the obesity epidemic started. Our emphasis here is on the reduction of sedentary activity. Encouraging physical activity and, especially, avoiding inactivity, are key challenges in the prevention of future obesity.

Being physically active has several advantages:

* easier control of body weight;
* improved physical fitness;
* lower blood pressure;
* improved metabolic status, for example insulin sensitivity and HDL/LDL (high-density-lipoprotein/low-density-lipoprotein) cholesterol ratio;
* increased bone mineralization;
* improved sense of well being.

12.3.2 Reduce energy intake

The second plank of a prevention strategy is lowered energy consumption, but this oversimplifies the health education message and makes it sound unnecessarily negative. The very positive aim is much wider than this: healthy eating. This should lead to diets where *all* nutrients, not just energy, are appropriate for children's needs, leading to increased micronutrient intakes in addition to re-duced intakes of energy and fat. Healthy eating involves not only attention to the quality of foods but also to the circumstances under which foods are eaten. Eating meals as a family should be an important part of family life and contribute to the development of sound dietary practices.

> *'Oh, my friends, be warned by me,*
> *That breakfast, dinner, lunch and tea*
> *Are all the human frame requires...'*
> *(With that, the wretched child expires).*[1]

Regular meals are important not only in terms of the quality and quantity of food provided, but also in the frequency of eating and the social ambience in

---

[1] Hilaire Belloc. The chief defect of Henry King was chewing little bits of string. *Cautionary Tales* quoted in *The Oxford Dictionary of Quotations* (2nd edition), London, Oxford University Press: 1959: p. 41.

which eating takes place. Regular meal patterns ensure cycles of appetite followed by satiety, which train children to recognize when intakes are sufficient. The alternative of snacking throughout the day ('grazing' or 'eating on the hoof'), means that the hunger–appetite–satiety cycle does not operate in the same way, making it harder for children to regulate their intakes.

In general, three main meals and two or three, modest in energy terms, snacks during the day are recommended for children.

The separate components of a healthy diet are well known and many countries have their own sets of recommendations. These may differ slightly in the quantities of particular foods recommended but the overall recommendations are very similar. Denmark for example has seven official dietary recommendations:
- eat plenty of bread and cereals;
- eat six portions of fruit and/or vegetables per day;
- eat potatoes, rice and/or pasta every day;
- eat fish frequently, and vary between fish with low and high fat content;
- choose milk and milk products with low fat content;
- choose meat with low fat content;
- use butter, margarine and oil sparingly, and use as little sugar and salt as practical in terms of palatability.

An important aspect of obesity prevention is encouraging eating habits which follow these principles.

12.3.3 Reduce television watching

If there is one social practice which has paralleled the development of the obesity epidemic, it must be the increase in time spent watching television. This creates particular environmental risks for obesity, since it encourages positive energy balance: physical activity is reduced whilst energy intake is boosted through snacking.

Children in many westernized countries spend around 23 hours a week on average watching television (Lipman, 1991). Dietz & Gortmaker (1985) showed that the hours children watch television are significantly related to the development of obesity. Children studied in cycles II and III of the US National Health Examination Survey were asked about the time spent watching television each day. Prevalences of obesity and super-obesity showed clear dose–response relationships with the hours spent watching television. Further, in those subjects seen in both cycles, hours watching television in cycle II correlated positively with obesity in cycle III four years later, demonstrating the long-term effects of television viewing on obesity. In Brussels, the most severely obese children attending an outpatient clinic spent at least 20 hours a week watching television whilst they spent only 35 hours a week at school (Burniat & Van Aelst, 1993).

The effects of television viewing on nutritional status seem to vary with social circumstances. In Pennsylvania, time spent watching television correlated positively with fatness in children from lower socioeconomic districts, but not in children from more advantaged districts (Shannon et al., 1991).

12.3.4 Side effects of prevention

Eating disorders

An increasing prevalence of eating disorders such as anorexia and bulimia has accompanied an emphasis on the perceived attractions of slimness to many societies. In Denmark, the prevalence of underweight (BMI < 20) in young women aged 16–25 years rose by 30% from 1987 to 1994, while the prevalence of obesity (BMI > 30) in the same age-group doubled over this period (Kjøller et al., 1995). It seems inevitable that a minority of young people, mainly women, with distorted self-image, will develop eating disorders as a direct result of society's emphasis on looking slim. As community problems, eating disorders and obesity are probably directly linked.

Interventions aimed at preventing obesity might thus precipitate the development of eating disorders associated with undue fear of fatness, especially among young adolescent girls. However, this is unlikely if interventions focus on healthy eating rather than reduced energy intake. There is no evidence that encouraging healthy eating makes eating disorders more likely.

Smoking

People may adopt harmful behaviours such as smoking because they believe these will control their weight (WHO, 1998; Wiseman et al., 1998). This may be one reason why young women now smoke more than previously (Friestad & Klepp, 1997; Lloyd et al., 1997). There is no doubt that smoking does reduce weight, but at the same time it reduces life expectancy, and to a much greater extent (Basvaraj, 1993; Prescott et al., 1999). The important message for young people who smoke in order to regulate their weight is – Stop! The potential risk to future health from the small increase in weight is minute compared to the overall risk to health from smoking.

12.4 Responsibilities for prevention

If prevention is to be effective, interventions need to be targeted appropriately, focusing on those individuals or institutions best placed to effect change. There are essentially five relevant groups: family (i.e. child, siblings, parents), school, health professionals, government (local and national) and industry. Each group has different roles and responsibilities which are expanded below.

12.4.1 Family
Parent(s)

Parents have a strong influence on their children's lifestyles through the example they set and through education. Their own attitudes to their children's nutritional status will be coloured by their socioeconomic status and their own nutritional state.

Children with obese parents have increased risk of obesity. The odds ratio of becoming obese by early adult life for US children with both parents obese are 14 for children aged 1–2 years and 22 for children aged 10–14 years (Whitaker et al., 1997). Growing up with obese parents means that children who are genetically predisposed to obesity are also exposed to environments likely to encourage obesity. Obese parents may accept obesity in their children more readily than lean parents and consequently do less to change eating habits and patterns of physical activity, thus transferring obesity-promoting habits to their offspring. Obesity hampers easy movement and so inactivity may be environmentally determined, but relative inactivity could also be determined by an inactivity-predisposing genotype. Whatever the explanations for familial obesity, high risk group strategies must prioritize children of families with obesity in close relatives.

Articles from Denmark (Lissau & Sørensen, 1992, 1994; Lissau et al., 1993) have drawn attention to the significance of care in children's environments for the development of obesity. A prospective study of a randomly selected cohort of children showed that parental neglect, whether assessed by the school health service, the class teacher or indirectly by the mother herself, significantly increased the risk of obesity in young adulthood independently of body mass index in childhood and social background. Families where nurturing is recognized as a problem may benefit from systematic family therapy (Chapter 16).

Child

The degree of responsibility expected of children towards control of their dietary intakes and patterns of exercise depends largely on their age. Preschool children, although understanding at the time of explanation why they are encouraged to eat or to do certain things, and, although sometimes pointing out where parents are taking wrong decisions in this respect, cannot be expected to show consistently appropriate decision making when confronted with choices. Parents must involve their children in choices as far as possible but need to guide their choice towards healthy living. As children grow up, they learn what is involved in choosing and can understand reasons for choice better, as well as recognizing the need to 'resist temptation'. However, as children mature, the influences of peer groups become more important and, in adolescence, parents who try to impose dietary habits or activity on their children are likely to find themselves in undesirable and noncontributory confrontational situations. The importance of peer-group attitudes makes healthy-living education, in schools and in the community, critically important.

12.4.2 School

Schools have an important role in many aspects of health promotion. When involving schools in obesity prevention, it should not be necessary to cut other aspects of health promotion, since the messages for obesity prevention are essentially those for prevention of cardiovascular disease, reduction of cancer risk, maintenance of bone health, mental health and so on. Education to prevent obesity has to include not only education of what is 'right' in terms of foods, eating and activity, but also the ability to be critical of advertising and media influences and to learn how to withstand the commercial pressures within society (Casado Gorriz et al., 1999).

The school usually occupies a significant place in its community. Thus schools can provide an impetus to community efforts to implement 'healthy living'. Such efforts might be encouraging or developing advocacy for safe roads, schoolchild friendly public transport, better food choices in 'corner' shops near schools, safe parks and playgrounds.

Guidelines have recently been produced in the United States (Anon, 1997) for school health programmes to promote healthy eating. Recommendations cover seven aspects of a school-based programme and could cover aspects of healthy living broader than just eating, as shown by the very similar recommendations to promote physical activity (see later). The recommendations are:
- a school policy on nutrition;
- a sequential coordinated curriculum;
- appropriate instruction for students;
- integration of school food service and nutrition education;
- staff training;
- family and community involvement;
- programme evaluation.

In our view most schools would react in horror if suddenly presented with such a wide-ranging programme. We can sympathize. However, if the present epidemic of obesity is to be controlled, it is our firm belief that multifaceted lifestyle changes are required within societies. Somehow, the already overburdened schools need to take a leading role in effecting these changes.

12.4.3 Health professionals

The health profession is central to the provision of informed support, detailed knowledge, and professional attitudes which can encourage others' efforts in the prevention of obesity. Too often families' concerns about their children's increasing weight have been 'fobbed off' with comments such as 'it's only puppy fat' or 'nothing can be done anyway'. Often, the education of other health professionals about the importance of obesity-prevention policies and activities and about seeing these in a positive light is the first duty of health professionals towards implementing healthy eating. Health professionals should be able to advise their clients on healthy eating – and, hopefully, take a lead in this respect in their own lives. In addition, it may be relevant for professional societies and voluntary organizations dealing with nutritional problems and with children to review how their relationships with food companies, commercial sponsors and so on might be interpreted by 'outsiders' (Tobin et al., 1992).

12.4.4 Government

Much of what is discussed here, particularly in relation to schools, will be difficult to implement and will have little impact without being underpinned by larger community-wide or nationwide programmes for improving diets and increasing opportunities for healthy levels of activity for all. Local governments are likely to be the most involved in town-planning measures and local environment improvement, road-safety measures, provision of areas for activity and sport and provision of entertainments which divert children from the television screen. Adults have the power to influence local (and national) government activities in these areas through lobbying and ultimately through the ballot box.

At the national level, governments should heed the advice of health professionals and families in determining priorities. Their support for healthy-living programmes must be financial and physical and not just verbal. If necessary, the importance of obesity prevention in childhood must be made plain through economic arguments on the cost of obesity through loss of physical and – perhaps particularly – mental health, underachievement at school, incapacity to work, as well as the costs to society of providing larger seats on public transport, larger desks in schools and so on.

12.4.5 Industry

It may be difficult to convince industry that it has a responsibility for the prevention of childhood obesity. Industry must see its success in terms of tangible monetary profit. Yet, industry in many countries is beginning to recognize that it has a role in benefiting communities around factories and benefiting those who buy its goods as well as realizing the importance of having a workforce which is healthy and has healthy families. More specifically, within the food manufacturing companies there is now some – probably increasing – recognition that there are ethical issues in marketing and advertising foods which may be turned to a company's disadvantage if a strong 'protest' movement sees reason to develop.

12.5 Reduce sedentary activity

12.5.1 Family

Several behavioural factors influence physical activity in children and adolescents (US Centers for Disease Control and Prevention, 1996, 1997):

- *Parental activity* relates positively with the physical activity of preschool children. The physical activity of friends and siblings is also positively related to levels of physical activity in older children and adolescents. Parents' activity influences that of their children (Anderssen & Wold, 1992; Wold et al., 1994). Habits of activity developed during childhood are commonly maintained in adulthood. The Framingham study has shown that children of active mothers are twice as likely to be active as children of inactive mothers (Moore et al., 1991).
- *Parental support* is positively related to physical activity amongst preschool children and adolescents. Parents organizing activities or providing transport encourage physical activity amongst older children and younger adolescents if the use of play spaces and play facilities is open to all age-groups (Garcia et al., 1995; Zakarian et al., 1994). Girls' activity seems more related to equipment availability than that of boys who exercise anyway in open spaces (Butcher, 1986; Stucky-Ropp & DiLorenzo, 1993). Time spent outdoors correlates positively with physical activity in both sexes and at all ages (Sallis et al., 1993).
- *Demographic factors*, which include gender, age and ethnicity.
- *Self-efficacy*, a construct from social cognitive theory, is an attitude which has been positively associated with physical activity amongst older children and adolescents (Bandura, 1998). Self-efficacy in relation to exercise includes confidence in one's ability to engage in exercise. Boys, who believe in themselves and their skills more than girls do, have higher self-efficacy.
- *Expectations* for the outcomes of physical activity are associated with the level of physical activity of preadolescents and adolescents.
- *Perceived benefits* are positively associated with physical activity, whereas *perceived barriers* are negatively associated. The intention to be active, a construct from the theory of reasoned action and the theory of planned behaviour (Ajzen & Fishbein, 1980), has been consistently and positively related to physical activity amongst older children and adolescents.
- *Perceived competence* in physical sport.
- *Positive attitudes* towards physical education.
- *Enjoyment*, the major reason young people engage in physical activity (Borra et

al., 1995), has been positively associated with physical activity in both children and adolescents.

- *Social influences*, such as physically active role models and role-model support for physical activity, are important determinants of activity amongst young people.
- *Competition* motivates boys more than girls, whereas the desire to control weight motivates girls more than boys (Tappe et al., 1990; Kelder et al., 1995).

Daily physical activity can both help prevent obesity and maintain fitness. To encourage physical activity, a variety of opportunities for energy expenditure, selected according to children's ages, should be available. Adolescents, particularly girls, often become less active at puberty. Promoting habitual physical activity in adolescence is thus important for obesity prevention (Kemper et al., 1999). So far, only a few health-promotion programmes have been evaluated, mainly in the United States (US Centers for Disease Control and Prevention, 1997). Some simple aims for the family to reduce inactivity are:

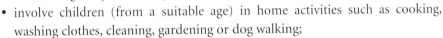

- encourage physical activity in children;
- walk or cycle to school;
- exercise regularly as a family;
- involve children (from a suitable age) in home activities such as cooking, washing clothes, cleaning, gardening or dog walking;
- encourage hobbies and interests which divert children from the pastime of television.

12.5.2 School

Schools present almost ideal settings for the prevention of obesity. All individuals can be reached, regardless of background. In addition, the amount of time set aside for mandatory physical education can be part of the National Curriculum, where this exists, and thus be regulated by government. However, forcing children to take exercise may put them off formal activity. Competitive sports are unpopular with less sporty children. Emphasis on noncompetitive activities is likely to be more effective in the long term.

Every school should have
- a policy on physical activity,
- at least one hour daily of mandatory physical activity for each child.

12.5.3 Health professionals

The health profession is in a unique position for emphasizing the immediate and long-term benefits of activity and exercise. A health visitor will see the mother soon after the child's birth and can thus encourage an active lifestyle from an early age. Health visitors may also be able to advise anxious parents about matters such as child safety outside the home: teaching children how to cross roads safely; when they can be left to swim relatively unsupervised; when they are safe cycling by themselves or playing outside without close parental supervision and so on.

The health profession is also central in the assessment of child nutrition and in the documentation of nutritional status in groups and communities. It will be impossible, for example, to evaluate whether the suggestions in this chapter, if implemented, have any impact on the epidemic of childhood obesity unless there is 'before and after' documentation of nutritional status. Such documentation itself provides important material for further preventive programmes by quantifying the impact of activity (for example) on health, and using the findings to lobby government to implement further change.

12.5.4 Government

Local government

There is much to be done at local-government level to effect the changes which might facilitate greater activity over obesity prevention by the local population, particularly the children. For example, local governments should:

* provide information on physical activity, giving priority to activities that families can do together;
* provide a variety of sporting facilities such as supervised swimming baths and football pitches to meet the different needs, interests and skills of the community;
* improve facilities and opportunities for walking and cycling, for example traffic calming, cycle lanes and pedestrian precincts;
* ensure families with young children in high-rise flats are housed at ground or first-floor level, so mothers homeworking in the flats can supervise their children playing outside – preferably in garden areas;
* give prominence to staircases rather than lifts in public buildings.

Society has to ensure that children and adults are safe as well as active. This involves dealing with neighbourhood crime, traffic safety and pollution. There are many good policies for increasing the activity of children – but they must be safe. Cycle tracks, car-free play streets and swimming baths are excellent opportunities for urban children to have enjoyable activity provided they are adequately protected and supervised.

National government

There is much national governments can do to introduce and promote prevention of childhood obesity measures. National transport policies which are user friendly in terms of frequency, cost, safety and reliability could do much to encourage walking and cycling as realistic alternatives to using the car. Recommendations to schools could expand the place of physical activity in the curriculum. Financial support could be provided for further sports centre development.

One important activity for a national government should be the development and dissemination of guidelines for healthy living. For example, the Health Education Authority in Britain has proposed guidelines for physical activity in children and youths (Biddle et al., 1998). These are not directed specifically at preventing obesity as such but can, nevertheless, be effective in this.

- All children and youth should participate in physical activity that is of at least moderate intensity for an average of 1 hour per day. While young people should be physically active nearly every day, the amount of physical activity can vary from day to day in type, setting, intensity, duration and amount.
- All children and youth should participate at least twice per week in physical activities that enhance and maintain strength in the musculature of the trunk and upper-arm girdle.
- All children and youth should meet physical activity recommendations 1 and 2 participating in types, intensities and duration of physical activity that are developmentally appropriate from both physiological and behavioural perspectives.

The US Department of Health and Human Services has come up with guidelines for school and community programmes to promote lifelong physical activity among young people (US Centers for Disease Control and Prevention, 1997):

- *Policy:* establish policies that promote enjoyable, lifelong physical activity among young people.
- *Environment:* provide physical and social environments that encourage and enable safe and enjoyable physical activity.
- *Physical education:* implement physical education curricula and instruction that emphasize enjoyable participation in physical activity and that help students develop knowledge, attitudes, motor and behavioural skills, and the confidence needed to adopt and maintain physically active lifestyles.
- *Health education:* implement health education curricula and instruction that help students develop the knowledge, attitudes, behavioural skills, and confidence needed to adopt and maintain physically active lifestyles.
- *Extracurricular activities:* provide extracurricular physical activity programmes that meet the needs and interests of all students.
- *Parental involvement:* include parents and guardians in physical training and in extracurricular and community physical activity programmes, and encourage them to support their children's participation in enjoyable physical activities.
- *Personnel training:* provide training for education, coaching, recreation, health-care and other personnel that imparts the knowledge and skills needed for the

effective promotion of enjoyable, lifelong physical activity among young people.

- *Health services:* assess physical activity patterns among young people; counsel them about physical activity; refer them to appropriate programmes; and advocate for physical activity instruction and programmes for all young people.
- *Community programmes:* provide a range of developmentally appropriate community sports and recreation programmes that are attractive to all young people.
- *Evaluation:* evaluate school and community physical-activity instruction, programmes and facilities regularly.

12.5.5 Industry

Industry should be encouraged to sponsor environmental changes such as upgrading footpaths, maintaining parks and gardens, or funding sports stadia. However, questions over which industries are acceptable as named supporters or sponsors can present tricky ethical and political issues with which potential recipients may not wish to become involved (Tobin et al., 1992).

One rather specific recommendation to industry would be that the travel industry should be encouraged or cajoled to make cycling easier by simplifying the transport of cycles on trains or buses.

The advertising industry has its own role to play in encouraging activity. Advertising can fund projects like the Citybike initiative in Copenhagen, where a pool of bicycles, each with advertisements pasted on the frame, can be collected and later returned for a small fee. Advertising on the cycles makes the project financially viable.

The advertising industry can also influence activity by projecting positive images of individuals and families following healthy lifestyles in their advertisements.

12.5.6 Television

Previous sections have focused mainly on encouraging physical exercise in various forms. By contrast, television is an important component of *sedentary* activity. Parents have the main responsibility to restrict watching, both negatively (by rationing viewing time) and positively (by encouraging other interests and hobbies, which may or may not involve physical exercise).

Television watching is not just sedentary. It actually leads to a fall in metabolic rate recorded as even below basal metabolic rate (BMR) (Klesges et al., 1993). Further, children watching television excessively miss opportunities for developing social and cultural interests with friends and family.

Parents need to be careful that television viewing does not become integrated into the daily routine of their children. Television may be used as a surrogate baby sitter when children are small and, gradually, viewing becomes a habit with older children. Later on, when parents decide to provide children with their own televisions, they surrender any remaining control over their children's viewing. Televisions in children's rooms should be postponed for as long as possible.

Metabolic rates do not fall quite as low with computer games as with television watching. In Mexico City, obesity prevalence showed no relation to video use although obesity level did relate to low levels of activity and to television viewing (Hernandez et al., 1999). Nevertheless, these games pose similar risks to television in terms of sedentary behaviour and diminished social contact.

The role of television is not entirely negative. Programmes can be planned with health promotion and obesity prevention in mind. For example, they can portray positive images of activities which are practical and feasible and to which children can relate. Exploration of the polar icecaps or swimming the Channel may in themselves be wonderful examples of human achievement, but they do not reflect activities the average child might feel he or she could accomplish.

12.6 Reduce poor dietary habits

12.6.1 Family

Families must take the lead in providing guidance for children in healthy eating. Habits learnt early in life are likely to carry through to adulthood. However, healthy eating is not just about what is eaten but also about the environment in which eating takes place: meal patterns and the social setting for meals. Teaching children to cook at home encourages an interest in food, leads to knowledge of food ingredients and composition of meals and provides skills which may facilitate healthy eating in later life. The increase in childhood obesity seems to have more or less paralleled the decline in cooking skills and rise in the use of prepared-before-sale, precooked and 'take away' foods together with the increase in 'eating out' by families.

Mealtimes are important for family communication. When both parents are working, children spend much of the day outside the home with other adults taking responsibility for them. Then parents share responsibility for children's eating habits with other adults. Nevertheless, the family meal at the end of the day and at weekends can be an important bonding experience with opportunity for developing interpersonal skills. It can also create a meal when food is eaten fairly slowly and satiety may come from the time spent socializing as much as from the quantity of food consumed.

Avoid meal skipping

The effects of skipping breakfast have been studied widely – much more than the effects of skipping other meals. This may be because breakfast is a meal which is easy to record as taken or not taken. It may be no more specific than documentable evidence of meal skipping in general. However, eating breakfast does seem to improve cognition (Benton & Parker, 1998; Murphy et al., 1998) and reduce snacking later in the day (Schlundt et al., 1992). Despite this, an increasing number of children now skip breakfast. Among Dutch children aged 4–15 years, 5% of those in primary school and 13% in secondary school skip breakfast (Brugman et al., 1998). Skipping breakfast is more common amongst children in large city schools, girls, older children, children from single-parent families, and children of fathers with low educational achievements. In Copenhagen, 10–20% children do not eat breakfast daily (Lissau et al., 2001). Between 1965 and 1991 there was a decline in breakfast consumption among US children and adolescents (Siega-Riz et al., 1998).

Regular organized eating seems important for the development of satiety and appropriate nutrient intake. Health-education programmes need to encourage breakfast eating, targeting groups at special risk. Programmes should take into account possible reasons for skipping breakfast, such as single parents who are too busy to prepare breakfast. School Breakfast programmes have been instituted in the United States and in some other countries. These are mainly designed to help disadvantaged children but it is of interest that they are associated with reduced simple sugar and increased starch and complex carbohydrate intakes (Worobey & Worobey, 1999), thus theoretically contributing to the prevention of obesity. Further, where nutrition has been assessed, breakfast programmes – but not lunch programmes which have small but significant positive effects on fatness – have been associated with shifts in the nutrition of participants towards the middle of the weight distribution and away from the extremes (Vermeersch et al., 1984).

Attention should also be paid to other meals, which are just as important as breakfast, though they are probably less easy to document if skipped. The goal should be to eat regular meals.

- Encourage meals as a family where time is taken eating, and satiety may come from a pleasant experience rather than overeating.
- Discourage undisciplined eating, that is snacking throughout the day rather than at defined 'snack' periods.
- Avoid snacking whilst watching television or playing on the computer.
- Avoid snacks with high refined carbohydrate and high fat content.
- Encourage snacks of whole fruit, raw carrots, celery or similar items.

Eat good food

Try to eat foods of known origin, that is home-prepared foods or foods whose nutrient content is known and:

- discourage food between meals,
- discourage food as reward,

- discourage sweetened commercially produced drinks;
- discourage added sugar in hot drinks;
- use added sugar sparingly;
- grill rather than fry, and add oil/butter/margarine to foods sparingly.

However:

- encourage plain water as a drink;
- consume whole fruit instead of fruit juice;
- eat wholemeal bread and cereals rather than white bread and refined cereals;
- teach children to read and understand the significance of food labels.

For children over 5 years, semi-skimmed milk can reduce energy intakes without having much effect on other nutrient intakes. However, semi-skimmed milk is not recommended for children under 5 years unless they take it as part of a balanced diet. Normal-weight children may depend significantly on the energy and micronutrient content of whole milk and thus find their overall energy and fat-soluble vitamin intakes reduced to marginal levels. Semi-skimmed milk is not advised for children less than 2 years old (Department of Health, 1994).

As a guide to the relative proportions of types of foods to be consumed at a meal, the plate model is easy to explain to children. Vegetables and fruit should cover about half the plate. Rice, pasta, bread and potatoes should cover a quarter of the plate. Fish, meat or eggs should cover a quarter of the plate.

12.6.2 School

Every school should have a policy on diet and nutrition. For instance a recent survey of state and public schools in Denmark showed that 5% of schools have installed carbonated drinks machines (Lissau & Poulsen, 2000). Healthier alternatives might have been cold-water dispensers.

Efforts to improve the quality of foods available in schools need supporting with nutrition education and cookery classes for both boys and girls. Nutrition education should encourage good nutrition for normal-weight as much as for obese children so that the focus is on *healthy eating* rather than *slimming*.

Nutrition education should also encourage children to read nutrient content tables on packaging, and should give children some understanding of the variation in nutrient content and energy density of foods, as well as of their own daily requirements. Then children may be able to interpret terms such as 'only 10% fat' in relation to the context under which they are quoted.

One area where schools may need dramatic change to put healthy living into practice is the school canteen. Many countries have had campaigns to improve the quality of food available in schools. 'Tuck' shops traditionally exist for sale of crisps (chips), sweets and sugary, carbonated drinks. Fresh fruits do not have the same shelf life and may not be eaten as easily. Thus, change can have significant cost implications which are not easily resolved. School dinners have often been planned with the nutrition of children who do not have enough to eat at home in mind. Such children may still benefit from a good school dinner in terms of energy, but the overall quality of many typical school meals leaves much to be desired, particularly in terms of the ratio of energy from fat and carbohydrate or from saturated and unsaturated fats.

Where they exist, recommendations for energy and fat intakes in school dinners should be reviewed, with concern for the epidemic of obesity amongst children as a high priority. In Norway, for example, the National Nutrition Council promotes well-organized school meals with increased fruit and vegetable consumption through national guidelines for school meals, supports research into best practice in running school cafeterias, promotes the traditional Norwegian packed lunch and has introduced a fruit and vegetable purchasing scheme in schools. All these activities have been backed by community and media propaganda exercises (Klepp et al., 1998). Schools need not only to *teach* healthy living but to *implement* healthy living (Snyder et al., 1999). This requires imaginative but effective programmes. Total and saturated fats in school meals were reduced by the CATCH (Child and Adolescent Trial for Cardiovascular Health) Eat Smart intervention in the USA, without effect on the total energy content of the meals (Osganian et al., 1996). Impressively, the effect remained after 3 years (Nader et al., 1999). This approach could solve the concerns of those who expect school meals to help the poorly nourished as well as the overnourished.

The quality of the diet and its energy density may impact on the effect of a meal as much as the total energy content. However, change will not be easy and, given prevailing societal attitudes to school meals and restrictions imposed by finite budgets, it will require the imagination, initiative and extraordinary willingness of all school staff, as well as the resources of parents, the wider community and local government to make these programmes effective.

12.6.3 Health profession

It is only relatively recently that nutrition, other than advice on infant feeding and the prevention of vitamin deficiencies such as rickets, has received much attention from health professionals. Recognition of the major health risks of overnutrition in adult life and other health concerns relating to 'westernized diets' has changed this. Good nutrition, beginning before conception, is now seen as protection against many conditions in later life. Health professionals, as those with the earliest opportunities to provide dietary advice for young children, need to promote all aspects of healthy lifestyles to families from their earliest contacts. Further, they should be lobbying governments on measures to improve national nutrition. They should be prepared to participate in policy-forming organizations, to advise governments and industry and to monitor progress and evaluate new initiatives in obesity prevention, particularly with children and young people.

12.6.4 Government

'Good' food is often perceived as expensive or difficult to obtain. This is particularly true for those living in deprived areas and without transport to reach large supermarkets. If governments and communities are genuine in their interest to improve the health of all through preventive measures, action needs to be taken to make good food more available to those who most need it and can least afford it. Local government should encourage local shops that are selling good food at reasonable prices. It should examine ways of facilitating access to fresh fruit, vegetables, wholemeal foods and low-energy forms of foods for those in poorer areas where choice in shops may be limited. This may necessitate either some form of support so that quality shops can move into an area, or the provision of supplemented transport to more distant supermarkets. What is needed will vary from country to country and from town to town within a country.

At the national level, governments can legislate on food labelling, food advertising and school food policies. They can encourage nutrition education and produce educational materials on healthy living and obesity prevention. They can sponsor research into obesity in childhood and its prevention.

Working women may need help in providing quality meals for their families. Subtle measures may be necessary to enable all busy carers to provide healthy lifestyles for their families. Somehow, governments should develop and support policies that will increase the opportunities for parents and children to make healthy food choices.

Food advertising is another area where governments may have a role which could be relevant in the fight to prevent obesity. This is perhaps an area where, within Europe, there could be international political consensus on what is ethical and acceptable in food advertising.

Through a similar wide-reaching concept, the European Union might be able to develop healthy-eating programmes and even legislation that could promote obesity prevention. The Common Agricultural Policy currently subsidizes farming to a considerable extent within Europe. In some countries, this has led to anomalies such as subsidized full-fat milk being cheaper than semi-skimmed milk – a disaster for policies to reduce fat intakes and to reduce overall energy intakes. A food policy more focused on healthy eating than on the financial success of the farming industry could make a real difference to patterns of eating throughout the Union and might also alter farming policies to general benefit.

12.6.5 Industry

The industry most involved in children's diets is, not surprisingly, the food industry. Children are an important market for food-marketing companies. According to the American Academy of Pediatrics, children and adolescents spent US$14.3 billion in 1991 and caused their families to spend US$128 billion on their behalf (Lipman, 1991). Opportunities for advertising through the media, particularly television, are immense. In the United States, 45% of children have their own television and 79% usually snack when viewing. There are 40 000 food related advertising spots per year (Lipman, 1991).

12.6.6 Television

As well as encouraging sedentary behaviour, television watching can also lead to snacking of high-fat foods. Most children eat when watching – mainly products advertised on television (Jeffrey et al., 1982). Parents should not let children eat while they are watching television, and instead should recommend them water to drink. Any food eaten should be low in fat, such as fruit and vegetables.

An additional disadvantage of television viewing is that children are assailed by advertisements for soft drinks and energy-rich foods, especially those rich in fat. A 1994 study analysed food advertising on five major television networks in the United States (ABC, NBC, CBS, Fox and Nickelodeon) during the Saturday-morning children's programmes (Kotz & Story, 1994). Between 8 a.m. and 12 noon, over the five networks, 564 food commercials appeared: 44% were for products that could be described as 'junk' foods, high in fat and/or sugar; 38% presented bread, cereals, rice or pasta; and 11% advertised fast-food restaurants. Only 4% of advertisements described milk, cheese or yoghurt and 1.4% concerned meat, poultry, fish or eggs.

The Food Pyramid suggested by the Saturday-morning children's programmes was compared with the US Department of Agriculture Food Guide Pyramid. The Saturday-morning Food Pyramid contained no vegetables or fruit, while fats, oils and sugars provided more than 50% of the energy. Bread, cereals, rice and pasta were also present, but were usually associated with sausages and fat. Dietz & Gortmaker (1993) emphasized the predominance of high-fat products in television food advertising.

Besides direct food advertising, some advertising messages come indirectly through films part-sponsored by commercial companies. The US Center of Study of Commercialism found that in 1990, more than 100 brand name products appeared in five top-grossing films (*Ghost, Pretty Woman, Home Alone, Total Recall* and *Teenage Mutant Ninja Turtles*) (Williams et al., 1993).

A second product-promoting industry has arisen from films and television. This is related to the first media advertising industry and uses products which are essentially the same but in different forms or wrappings representing familiar heroes, actors and pictures. For example, Dinosaur Candies were inspired by *Jurassic Park.* These products are widely promoted in supermarkets through mailing and television campaigns.

The pernicious influence of the food industry on child eating habits through television and film is a real concern, and television poses other problems as well. Health professionals need to publicize the dangers posed by the media and advertising and to press for government action to control this.

The American Academy of Pediatrics Committee on Communications (AAP, 1990) delivered a statement on the potentially negative influence of television viewing on the promotion of early sexual activity, drug and alcohol use, violent behaviour and obesity. The Academy proposed limiting television watching to a maximum of 1 or 2 hours per day. Food advertising and promotion programmes which targeted children and adolescents were blamed for the development of obesity. The Academy called for a ban on television food advertisements aimed at children because 'they exploit young minds and contribute to obesity' (Lipman, 1991).

In practice, it is doubtful whether an isolated measure like this could be expected to impact on such a massive health problem. Advertising reaches adults and children in many different ways.

12.7 Prevention programmes

Widespread changes in nutrition and lifestyle require long-term work, and are difficult to achieve. Successful community-health programmes on nutrition and fitness have been developed in the past in the United States and Finland (Puska et al., 1979; Leventhal et al., 1980). Can similar approaches still be effective in reducing the childhood obesity epidemic? One interdisciplinary obesity prevention programme has recently been tested in the USA (Caballero, 1999). Targeting American Indian children, the programme involved physical activity, dietary behaviour, classroom curricula and family involvement. It involved more than 2000 third-grade children in 41 schools in seven Amero-Indian communities. The 5-year full-scale phase has now been initiated and the project will be evaluated.

Too few programmes are soundly monitored. Where they are, it still seems that the impact of even soundly based programmes for the prevention of childhood obesity is, so far, very limited (Campbell et al., 2001).

12.8 Monitoring and evaluation

Monitoring overweight and obesity in children requires measuring height and weight and calculating body mass index regularly, as well as monitoring the areas of diet and activity which might have changed as a result of interventions. Without objective monitoring, changes could be due to universal changes over time rather than those resulting from programme interventions.

As understanding of the range of nutritional problems remaining or arising in westernized societies has increased, growth monitoring in childhood has also received increased prominence. Documentation of obesity, or of trends towards obesity, needs weight and height converting into relative BMI (or some other formula) and related to age/sex 'normal' values. This makes assessment more complicated than simply following whether children are gaining – or not gaining – weight. It becomes particularly difficult when children move into puberty, since expected size depends considerably on the individual's pubertal development at a particular age. It will need training and experience on the part of those who currently measure children in schools and clinics before screening for obesity or trends towards obesity is a valid process. However, there is currently no method of treatment which can guarantee cure or prevention of obesity. Moreover, compliance with treatment is poor even amongst those who recognize they have significant problems with obesity. Annual (for example) measurements of children may be valuable as a method of keeping track of changing prevalences in obesity and overweight, but *screening* for obesity is probably unwise since it is likely to lead to increased numbers of self-conscious obese children who are frustrated by treatment failures. Thus, we return to our view at the beginning of this chapter that programmes for prevention should be community-wide, multifaceted and involving lifestyle changes across societies.

12.9 Conclusions

Throughout this chapter we have tried to focus not solely on the '*what?*' of actions that can be taken to prevent obesity, but also on the '*how?*' and '*by whom?*' relating to such actions. This has highlighted the wide variety of people and groups who could be considered as having responsibilities for the prevention of obesity in children, if the more-or-less world-wide increase in childhood obesity is to be arrested. Apart from people to run them, programmes will require clear visions and goals. Initial programmes as small, manageable enterprises may be the most effective. Too often, the vision of a programme is seen in terms of preventing *all* childhood obesity. Yet, even a small reduction in the fatness of children across a community could have dramatic effects on health and on the prevalence of adult obesity, particularly if the preventive methods could be carried forward into adult life. The prevention of obesity should be recognized for what it is: a positive message to develop a healthy enjoyable lifestyle which provides greater physical and social well-being. In other words: 'Get a better life!'

It is our belief that the prevention of childhood obesity will only be achieved through wide-ranging community schemes which impact both on families and on the national consciousness. The first goal in this respect must be raising awareness, understanding, and public concern for the issue of childhood obesity. This book is our contribution towards that goal.

12.10 REFERENCES

Ajzen, I. & Fishbein, M. (1980). *Understanding Attitudes and Predicting Social Behavior*. Englewood Cliffs, NJ: Prentice Hall.

American Academy of Pediatrics Committee on Communications (1990). Children, adolescents, and television. *Pediatrics*, **85**, 1119–20.

Anderssen, N. & Wold, B. (1992). Parental and peer influences on leisure-time physical activity in young adolescents. *Research Quarterly for Exercise and Sport*, **63**, 341–8.

Anon (1997). Guidelines for school health programs to promote lifelong healthy eating. *Journal of School Health*, **67**, 9–26.

Bandura, A. (1998). *Self-Efficacy. The Exercise of Control*, pp. 79–111. New York: W.H. Freeman.

Basavaraj, S. (1993). Smoking and loss of longevity in Canada. *Canadian Journal of Public Health*, **84**, 341–5.

Benton, D. & Parker, P.Y. (1998). Breakfast, blood glucose, and cognition. *American Journal of Clinical Nutrition*, **67**, 772S–8S.

Biddle, S., Sallis, J. & Cavill, N., eds. (1998). *Young and active? Young people and health-enhancing physical activity – evidence and implications*. London: Health Education Authority.

Borra, S.T., Schwartz, N.E., Spain, C.G. & Natchipolsky, M.M. (1995). Food, physical activity, and fun: inspiring America's kids to more healthful lifestyles. *Journal of the American Dietetic Association*, **7**, 816–8.

Brugman, E., Meulmeester, J.F., Wekke, S.V.D. & Verloove-Vanhorick, P.S. (1998). Breakfast-skipping in children and young adolescents in the Netherlands. *European Journal of Public Health*, **8**, 325–8.

Burniat, W. & Van Aelst, C. (1993). Therapeutic approach to childhood obesity. *Nutrition Research*, **13**, 117–32.

Butcher J. (1986). Longitudinal analysis of adolescent girls' aspirations at school and perceptions of popularity. *Adolescence*, **21**, 133–43.

Caballero, B (1999). Obesity in American Indian Schoolchildren: pathways. *American Journal of Clinical Nutrition*, **69**, 745–815.

Campbell, K., Waters, E., O'Meara, S. & Summerbell, C. (2001). Interventions for preventing obesity in children (Cochrane Review). In *The Cochrane Library*, Issue 1, 2001. Oxford, Update Software.

Casado Gorriz, M.R., Casado Gorriz, I. & Diaz Gonzales, G.J. (1999). *Revista Espagna Salud Publica*, **73**, 501–10.

Department of Health (1994). *Weaning and the weaning diet*. London: HMSO, p. 54.

Dietz, W.H. & Gortmaker, S.L. (1985). Do we fatten our children at the television set? Obesity and television viewing in children and adolescents. *Pediatrics*, **75**, 807–12.

Dietz, W.H. & Gortmaker, S.L. (1993). TV or not TV: fat is the question. *Pediatrics*, **91**, 499–501.

Friestad, C. & Klepp, K.I. (1997). Roking, kroppsbilde og slankeatferd. Tre ars oppfolgning av ungdom I alderen 15–18 ar. *Nordic Medicine*, **117**, 334–8.

Garcia, A.W., Broda, M.A., Frenn, M., Coviak, C., Pender, N.J. & Ronis, D.L. (1995). Gender and developmental differences in exercise beliefs among youth and prediction of their exercise behavior. *Journal of School Health*, **65**, 213–9.

Hernandez, B., Gortmaker, S.L., Colditz, G.A., Peterson, K.E., Laird, N.M. & Parra-Cabrera, S. (1999). Association of obesity with physical activity, television programs and other forms of video viewing among children in Mexico city. *International Journal of Obesity*, **23**, 845–54.

Jeffrey, D.B., McLellarn, R.W. & Fox, D.T. (1982). The development of children's eating habits: the role of television commercials. *Health Education Quarterly*, **9**, 174–89.

Kelder, S.H., Perry, C.L., Lytle, L.A. & Klepp, K.I. (1995). Community-wide youth nutrition education: long-term outcomes of the Minnesota Heart Health Program. *Health Education Research*, **10**, 119–31.

Kemper, H.C., Post, G.B., Twisk, J.W. & van Mechelen, W. (1999). Lifestyle and obesity in adolescence and young adulthood: results from the Amsterdam Growth And Health Longitudinal Study (AGAHLS). *International Journal of Obesity*, **23** Suppl. 3, S34–40.

Kjøller, M., Rasmussen, N.K., Keiding, L., Petersen, H.C. & Nielsen, G.A. (1995). Sundhed og sygelighed i Danmark – og udviklingen siden 1987: rapport fra DIKEs repraesentative undersøgelse blandt voksne danskere [The Danish Health and Morbidity Survey 1994. A report from DICE's representative survey among adults in Denmark]. Copenhagen: Danish Institute for Clinical Epidemiology (DICE).

Klepp, K.I., Andersen, L.F., de Paoli, M., Halvorsen, M. & Bjornboe, G.E. (1998). Tiltak for a fremme sunne kostvaner blant skoleelever. *Tideskrift Norvege Laegeforen*, **118**, 3306–9.

Klesges, R.C., Shelton, M.L. & Klesges, L.M. (1993). Effects of television on metabolic rate: potential implications for childhood obesity. *Pediatrics*, **91**, 281–6.

Kotz, K. & Story, M. (1994). Food advertisements during children's Saturday morning television programming: are they consistent with dietary recommendations? *Journal of the American Dietetic Association*, **94**, 1296–300.

Leventhal, H., Safer, M.A., Cleary, P.D. & Gutmann, M. (1980). Cardiovascular risk modification by community-based programs for life-style change: comments on the Stanford study. *Journal of Consulting and Clinical Psychology*, **48**, 150–8.

Lipman, J. (1991). Pediatric academy prescribes ban on food ads aimed at children. *Wall Street Journal*, July 24, B82.

Lissau, I. & Poulsen, J. (2000). En Landsdaekkende undersoøgelse af vilkår ogrammer for mad og måltider i skoler og fritidshjem/SFO'er. [A national survey of nutrition and meals in public and state Schools and in after school care. A national survey in Denmark.] National Institute of Public Health and National Board of Health.

Lissau, I. & Sørensen, T.I. (1992). Prospective study of the influence of social factors in childhood on risk of overweight in young adulthood. *International Journal of Obesity*, **16**, 169–75.

Lissau, I. & Sørensen, T.I.A. (1994). Parental neglect during childhood and increased risk of obesity in young adulthood. *Lancet*, **343**, 324–7.

Lissau, I., Breum, L. & Sørensen, T.I.A. (1993). Maternal attitude to sweet eating habits and risk of overweight in offspring: a ten-year prospective population study. *International Journal of Obesity*, **17**, 125–9.

Lissau, I., Thoning, H., Poulsen, J. & Rasmussen, N.K. (2001). Copenhagen Municipality's Health Profile 2000. National Institute of Public Health, Denmark.

Lloyd, B., Lucas, K. & Fernbach, M. (1997). Adolescent girls' construction of smoking identities: implications for health promotion. *Journal of Adolescence*, **20**, 43–56.

Moore, L.L., Lombardi, D.A., White, M.J., Campbell, J.L., Oliveria, S.A. & Ellison, R.C. (1991). Influence of parents' physical activity levels on activity levels of young children. *Journal of Pediatrics*, **118**, 215–9.

Murphy, J.M., Pagano, M.E., Nachmani, J., Sperling, P., Kane, S. & Kleinman, R.E. (1998). The relationship of school breakfast to psychosocial and academic functioning: cross-sectional and longitudinal observations in an inner city school sample. *Archives of Pediatric and Adolescent Medicine*, **152**, 899–907.

Nader, P.R., Stone, E.J., Lytle, L.A., Perry, C.L., Osganian, S.K., Kelder, S., Webber, L.S. et al. (1999). Three-year maintenance of improved diet and physical activity: the CATCH cohort. Child and Adolescent Trial for Cardiovascular Health. *Archives of Pediatric and Adolescent Medicine*, **153**, 695–704.

Nicklas, T.A., Webber, L.S., Srinivasan, S.R. & Berenson, G.S. (1993). Secular trends in dietary intakes and cardiovascular risk factors of 10-y-old children, the Bogalusa Heart Study (1973–1988). *American Journal of Clinical Nutrition*, **57**, 930–7.

Osganian, S.K., Ebzery, M.K., Montgomery, D.H., Niklas, T.A., Evans, M.A., Mitchell, P.D., Lytle, L.A. et al. (1996). Changes in the nutrient content of school lunches: results from the CATCH Eat Smart Food Service Intervention. *Preventive Medicine*, **25**, 400–12.

Parsons, T.J., Power, C., Logan, S. & Summerbell, C.D. (1999). Childhood predictors of adult obesity: a systematic review. *International Journal of Obesity*, **23** Suppl. 8, S1–107.

Power, C., Lake, J.K. & Cole, T.J. (1997). Measurement and longterm health risks of child and adolescent fatness. *International Journal of Obesity*, **21**, 507–26.

Prescott, E.I., Osler, M., Heim, H.O., Borch-Johnson, K., Schnohr, P. & Vestbo, J. (1999). Rygning middellevetid blandt danske maend og kvinder. *Ugerskr Laeger*, **161**, 1261–3.

Puska, P., Tuomilehto, J., Salonen, J., Neittaanmaki, L., Maki, J., Virtamo, J., Nissinen, A., Koskela, K. & Takalo, T. (1979). Changes in coronary risk factors during comprehensive five-year community programme to control cardiovascular diseases (North Karelia project). *British Medical Journal*, **2**, 1173–8.

Sallis, J.F., Nader, P.R., Broyles, S.L., Berry, C.C., Elder, J.P., McKenzie, T.L. & Nelson, J.A. (1993). Correlates of physical activity at home in Mexican-American and Anglo-American preschool children. *Health Psychology*, **12**, 390–8.

Schlundt, D.G., Hill, J.O., Sbrocco, T., Pope-Cordle, J. & Sharp, T. (1992). The role of breakfast in the treatment of obesity: a randomized clinical trial. *American Journal of Clinical Nutrition*, **55**, 645–51.

Shannon, B., Peacock, J. & Brown, M.J. (1991). Body fatness, television viewing and calorie intake in a sample of Pennsylvania sixth grade children. *Journal of Nutrition*, **23**, 262–8.

Siega-Riz, A.M., Popkin, B.M. & Carson, T. (1998). Trends in breakfast consumption for children in the United States from 1965 to 1991. *American Journal of Clinical Nutrition*, **67** (suppl.), 748S–56S.

Snyder, P., Anliker, J., Cunningham-Sabo, L., Dixon, L.B., Altaha, J., Chamberlain, A., Davis, S. et al. (1999). The Pathways study: a model for lowering the fat in school meals. *American Journal of Clinical Nutrition*, **69** (suppl.), 810–5S.

Stucky-Ropp, R.C. & DiLorenzo, T.M. (1993). Determinants of exercise in children. *Preventive Medicine*, **22**, 880–9.

Tappe, M.K., Duda, J.L. & Menges-Ehrnwald, P. (1990). Personal investment predictors of adolescent motivational orientation toward exercise. *Canadian Journal of Sports Science*, **15**, 185–92.

Tobin, D.S., Dwyer, J. & Gussow, J.D. (1992). Cooperative relationship between professional societies and the food industry: opportunities or problems? *Nutrition Reviews*, **50**, 300–6.

US Centers for Disease Control and Prevention (1996). *Physical activity and health*. Atlanta, GA: International Medical Publishing, p. 1.

US Centers for Disease Control and Prevention (1997). Guidelines for school and community programs to promote lifelong physical activity among young people. *Morbidity & Mortality Weekly Report*, **46**, 1–36.

Vermeersch, J., Hanes, S. & Gale, S. (1984). The national evaluation of School Nutrition Programs: program impact on anthropometric measures. *American Journal of Clinical Nutrition*, **40** Suppl. 2, 414–24.

Whitaker, R.C., Wright, J.A., Pepe, M.S., Seidel, K.D. & Dietz, W.H. (1997). Predicting obesity in young adulthood from childhood and parental obesity. *New England Journal of Medicine*, **337**, 869–73.

Williams, J.D., Achterberg, C. & Sylvester, G.P. (1993). Target marketing of food products to ethnic minority youth. *Annals of the New York Academy of Sciences*, **699**, 107–14.

Wiseman, C.V., Turco, R.M., Sunday, S.R. & Halmi, K.A. (1998). Smoking and body image concerns in adolescent girls. *International Journal of Eating Disorders*, **24**, 429–33.

Wold, B., Øygard, L., Eder, A. & Smith, C. (1994). Social reproduction of physical activity. *European Journal of Public Health*, **4**, 163–8.

World Health Organization (1998). *Obesity. Preventing and managing the global epidemic.* Report of a WHO Consultation on Obesity, Geneva, 3–5 June 1997. Geneva: World Health Organization, p. 1 (document WHO/NUT/NCD/98.1).

Worobey, H.S. & Worobey, J. (1999). Efficacy of a preschool breakfast program in reducing refined sugar intake. *International Journal of Food & Science Nutrition,* **50**, 391–7.

Zakarian, J.M., Hovell, M.F., Hofstetter, C.R., Sallis, J.F. & Keating, K.J. (1994). Correlates of vigorous exercise in a predominantly low SES and minority high school population. *Preventive Medicine,* **23**, 314–21.

13

Home-based management

Elizabeth M.E. Poskitt

International Nutrition Group, London School of Hygiene and Tropical Medicine

13.1 Introduction

The treatment of obesity has a depressing reputation. The reported levels of success are low at all ages (Serdula et al., 1993; Lake et al., 1997) with many obese children continuing life as obese adults. Yet, most of us know overweight or obese individuals, both adults and children, who slimmed successfully without formal 'treatment' and who have continued to maintain normal physique. Data suggest that, particularly amongst younger obese children without an obese parent, spontaneous slimming is a frequent occurrence (Whitaker et al., 1997). Thus there seems something anachronistic about the effect of treatment in obesity.

13.1.1 Goals of slimming

One of the reasons why the outlook for the treatment of obesity has such a poor reputation is a lack of definition of what is perceived as successful treatment. Ideally, the return to, and maintenance of, normal fatness would be the goal of all treatment. However, many children and adults are so obese before they embark on treatment that to return to normal fatness may be an impossible dream. Too often, clinicians are confronted by totally unrealistic expectations: the social and nutritional crisis created by an obese girl's appointment as bridesmaid in 8 weeks time, for example. Failure to achieve normal body weight in time is seen as total failure of the slimming process. Yet ... Mission Impossible?

The goal of all weight-control programmes should be some reduction in excess fat even if this does not result in normal nutrition. Evidence suggests that even modest reductions in excess fat can reduce health risks (Epstein et al., 1989; Pidlich et al., 1997). However, fat reduction needs to be achieved through sustainable programmes compatible with normal social interaction. This is especially true with obese children and adolescents, where the development of healthy lifestyles which continue after contact with clinic and/or practitioner have ceased should be the highest priority in management. To achieve slimming which is transient and introduces children to lifetimes of 'yo-yo' type weight cycling is not helpful.

13.1.2 Can we do any good by formalizing slimming?

There have been suggestions that the more the obese are involved in formal slimming programmes, the less likely they are to be successful slimmers (National Task Force on the Prevention and Treatment of Obesity, 1994; Wardle, 1996). However, the poor reputation of weight-loss programmes may have a simpler explanation. The concept that obesity and overweight result from too much food and too little exercise is quite well understood in most of the westernized world. Many people also have some understanding of the foods which contribute significantly to the energy content of their diets. Efforts to slim frequently begin without any professional involvement and some, perhaps even many, of these 'self-help' slimmers succeed in their aims to lose weight – and seek no further advice. Thus, those *seeking* help could be predominantly those who have difficulty complying with well-known recommendations for weight reduction (reduced energy intake, increased activity etc.) or those who have obesity which is, for one reason or another, relatively unresponsive to simple slimming measures. If this is so, the obese subjects seeking help for weight reduction will then be, almost by definition, those for whom success with treatment is least likely.

Data on the prevalence of obesity and overweight in childhood support the view that many obese children do slim successfully, either spontaneously during the physiological changes in body composition which take place with growth, or as the result of family instituted measures. Correlations between obesity in young children and in adult life are not very strong (Whitaker et al., 1997). Physiological slimming – normal growth-related reduction in the proportion of body weight which is fat – occurs most markedly between 1 and 5 years and during the male pubertal growth spurt. It is likely that some obese children lose their excess fat during these periods. Indeed, the bad prognosis for obesity which *develops* between 1 and 5 years – the 'early adiposity rebound' (Rolland-Cachera et al., 1984) – may only indicate that children who fatten at ages when the physiological tendency is to *reduce* the proportion of body fat are subject to unusually strong environmental and/or genetic pressures to become obese and are thus highly likely to develop intractable obesity.

The corollary to the suggested association between failure to slim and slimming programmes might seem that the less children are involved in the slimming process, the more successfully they will slim. We cannot support this assumption. The significant point may be that relatively modest but sustainable changes in lifestyles may have more long-term impact on obesity than radical regimens which achieve rapid change but which make long-term adherence difficult.

13.1.3 The part played by the family

Families of children who are significantly obese should be encouraged to seek nutritional help and advice. It is usual to involve obese children in the slimming process and to develop their commitment to the programme of management as much as their age and maturity allow. This is very necessary with children of secondary school age (11 + years) whose lifestyles offer them plentiful access to food outside the home and who must therefore exercise dietary self-control. Indeed, information from school may even be brought back to educate the parents in nutrition (Basdevant et al., 1999). However, Golan et al. (1998) have shown, with obese children aged 5–11 years, that directing the education and management advice at the parents is more effective, in terms of weight loss and slimming, than directing the education at the children. So, how much should parents be involved in their children's slimming?

Parents will need to initiate changes in diets and lifestyles with young preschool children. The obese adolescent, at the other end of the childhood spectrum, has plenty of opportunity, both at home and away from home, to access food without parental involvement. In adolescence, particularly, parental strictures on diet and lifestyle may be greeted with unhelpful antagonism and refusal to comply (Birch & Fisher, 1998). Truswell & Darnton-Hill (1981) have characterized what they view as the particular features of adolescent food habits. They suggest common features which differ either in kind or in degree from children at other ages:

• missing meals and generally erratic meal patterns;
• snacking (especially high sweet consumption);
• unconventional meals;
• beginnings of alcohol consumption;
• excessive consumption of cult soft drinks;
• strong likes/dislikes of socially popular foods – often of very high energy content;
• frequent low micronutrient intakes;
• fashion for self-designed 'diets' which may be nutritionally inappropriate.

Clearly many of these habits do not fit easily with a healthy lifestyle. Adolescents will need to make their own decisions on diet and lifestyle changes. It is however important that parents have knowledge and understanding of obesity and its control, so they can advise, support and encourage their adolescent children by whatever means appropriate. Family shopping must make low-energy-density foods available – so as to encourage moderated intakes by children helping themselves from cupboards and refrigerators. In many families of obese children, the whole family will benefit from adopting 'healthy' lifestyles to support their obese children's efforts.

Much can be done safely without recourse to medical services, private groups or clinics. With the current epidemic of obesity overwhelming several westernized countries (Livingstone, 2000), societies will need to develop 'self-help' skills in obesity management.

13.1.4 Risks of treatment

Another anachronistic attitude to slimming suggests that it is dangerous to slim obese children because they are at risk of anorexia nervosa, a condition carrying a significant mortality risk. If the prognosis for the cure of childhood obesity is as poor as reported, anorexia nervosa must be a rare complication *of obesity*. Over many years of running obesity clinics, I have not encountered any anorexic children, or even children seeming to be close to anorexia, amongst the hundreds of obese children we have advised. The determination with which the typical anorexic pursues dietary restraint seems very alien to obese children who diet – and lose weight – with great difficulty. However, the concern for the development of anorexia nervosa in some children because of introducing children to dieting is a serious one. A characteristic of anorexia nervosa is abnormal body image. The abnormal perceptions of children developing anorexia nervosa and envisaging themselves obese when, at the most, they are of normal fatness may have led to histories of fat children slimming into anorexia. Inappropriate programmes for the prevention or treatment of obesity may strengthen disturbed children's desires for unnecessary slimming. There is a very real risk that societal overconcentration on slimness, thin body image and diet will precipitate anorexia in nonobese children who already have distorted body images and some anorexic traits. This is a further reason to develop slimming programmes which adopt family-based lifestyle changes, which avoid undue emphasis on dieting, and which are compatible with normal health and weight maintenance in the nonobese members of the family.

13.2 Principles of modifying lifestyles to encourage slimming in obese children

All this presumes that there are effective ways of slimming children which can be applied effectively by the families of obese children without recourse to medical or nutritional advice. It is my belief that there are effective family-led or primary-care measures which could be successful in many cases. How successful they are remains unknown since, by definition, those adopting these practices are usually acting outside research or other documented programmes. The recommendations in this section of the book are thus based more on logical speculation and – it is hoped – common sense rather than on evidence-based practice. Our methodology may be unfashionable, but it could possibly be helpful!

13.2.1 What are the aims of slimming programmes?

Energy expenditure must exceed energy intake

The basis of all slimming recommendations must be to alter the energy balance of obese individuals so that energy expenditure exceeds energy intake. Negative energy balance must continue for a significant period of time, in many cases for months or years, if it is to succeed in reducing obese individuals to normal fatness.

Success is *some* fat loss rather than loss of *all* excess fat

Normal fatness may be an almost impossible goal for the significantly obese. However, any reduction in fatness, if sustained, should improve health, fitness and longevity (Epstein et al., 1989; Pidlich et al., 1997). Thus, success can be perceived as either the attainment of a body of normal fatness or as achieving sufficient reduction in body fatness to enhance well-being, self-esteem and physical fitness.

Slimming is fat loss but not always weight loss

Slimming is almost universally equated with weight loss. For adults, weight loss is almost invariable with slimming. However, children grow and at certain stages in life (early infancy, the preschool years and during the adolescent growth spurt) grow very rapidly. Fat loss can thus be compatible with no loss of weight or even slight weight gain. Many slimming recommendations for children do recognize this by aiming for no weight gain, rather than for weight loss. Such an outcome is acceptable, provided parents and children understand and accept no weight gain as a goal, and provided obese subjects are not close to, or already over, ideal weight for their expected adult height.

Avoid overindulgence in weighing

Weighing, although a traditional component of obesity management, should be used very sparingly. It is a great boost to a child's morale if weighing shows weight loss. However, this has to be balanced against the potential for distress and demoralization if the scales report 'no change', or even weight gain, when a child has been struggling with diet and increased activity.

Home scales are rarely very accurate. Weighing should be done at the same time of day (preferably early morning before breakfast) and in the same light clothing, with weights written down each time so that memory does not 'cheat'. Weighing once a week is the maximum frequency we can recommend and weighing once a month may be more realistic in terms of evaluating what is being achieved by slimming practices. Without all these provisos, weight changes may mislead. Parents can often guess how successful their young children are with slimming by observing lifestyle changes carefully. However, parents may be misled by the very different lifestyles children may adopt at school. Also, parental skills in objective assessment of children's progress vary.

'Slimming' should not damage family dynamics

Slimming practices should interfere as little as possible with normal life. Fat loss is likely to be more sustainable if achieved slowly, since gradual changes in body mass index (BMI) are more likely to be due to loss of fat mass than loss of lean tissue. However, body composition changes which take place very slowly are likely to lead to disillusion since 'slimming' is usually equated with weight loss, and children may feel the efforts they have put into slimming are not rewarded. There is a fine balance – varying from individual to individual – between lifestyle changes which interfere little with daily life but which, nevertheless, have positive effects on nutritional status, and changes which have more marked effects on nutritional status but which create unsustainable fat loss and/or intervene awkwardly with normal family life.

13.3 What can be recommended?

13.3.1 Activity

For many, an instruction to increase exercise and activity is interpreted as taking up vigorous sporting exercise: running, tennis, football, squash. However, the current epidemic of obesity in the westernized world has not arisen simply because we have stopped playing these sports but because we are less active than previous generations in many aspects of daily life. We walk less. We do less physical work in our employment or at home in house and garden. We spend more of the day sitting. In addition, we live in much warmer homes and work environments. Children walk less in order to get to school or play with friends. Much out-of-school activity now involves television, video or computer games. The home environment does not allow children to visit friends or play in the streets as safely as in the past. Thus, changes in activity must try to restore some of the background activity that was part of life in previous generations. Formal physical activity rarely occupies more than an hour or so each day at the most and, if it is taken in short sharp bursts of vigorous exercise, may involve anaerobic metabolism which has less fat-mobilizing effect than prolonged sustained activity (Saris, 2000). Thus, modest increases in activity which are 'around the clock' can be as effective, or more effective, in producing fat loss than formal sports sessions. For those obese individuals with poor cardiorespiratory fitness, moderate increases in activity are likely to be more acceptable than what is often, to them, the misery of under-achieving on the football field or in the gym.

Some obese children are quite 'sporty' and are neither embarrassed by, nor bullied about, their appearance, but many are very self-conscious. The need to undress in order to participate in school sports, particularly swimming, may inhibit them. Fat arms and thighs rubbing together under the sweaty conditions of 'sport' may be physically very uncomfortable. Thus, whilst all efforts to increase activity in slimming programmes are important, obese children may only begin to show interest in sport when they have lost some fat, have developed a sense of achievement by slimming, and have also improved cardiorespiratory fitness, so it is physically more comfortable to exercise. If children have dropped out of participation in sport, it is unkind, and likely to be unhelpful, to force them to participate in what may be utter misery to them. Explaining to teachers that these children need positive and supportive comments on their sporting efforts can encourage full sports participation by obese children.

13.3.2 Suggestions for increasing energy expenditure without dramatic lifestyle changes

Epstein and his team (Epstein et al., 1995; Epstein & Goldfield, 1999) in Buffalo, USA, have been in the forefront of developing programmes which aim to control or reduce adiposity in childhood by reducing sedentary activities. The concept of *decreasing inactive behaviour*, rather than *increasing physical activity*, may be helpful to obese children who have recognized their physical unfitness and are consequently shy about joining their peer groups in formal physical activity. However, attempts to reduce obesity through reduced sedentary activity are most likely to be successful if at least one parent is involved in the slimming programme and if that parent, and others, contribute to positive reinforcement of those behavioural changes which reduce inactive and sedentary behaviours (Epstein, 1996). The following are possible ways in which energy expenditure in exercise may decrease sedentary behaviour in obese children:

- Use public transport in preference to family cars, since public transport usually involves at least a little walking to and from bus stops.
- Cycle, if it is safe on the roads, rather than use a car for longer distances (cycling can be quite awkward for the very obese and sympathetic support may be needed to get children on to bicycles).
- Use stairs rather than lifts (elevators), or walk up escalators. If the number of floors which must be ascended is impractical by stairs, walk some of the flights. If this is a regular climb, try to increase gradually the number of flights walked – walk up three flights and then four flights next time. Always walk downstairs.
- Encourage helpful attitudes which can lead to activity. The obese children need to become the children who willingly jump up to fetch and carry for others. They should be encouraged to go up and downstairs frequently, rather than delaying actions until there are several reasons for going upstairs.
- Perhaps be more tolerant of fidgeting?

- Encourage children to participate in family domestic activities: washing up, bed making, tidying the bedroom.
- Encourage gardening and interest in growing vegetables. Encourage lawn mowing if the mower and age of the child are suitable.
- Encourage hobbies. Ideally, hobbies should be active and energy consuming. However, any hobby is helpful if it diverts children's attention from food and from watching television (an activity recognized as a major risk for 'grazing'), and if it leads to improved self-confidence and self-esteem through achievement, constructive activity and perhaps succeeding with something others cannot do.
- Reduce home heating levels. If this is done very gradually – by a few degrees at a time – it will not be very noticeable. It not only encourages individual energy expenditure in heat generation but also saves money and helps preserve the environment.
- Consider restricting time spent watching television or allowing television/video watching and computer time only after certain active tasks (Saelens & Epstein, 1998; Goldfield et al., 2000).

13.4 Eating and diet

The development of a healthy lifestyle must include changes in both what is eaten and how it is eaten. Children should become more aware of what they eat and when they eat. If eating takes time and if it takes place in association with other 'satisfying' events, satiety may be achieved at lower energy intakes. Food should become something consumed in family meals and recognized snack periods rather than something used to combat 'boredom'.

13.4.1 Lifestyle changes in feeding patterns which may help fat reduction

- Plan eating so that food is eaten to avoid hunger rather than as a time-filling event.
- Eat only at mealtimes and recognized snack periods.
- Eat, if possible, as a family so there is social intercourse and time is spent during the meal waiting for others to be served. This may contribute to satisfaction from a meal and psychophysiological satiety.
- Discourage eating in front of the television, or snacking when playing/working with the video or computer.
- Select 'whole foods' or raw unprocessed foods whenever possible and prepare and cook meals at home.
- Raw ingredients, rather than foods bought already prepared, make it easier to see what is being consumed. Many prepared foods are cheaper than their raw ingredients due to supplementation with starches and fats.

- It is more time consuming to eat whole foods, for example apples compared with apple juice or apple puree. This helps satiety. Wholemeal bread is of similar energy content to white bread, but may have greater satiety effect and can be a little more substantial to chew.
- Drink water rather than fruit juices, or carbonated drinks. Drinks with 'sweeteners', even though lower in energy than those with sugar, may encourage a 'sweet tooth' and should be avoided.

13.4.2 Changing the family diet

There are a number of changes which can be made to the family diet without necessarily reducing the volume of food eaten and which may not make the reduced-energy nature of a diet very noticeable. However, changes which involve more wholefoods can be difficult for some children to accept if they have become obese partly because of strong dislikes of vegetables, fruit, wholemeal bread or unsweetened drinks. In my experience, such 'faddy' children are very common amongst the obese and quite difficult to help unless they are prepared to make some dietary concessions.

It is important that children have the significance of dietary changes explained to them. Many will be prepared to try to cooperate, particularly if dietary changes are introduced gradually and in ways which make them attractive. Dietary changes are unlikely to be successful, particularly with older children, if they are imposed forcefully. They are also unlikely to be successful if they are regarded as something special for the obese child and not part of more general changes in the family diet. Children – quite correctly – have difficulty understanding why they are denied certain foods which their obese parents eat unrestrainedly in front of them.

In some parts of Europe, perhaps most notably the UK, cooking at home is largely confined to deep frying or heating prepared meals in the microwave. The ability to create attractive salads without drenching them with oily dressings, to cook vegetables so they are pleasant to eat, to know how to boil, grill or steam foods instead of heating them in the microwave or deep frying, are skills which many of today's mothers have never learnt. They are also skills which may determine whether a family adopts happily to 'healthy' eating or eats healthily only under pressure.

13.4.3 Changes in the energy content of diets which have little impact on the volume of food consumed

- Avoid sweetened drinks. Try to encourage drinks which have no sweet taste rather then 'low calorie' drinks sweetened with artificial, calorie-free sweeteners, which may encourage sweet tooth and can cause diarrhoea because of the side effects of some sweeteners.

- Recognize that 'whole' fruit juice contains a lot of energy in one glass.
- Use semi-skimmed milk. This is not usually recommended for normal children under 2 years but is probably safe for overweight and obese children, even those under 2 years, since the main concern for young children drinking semi-skimmed milk lies in its low energy content. This milk is also only recommended for children between 2 and 5 years as part of a balanced diet. The low fat content of semi-skimmed milk makes it a less good source of fat soluble vitamins than full-cream milk. It is important to make sure children on semi-skimmed milks are receiving other sources of fat-soluble vitamins (such as fortified low-energy margarines).
- Use low-fat margarines and spreads.
- Use low-fat yoghurts, salad creams, soups and so on. Make sure they are not only low in fat but also lower in total energy than the normal versions of the food. Some low-fat foods (e.g. some low-fat yoghurts) have extra carbohydrate and, although different in composition, are no less energy dense than the original foods.
- Avoid sugared or chocolate-coated cereals. Encourage wholemeal cereals (their fibre content may be beneficial) but recognize that they may be quite energy dense. Muesli, with dried fruit and nuts, can be surprisingly energy dense, given its 'healthy' image.
- Use wholemeal breads and flours. They are not lower in energy than more refined flours but low-energy diets are sometimes perceived as constipating. Wholemeal flours and breads should help prevent this.
- Grill, boil or steam foods rather than fry. Avoid adding butter or other fats and oils to cooking.
- Avoid thickening gravies and stews.
- Discuss school dinners with child and school. Aim for meat and vegetables, but no chips and no fried foods, or choose salads without oily dressings. Fresh fruit and low-energy yoghurts are useful as 'puddings'.
- Stew fruit without added sugar. Very, very small amounts (tip of a teaspoon) of sodium bicarbonate added to fruit before cooking may remove some of the 'acidity' of soft fruits such as rhubarb, gooseberries and even stewed apple. Sweetening agents dissolved in warm water can be added to the cooked fruit but it is probably better to avoid encouraging a desire for sweetness.
- Avoid biscuits, chocolate bars, crisps and other energy-dense snacks at break (and other) times. Changing snacks may be the most difficult aspect of the whole slimming effort and needs handling sympathetically, particularly since peer-group pressure to eat, or unkind teasing, may accompany snack avoidance. Snacks of apples or oranges (bananas are of quite high energy content) or even of raw carrot and celery strips are helpful (if acceptable!).

- Avoid using food as reward – especially energy-dense treats as reward for keeping to some aspect of the diet.
- Encourage the child to persist in dietary modification but supportively. Recognize how difficult dietary modification can be. Parents should be encouraged to acknowledge that if they cannot pursue a diet themselves, they should not blame their children for also failing – even if the children have the more severe obesity.

13.5 Conclusions

Successful slimming requires imagination in order to make the subtle changes which are acceptable to families but which do make sustainable and effective changes to diet and lifestyle. Unfortunately, costs and availability of some foods, particularly fresh fruit and vegetables, vary around countries and according to the time of year. Whilst the initial efforts to reduce the current epidemic of obesity lie in individual choice, it is essential that local and national governments, schools, supermarkets and local shops make healthy diets and active lifestyles accessible, practical and affordable for families. Governmental and private enterprises need to create more consumer outlets for healthy living, as well as helping individual choice through health and nutrition education, if the current epidemic of obesity sweeping the western world is to be contained and conquered.

13.6 REFERENCES

Basdevant, A., Boute, D. & Borys, J.M. (1999). Who should be educated? Education strategies: could children educate their parents? *International Journal of Obesity*, **23** Suppl. 4, S10–S13.

Birch, L.L. & Fisher, J.O. (1998). Development and eating behaviors among children and adolescents. *Pediatrics*, **101**, 539–49.

Epstein, L.H. (1996). Family based behavioral interventions for obese children. *International Journal of Obesity*, **20** Suppl. 1, S14–S21.

Epstein, L.H. & Goldfield, G.S. (1999). Physical activity in the treatment of childhood overweight and obesity: current evidence and research issues. *Medical Science of Sports and Exercise*, **31**, S553–9.

Epstein, L.H., Kuller, L.H., Wing, R.R., Valoski, A.M. & McCurley, J. (1989). The effect of weight control on lipid changes in obese children. *American Journal of Diseases in Children*, **143**, 454–7.

Epstein, L.H., Valoski, A.M., Vara, L.S., McCurley, J., Winiewski. L., Kalarchian, M.A., Klein, K.R. & Shrager, L.R. (1995). Effects of decreasing sedentary behavior and increasing activity on weight change in obese children. *Health Psychology*, **14**, 109–15.

Golan, M., Fainaru, M. & Weizman, A. (1998). Role of behaviour modification in the treatment of childhood obesity with the parents as the exclusive agents of change. *International Journal of Obesity*, **22**, 1217–24.

Goldfield, G.S., Kalakanis, L.E., Ernst, M.M. & Epstein, L.H. (2000). Open loop feedback to increase physical activity in obese children. *International Journal of Obesity*, **24**, 888–92.

Lake, J.K., Power, C. & Cole, T.J. (1997). Child to adult body mass index in the 1958 British birth cohort: association with parental obesity. *Archives of Disease in Childhood*, **77**, 356–81.

Livingstone, B. (2000). Epidemiology of childhood obesity in Europe. *European Journal of Pediatrics*, **159** Suppl. 1, S14–S34.

National Task Force on Prevention and Treatment of Obesity (1994). Towards prevention of obesity: research directions. *Obesity Research*, **2**, 517–84.

Pidlich, J., Pfeffel, F., Zwiauer, K., Schneider, B. & Schmindinger, H. (1997). The effect of weight reduction on the surface electrocardiogram: a prospective trial in obese children and adolescents. *International Journal of Obesity*, **21**, 1018–23.

Rolland-Cachera, M.F., Deheeger, M., Bellisle, F., Sempe M., Guilloud-Bataille, M. & Patois, F. (1984). Adiposity rebound in children: a simple indicator for predicting obesity. *American Journal of Clinical Nutrition*, **39**, 129–35.

Saelens, B.E. & Epstein, L.H. (1998). Behavioral engineering of activity choice in obese children. *International Journal of Obesity*, **22**, 275–7.

Saris, W.H.M. (2000). Athletics. In *Human nutrition and dietetics*, 10th edn., eds. J.S. Garrow, W.P.T. James & A. Ralph, pp. 471–80. Edinburgh: Churchill Livingstone.

Serdula, M.K., Ivery, D., Coates, R.J., Freedman, D.S., Williamson, D.F. & Byers, T. (1993). Do obese children become obese adults? A review of the literature. *Preventive Medicine*, **22**, 167–77.

Truswell, A.S. & Darnton-Hill, I. (1981). Food habits of adolescents. *Nutrition Reviews*, **39**, 73–88.

Wardle, J. (1996). Obesity and behaviour change: matching problems to practice. *International Journal of Obesity*, **20** Suppl. 1, S1–S8.

Whitaker, R.C., Wright, J.A., Pepe, M.S., Seidel, K.D. & Dietz, W.H. (1997). Predicting obesity in young adulthood from childhood and parental obesity. *New England Journal of Medicine*, **337**, 869–73.

Dietary management

Margherita Caroli[1] and Walter Burniat[2]

[1]Nutrition Unit, Department of Prevention, Brindisi. [2]University Hospital for Children 'Reine Fabiola', Free University of Brussels

14.1 Introduction

Why diet? Obesity is the consequence of a patchwork of environmental factors and specific genetic and biological features. Nutrition is only one environmental factor, albeit an important one (Chapter 4). In this chapter we:

- review studies presenting with dietary programmes from the 1950s;
- discuss and compare the evolution of the nutritional procedures;
- evaluate the positive and negative effects of dieting;
- propose nutritional guidelines related to different clinical situations.

14.2 History of dietary therapy

In 1957, Hoffman reported on the treatment of 60 obese children and adolescents, 30 boys and 30 girls (age range 5.4–16.3 years). The average excess weight was respectively, 47.9% and 42.9% above average for the age. The dietary instructions were those of a classic low-calorie diet. At 4 months, mean weight losses were 27% (range: 7.3–66.4%) body weight in boys and 18.3% (range: 3.5–51.8%) body weight in girls. The wide range in individual weight losses can be appreciated in this early paper and remains a feature of most more recent studies. Hoffman's 1957 paper can be considered a pioneering study but it is quite empirical and confused. The author limited fruit intakes with the aim of avoiding 'simple sugar'. Various anorexigenic drugs were prescribed. These were largely dexedrine sulphate and amphetamine but in some cases combined with amylobarbital. So, it is not clear how much the diet or the drugs were the main determinants of the weight losses observed. Further, there were no follow-up data.

Following Hoffman's paper and until the end of the 1970s, a number of other publications appeared presenting the effects of low-calorie diets (LCD) and/or simple nutritional counselling. On the whole, results were disappointing, with only a quarter of obese children treated with classical LCD as outpatients showing good short-term results.

In view of the poor results of LCDs, medical teams developed very-low-calorie diets (VLCDs) for young obese patients. Heyden & De Marsa (1973) reported on early results. VLCDs were used without any specific selection criteria. The use was based on the perceived benefits of rapid weight loss, the effects of ketonaemia in suppressing hunger, the effects of absence of hunger on improving compliance, the maintenance of weight loss, and reduced drop-out rates. However, most reports evaluated short-term results only, and others only after short-term treatment. Obesity was not considered a chronic condition and it was thought that rapid weight-loss would facilitate weight-loss maintenance. This latter was not the case. The consequent disappointment experienced by both patients and professionals stimulated new therapeutic approaches for use with, or instead of, diet and led to the current wide range of treatments and equally wide range of outcomes.

14.3 Aims of dietary treatment

The main aims of dietary treatment are to achieve healthy body weight, and to develop the eating habits which enable maintenance of healthy body weight during growth and in adult life.

In order to maintain healthy weight, energy intake and energy expenditure need to be balanced. Thus, we could outline a period of intensive dietary treatment, lasting usually less than 1 year, to produce suitable weight loss, followed by long-term dietary recommendations – a balanced diet – to be followed for life. However, as stressed earlier in this book (Chapters 3 and 5) energy balance equations are complicated by individual genetic and metabolic factors – as well as by variation in individuals' motivation.

Although weight loss is the most obvious outcome of successful obesity treatment, it is not the only desired outcome. Obesity is an important factor in the development of cardiovascular disease and other chronic noncommunicable disorders (Chapters 7 and 11). Most of these are benefited by even relative small losses of excess fat.

Dietary modifications which range from straightforward nutritional counselling to VLCDs, remain the cornerstone – however controversial – in the management of obesity. Finding 'the best solution' by comparing the reported results on different dietary regimens is not easy because of heterogeneity in dietary design and subject selection, lack of a common definition of obesity, lack of information on visit frequency, treatment duration, energy or nutrient intake, and, frequently, the absence of control groups or long-term follow-up.

14.4 Types of diet

The types of dietary approach in common use are:
- simple nutritional counselling (SNC) or balanced normal-calorie diet (BNCD);
- balanced low-calorie diet (BLCD);
- very-low-calorie diet (VLCD).

14.4.1 Simple nutritional counselling or balanced normal-calorie diet

The aim of SNC is to achieve energy and nutrient intakes appropriate for age, height and lifestyle (i.e. a BNCD). Although this should allow normal weight gain and growth in obese children it often leads to static weight, perhaps because basic energy requirements of large obese children are above the recommended average.

14.4.2 Balanced low-calorie diet

In BLCDs, the energy intakes assessed from Recommended Dietary Allowances (RDA) or Dietary Reference Values (DRV) are reduced by about one-third. Nutrient content remains balanced with 20%, 30–35% and 45–50% energy derived from protein, fat and carbohydrate respectively. An outline of such a daily regimen is presented in Table 14.1. Generally, BLCDs do not need supplementation with minerals and vitamins (Burniat & Van Aelst, 1993; Figueroa-Colon et al., 1993). These diets are used over widely varying periods of time: from 12 weeks (Figueroa-Colon et al., 1993) to more than 6 months (Burniat & Van Aelst, 1993). The duration of the treatment can influence results (the longer the treatment, the higher, we hope, the weight loss) and drop-out rates (the longer the treatment, the more subjects drop out). Burniat & Van Aelst (1993) have reported a large BLCD study with a long-period of follow-up. In this study the maximum decrease in body mass index (BMI) was observed between 6 and 12 months. Only 10% of children were still attending follow-up after 18 months, although this figure was 20% for those who attended at least three medical sessions. It was of interest that 75 children who followed the diet for more than 6 months and who successfully lost weight presented 3-day dietary records suggesting energy intakes lower than at entry to the study, although higher than prescribed by the clinician.

There is no general agreement on the definition of a BLCD. Some studies which state that a BLCD was used quote energy intakes which were reduced by more than one-third of the RDA (Di Toro et al., 1997; Epstein et al., 1985). Other studies in which BLCDs have been used omit specific information on the energy and nutrient content of the diet used (Becque et al., 1988).

Another method of approaching BLCD diets, and one which is widely used, is the 'traffic-light diet' (Epstein et al., 1985; Graves et al., 1988; Senediak & Spence,

Table 14.1. Outline of a typical balanced low-calorie diet (BLCD) for a school-age child

Daily food plan

Breakfast	Cereal, semi-skimmed milk, no extra sugar. Or slices of bread, bread rolls, thin scrape of low-energy margarine, ham or other low-energy delicatessen or low-fat cheese. Coffee, tea, semi-skimmed milk (if not added to cereal) or fruit juice.
Break	Fresh fruit or fruit juice.
Lunch	Soup or salad vegetables, slices of bread or sandwiches, low-energy delicatessen, vegetables, fresh fruit.
Home	Low-energy yoghurt or low-fat white cheese or cereal with semi-skimmed milk.
Supper	Soup or salad vegetables, lean meat (grilled or boiled), fish, chicken (skinned), vegetables (large amounts), no sauce, small portion of boiled potatoes, rice or noodles, fresh fuit or low energy pudding (home made).

Intended energy and nutrient intake

Energy	65% RDA for age
Protein	20% of energy
Fat	30% of energy
Carbohydrate	50% of energy
P/S ratio	0.8–1.0
Water	at least 1.5 ml/(kcal day)
Fibre	15–20 g/day

P/S ratio: ratio of polyunsaturated to saturated fat.

1985; Duffy & Spence, 1993). This groups foods into categories according to structured eating pattern to meet age recommendations. Green colour means 'go' – these foods may be consumed in unlimited quantities. Yellow means 'caution' and red, 'stop' – because of a particularly high fat or simple carbohydrate content. This approach is close to the widely used 'food-guide pyramid'. However, many papers reviewing traffic-light diets concentrate on psychological parameters and outcomes and pay little attention to nutritional intakes or nutritional outcomes.

The value of BLCDs is thought to be partly educational in view of the 'balanced' nutrition they are designed to provide. However, there are no data on subjects' change in long-term nutritional knowledge resulting from the use of BLCDs alone. Further, although BLCDs are claimed to be safe and nutritionally adequate, very few studies have examined their effects on lean body mass (LBM) and protein nutritional status (Caroli et al., 1991; Figueroa-Colon et al., 1993; Di Toro et al., 1997). No study has followed nitrogen balance during a BLCD. Since nutrient metabolism and, consequently, the adequacy of nutrient intakes can be modified by the reduced energy intakes of dieting obese subjects, the nutritional safety of a diet can only be determined by objective analysis of various parameters of nutritional status before, during and after dieting. This has been done only rarely with obese children following BLCD regimens. It is thus impossible to comment objectively on potential negative consequences of BLCDs in the treatment of childhood and adolescent obesity.

14.4.3 Very-low-calorie diet

Very-low-calorie diets provide 800 kcal/day or fewer (Wadden et al., 1983). They can be partially balanced (protein (P) 25%, fat (F) 30%, carbohydrate (CHO) 45%), or unbalanced (P 66%, F 24%, CHO 10%). This latter style of diet is described as a protein-sparing modified fast (PSMF) because it is supposed to spare lean body mass (LBM), while producing rapid loss of weight. The PSMF is the most widely used VLCD in the treatment of childhood obesity.

The protein-sparing effect can be explained using the metabolic fuel cycle regulatory system (Flatt & Blackburn, 1974). In physiological conditions, insulin decreases the release of free fatty acids (FFA) from adipocytes by reducing cyclic AMP (adenosine monophosphate) – mediated activation as well as by increasing glycerol phosphate availability for FFA re-esterification. During starvation the reduction of insulin serum level is associated with a high release of FFA from adipocytes, which can be utilized as metabolic fuel by several organs and tissues. The absence of carbohydrate intake, together with the increased fat catabolism, produces high levels of ketones which are utilized as metabolic fuel by the brain (which cannot utilize FFA as fuel). Due to these modifications, the consumption of glucose by the brain is reduced and, consequently, the need for gluconeogenesis from amino acids also declines. Thus, starvation ketosis is the main mechanism preserving body protein during fasting. If obese subjects are allowed some additional food, instead of being kept on total fast, the changes in fuel metabolism will differ according to the kind and the amount of food consumed.

An intake of additional protein will cause a very slight increase in serum insulin, which will not interfere with ketogenesis. A protein intake equal to requirements for age and sex will balance amino acid catabolism and reduce nitrogen losses.

The VLCD and, in particular, the PSMF (Table 14.2), can be composed of normal, natural protein-rich foods such as lean meat, fish, fowl or eggs (Merritt et al., 1980; Caroli et al., 1992; Figueroa-Colon et al., 1993). Alternatively, they can be prepared as special formulas which incorporate powdered protein from different sources (Brown et al., 1983; Widhalm & Zwiauer, 1987). When PSMFs are prescribed, vitamin and mineral supplements are usually added (Merritt et al., 1980; Caroli et al., 1992; Figueroa-Colon et al., 1993), although these diets do not seem to require the addition of all micronutrients (Di Toro et al., 1997). Initially,

Table 14.2. Outline of a standard protein-sparing modified fast (PSMF)

Daily food plan

Breakfast	Tea or coffee + artificial sweetener.
Lunch	Chicken or turkey, or lean beef, veal, lamb, or fish (roasted, boiled or baked); ham. Vegetables raw or boiled and dressed with lemon, vinegar, spices as desired.
Break	Raw vegetables such as tomatoes, salad etc.
Dinner	Chicken or turkey, or lean beef, veal, lamb, or fish (roasted, boiled or baked); ham. Vegetables raw or boiled and dressed with lemon, vinegar, spices as desired.

Intended energy and nutrient intake

Energy	10.6 kcal/(kg IBW day)
Protein	66% of energy
Fat	24% of energy
Carbohydrate	10% of energy
P/S ratio	0.6
Water	at least 1.5 litres/day
Fibre	15–20 g/day

IBW: ideal body weight; P/S ratio: ratio of polyunsaturated to saturated fat.

PSMFs were used for only 2 or 3 weeks, and then in metabolic wards (Pencharz et al., 1980, 1988). Now, use has been extended to periods of 2–3 months and to outpatient clinics with once-a-week or twice-a-week medical supervision and controls. Following PSMF, patients are advised on diets leading to a gradually increasing energy intake until they return to 'normal' balanced diets (Caroli et al., 1992; Figueroa-Colon et al., 1993). As with studies of BLCDs, comparisons of VLCD studies in terms of efficiency and safety are difficult to make. Studies vary in terms of sampling, duration of treatment, and quality and quantity of the diet (sources of calories, protein, supplementation or not with fat and/or carbohydrate and with minerals and vitamins).

When VLCD liquid formulas were first introduced adult deaths were reported amongst diet consumers, apparently because the formulas were not complete in all essential nutrients. No lethal accidents have been reported since introduction of new liquid formula nor in those taking VLCDs based on natural food (Wadden et al., 1983). VLCDs are generally prescribed only to extremely obese subjects but, since VLCD liquid formulas are available without medical prescription in many countries, there is a risk that they will be used by people who do not need such intensive energy restriction (Garrow, 1989). In Table 14.3 we review the results of studies in which BLCD and VLCD treatments were prescribed.

Table 14.3. Short term weight loss in clinical studies of obese children and adolescents using BLCDs and VLCDs in out patient settings

Authors	Subjects (n, sex, age)	Diet + other treatments	Time	Obesity initial	Obesity final	Weight lost (kg)	Drop out
BLCDs							
Burniat & Van Aelst 1993	571 (242M, 329F) M 11 ± 2.4 years F 10.3 ± 2.9 years	BLCD 65% of RDA (4.2 MJ/day)	6–12 mo.	M 156 ± 21% BMI F 151 ± 21% BMI	3 mo.: −5.0 ± 7.2% BMI 3 mo.: −5.0 ± 7.3% BMI	NR	241 (42.2%)
Caroli et al. 1991	10 (3M, 7F) 14.24 ± 2.17 years	4.2 MJ/day + systemic approach (1000 kcal/day)	9 wk	137.7 ± 12.7% EBW	119.7 ± 12.4% EBW	8.09 ± 1.8	NR
Deschamps et al. 1978	37 (20M, 17F) 6–16 years	4.2–6.3 MJ/day (1000–1500 kcals/day)	3mo.	+3.3 SD EBW	+1 SD EBW	NR	5 (13.5%)
Di Toro et al. 1997	33 (15M, 18F) 8.8 ± 3.1 years	BLCD 60% of RDA	13 wk	160 ± 20% EBW	137 ± 15% EBW	NR	NR
Endo et al. 1992	13 (6M, 7F) 12–14 years	5.1MJ (1200 kcal)/day + structured exercise	4 wk	143–710% EBW	−8.4 ± 2.5% initial BW	NR	0
Epstein et al. 1985	23 F 8–12 years in two groups	(A) TLD 3.78–5.1 MJ (900–1200 kcal)/day + exercise (B) ditto but no exercise	2 mo.	148 ± 23.2% EBW	130.7 ± 21.5% EBW	4.46	1
Figueroa-Colon et al. 1993	9 (4M, 5F) 11.3 ± 3.3 years	4.2 MJ (1000 kcal)/day	2 mo. 10 wk	148 ± 17.6% EBW 178 ± 19.6% EBW	136.2 ± 19% EBW −13.8 ± 7.7% initial wt	3.18 5.1 ± 4.1	NR
Hills & Parker 1988	10 (NR) age NR	Nutrition information + exercise	16 wk	51.6 ± 2.68 kg	46.1 ± 2.46 kg	5.05	NR
Valverde et al. 1998	245 (116M, 129F) 9.3 (1–17.1) years	Nutrition information	12 mo.	161.5% BMI	155.6% BMI	+4.6[a]	47 (19.2%)

VLCDs

Caroli et al. 1992	13 children 8.8 ± 1.4 years 11 adolescents 15.5 ± 2.4 years	PSMF + Echosystemic approach	8 wk	153.9 ± 17.2% EBW 147 ± 9.7% EBW	123.8 ± 14.4% EBW 126.7 ± 8.9% EBW	7.8 ± 2.2 9.8 ± 1.8	6 (18.7%) of the total
Caroli et al. 1994	27 children (12M, 15F) 9.2 ± 1.8 years 38 adolescents (13M, 25F) 14.3 ± 1.69 years	PSMF + echosystemic approach	9 wk	159.8 ± 20.3% EBW 161.9 ± 22.3% EBW	130.5 ± 18.6% EBW 136.3 ± 18% EBW	8.9 ± 2.2 11 ± 3.1	NR
Figueroa-Colon et al. 1993	10 (4M, 6F) 11.5 ± 2 years	PSMF (2.5–3.4 MJ/day) + exercise + behaviour modification	10 wk	182.2 ± 25.6% EBW	− 29.5 ± 7.4% initial wt	11.2 ± 4.4	NR
Stallings et al. 1988	17 (4M, 13F) 15 ± 1.4 years	PSMF	3 mo.	154.2 ± 15.3% EBW	125.2 ± 16.6% EBW	13 ± 0.3	NR
Stallings & Pencharz 1992	7 (2M, 5F) 13.8 ± 1.3 years	PSMF	8 wk	160 ± 13% EBW	142 ± 14% EBW	13.5 ± 4.7	NR

BLCD: balanced low calorie diet; TLD: traffic-light diet; VLCD: very-low-calorie diet; PSMF: Protein Sparing Modified Fast; EBW: Expected body weight; NR: not reported; BMI: body mass index; M: male; F: female.

[a] weight gain, but over the course of 1 year and loss in relative weight and percentage BMI.

14.5 Consequences of dieting

14.5.1 Positive consequences

The positive effects of dieting can be summarized as follows:
- fat mass reduction and healthier body fat distribution;
- reduced plasma lipid and apolipoprotein levels;
- enhanced insulin sensitivity and glucose tolerance;
- reduced blood pressure.

Fat mass reduction and healthier body fat distribution

The most obvious result of treatment for obesity is reduced fat mass. Table 14.3 presents clinical studies on obese children and adolescents treated with BLCD or VLCD programmes. We could presume that the lower the calorie intake, the higher the weight loss should be. Thus a logical conclusion is that VLCDs cause higher weight losses than BLCDs. However, there are also other factors which need to be considered as possible causes for the higher weight losses obtained with VLCDs. One factor could be the structure of the diet itself. Whilst the prescription of BLCDs is often based on a food exchange system in which the patients are free to choose their own daily food, VLCDs require stricter prescription of the kind and amount of food allowed daily. This could modify adherence to either diet and possibly affect weight losses (Wadden, 1993). Another consideration is that greater involvement with medical services through frequent check-ups can influence compliance positively and again affect short-term results (Valverde et al., 1998). Amongst the different groups treated with BLCDs, variations in the frequency of clinic visits could also be partially responsible for variations in weight loss. However, other reasons could also be variations in the age of subjects and in the tools other than diet (exercise, psychological approaches) used in the studies. Even the total number of obese children treated could be relevant (Epstein et al., 1985; Caroli et al., 1991; Endo et al., 1992; Burniat et al., 1993).

Weight losses obtained with VLCDs are more homogeneous than those observed amongst BLCD treated groups. However, as we have already stated, total weight loss is only one very short-term indicator of the benefits of the diet. For example, there are differences in fat mass distribution between subcutaneous and abdominal adipose tissue. Excess abdominal fat is well documented as associated with metabolic complications in obese adults. It is not known whether body fat distribution in obese children is also a significant risk factor for later morbidity. However, abdominal fat deposits in adolescents are associated with more frequent cardiovascular pathologies, hyperinsulinaemia and dyslipidaemia (Wabitsch et al., 1992; Flodmark et al., 1994; Caprio et al., 1995). Thus, the young obese with central adiposity should be particularly benefited by dieting and losing excess fat.

Moreover, it has been shown that adolescents with central adiposity, recognized by a high waist/hip ratio, lose more abdominal fat than subcutaneous deposits with dietary management. As a consequence they show significant metabolic improvements as well (Wabitsch et al., 1994). It is of interest that in a study by Ginsberg-Fellner & Knittle in 1981, only children with low total adipocyte number before dietary treatment showed stable lower body weight on 10-year follow-up.

Reduced plasma lipids and apolipoprotein levels

Abnormalities of serum lipids are often present in obese children and adolescents. Such abnormalities include high total cholesterol, low-density-lipoprotein cholesterol (LDL-C), triglycerides (TGL) and low high-density-lipoprotein cholesterol (HDL-C) serum levels. All these are more common in adolescents affected by central adiposity (Flodmark et al., 1994; Caprio et al., 1996). Falls in serum total cholesterol and TGL levels correlate with percentage weight loss. Epstein et al. (1989) also demonstrated that when weight is regained cholesterol and TGL serum levels return to the pretreatment values. Apolipoprotein B/A1 ratio is viewed as a marker for coronary artery disease. In children, it has also been speculated that this ratio could detect those prone to a higher probability of developing atherosclerosis later (Perosa et al., 1988). Thus an important positive result of a dietary treatment in obese children and adolescents is a fall in apolipoprotein B/A1 ratio even with only 4 weeks of dieting (Endo et al., 1992). A reduction in serum total cholesterol, LDL-C, and triglycerides levels, without reducing serum HDL-C is obtained with both BLCD (Epstein et al., 1989; Endo et al., 1992; Wabitsch et al., 1994) and VLCD regimens (Zwiauer et al., 1988; Caroli et al., 1992). Yet, the only aspects these diets have in common are reduced fat intakes. Certainly, in some of the more detailed studies, researchers have stressed the dietary importance of lowering total cholesterol consumption and enhancing the polyunsaturated to saturated fatty acid ratio. Such a diet design is well known as being effective in reducing total serum cholesterol, LDL-C and the TGL levels. However, it has never been proven that cholesterol-lowering diets, per se as opposed to global lowering of energy intakes, produce these positive changes in obese children and adolescents when they lose weight. Cholesterol levels are also dependent on the rate of natural production of cholesterol by the liver, which is only indirectly related to the diet.

Obesity in children and adolescents is often associated with enhanced insulin sensitivity and glucose tolerance (Chiumello et al., 1969). These findings are more common in children from families with a history of diabetes (Martin & Martin, 1973) and in adolescent females with central adiposity (Caprio et al., 1995). Falls in plasma insulin with weight loss show positive correlations with the degree of obesity before treatment, the severity of the hyperinsulinaemia, and the size of weight loss with treatment. In addition, weight loss with dieting has been positively correlated with the severity of both hyperinsulinaemia and obesity before dieting (Deschamps et al., 1978).

Both BLCDs (Deschamps et al., 1978; Knip et al., 1988; Wabitsch et al., 1994) and VLCDs (Brook & Lloyd 1973; Caroli et al., 1992) are effective in decreasing baseline serum levels and improving the glycaemic response to an oral glucose load. Even with long-term follow-up, provided the weight loss is maintained, serum insulin levels remain lower (Knip & Nuutinen, 1993). As with obese adults, weight loss improves insulin sensitivity and glucose tolerance in insulin-resistant obese children and adolescents. As these studies report various types of dietary management and different methods of evaluating insulin sensitivity, it is again impossible to assess which diet will lead to the best clinical and biochemical outcomes. Nevertheless, whatever the diet, loss of at least some excess fat seems to improve glucose–insulin metabolism.

Reduced blood pressure

Excess body weight correlates directly with both a high systolic blood pressure (SBP) and a high diastolic blood pressure (DBP) (Horswill & Zipf, 1991). As with adults, obesity in childhood and adolescence is accompanied by a significant prevalence of high blood pressure (Burns et al., 1989). Blood pressure tracks from childhood to adulthood and thus childhood obesity contributes to increased risk of cardiovascular disease in adult life (Lauer et al., 1991). Obese children and adolescents often show hyperinsulinaemia with alterations in the renin–angiotensin system with enhanced renal absorption of sodium and decreased natriuresis (Hall, 1997). Blood pressure in obese children and adolescents is thus highly sensitive to sodium intake. Obese adolescents do show significant reductions in blood pressure when they change from high- to low-salt diets, whilst blood pressure in normal-weight adolescents is largely unresponsive to changes in dietary intake of sodium (Rocchini et al., 1989). Many studies have demonstrated that weight loss, even if slight, improves blood pressure in the obese (Becque et al., 1988; Hoffman et al., 1995). Blood pressure remains lower at least 1 year later, provided weight loss is maintained (Brownell et al., 1983; Figueroa-Colon et al., 1993). However, if there is further weight gain, blood pressure will rise again (Brownell et al., 1983). Weight loss has more impact on the SBP than the DBP. The higher the blood pressure before dieting, the greater the reduction in SBP with weight loss (Brownell et al., 1983). Both BLCDs and VLCDs, when followed consistently, are effective in reducing the SBP of obese children and adolescents (Brownell et al., 1983; Becque et al., 1988; Figueroa-Colon et al., 1993). Nevertheless, the therapeutic approaches that include increased activity as well as reduced energy intakes, produce the best results by decreasing resting SBP and exercise

DBP (Rocchini et al., 1988). To some extent, this reaffirms our belief in the multi-faceted treatment of childhood obesity.

Reducing excess weight, even if it leaves young individuals still overweight, results in significant metabolic and clinical improvements. These are the consequences of fat loss rather than the benefits of specific diets, since several different dietary programmes are associated with improvements in the same aspects of health status.

14.5.2 Negative consequences

The negative effects of dieting can be summarized as follows:

- loss of lean body mass;
- slowing of linear growth;
- anorexia and binge eating;
- increased serum uric acid;
- gallstones.

Lean body mass loss

A major concern about the effects of dieting on obese children and adolescents, is loss of lean body mass (LBM) as a consequence of negative nitrogen and energy balance. Nitrogen balance and protein dynamics have been studied many times during treatment with VLCDs but rarely during treatment with BLCDs. Also, PNS (protein nutritional status) has rarely been compared for different groups of obese children using BLCDs and VLCDs (Caroli et al., 1991; Figueroa-Colon et al., 1993; Di Toro et al., 1997). The problems with evaluation are of the kind we have already mentioned: a variety of study protocols; variable intervals between pre- and postdiet evaluation; variation in the subjects studied. Table 14.4 lists studies which have evaluated PNS and LBM in overweight children. Table 14.5 shows the studies on the effects of treatment on PNS and LBM in obese children and adolescents treated with BLCDs or VLCDs. It cannot be claimed that BLCDs do not cause LBM loss but the extent to which they affect PNS and LBM in obese children and adolescents is not clear either. VLCDs produce both negative nitrogen balance and LBM loss in the first 2–3 weeks of dieting. On longer follow up, the few available data suggest that LBM and PNS stabilize rather than continue to decrease (Merritt et al., 1980; Brown et al., 1983; Stallings et al., 1988; Caroli et al., 1994). The percentage of loss in LBM is shown in Table 14.5. Differences could depend on the method applied (Archibald et al., 1983; Brown et al., 1983). Lean tissue estimations using TB^{40}K (total body ^{40}K potassium) show the highest percentage loss of LBM. However, all the potassium loss is presumed to originate in LBM, but potassium is also present in glycogen at the ratio of 0.45 mmoles of K to each gram

Table 14.4. Studies of protein nutrition and lean body mass following dietetic treatment in obese children and adolescents

Author	Subjects	Diet	Period	Methods	Results
Archibald et al. 1983	17 (M4 F13) 15 ± 1.3 years OW% 58 ± 16.3	PSMF 2 g P/(kg day)	3 mo.	1. Skinfolds: formula 2. TB[40]K 3. TB N (prompt γ-ray analysis)	1. 7.3% reduction in LBM 2. 13.2% reduction in LBM 3. No change
Brown et al. 1983	8 (M4 F4) 13.8 ± 3.7 years OW% 113 ± 27.9	PSMF Optifast 70 formula®	5 wk, follow-up at 5 mo.	1. TB[40]K 2. 3 Methylhistidine	1. 36% reduction after the first 5 wk 10% reduction between 5 wk and 5 mo. 2. No increase in basal values after 5 wk
Caroli et al. 1992	24 (24F) 11.9 ± 3.9 years OW% 51 ± 13.4	PSMF 1.8 g P/(kg day)	9 wk	1. Skinfolds: Frisancho formula 2. Serum protein	1. No change 2. No change in Alb and Som C Reduction in C3 and TTrans
Caroli et al. 1994	65 (25M 40F) 12.7 ± 3.8 years OW% 60.8 ± 21.4	PSMF 1.8 g P/(kg day)	9 wk	1. Skinfolds: Frisancho formula 2. Serum protein	1. 6% LBM loss in adolescents 2. No change in Alb and Prealb Reduction in C3 and TTrans at 15 days then stable to 9 wk
Caroli et al. 1998	31 (13M 18F) 14.6 ± 2.9 years	PSMF 1.8 g P/(kg day)	9 wk, control	1. Skinfolds: Slaughter–Lohman formula	1. Increase in LBM
Dietz & Schoeller 1982	9 (6M 3F) 14.6 ± 1.7 years OW% 86.7 ± 27.5	PSMF (a) 1.5 g P/(kg day) + Fat (b) 1.5 g P/(kg day) + C	3 wk	1. N balance 2. Serum protein	1. Nitrogen losses 39.5 g (a), 10.8 g (b) 2. (a) Alb, RBP no change, TTrans reduced (b) Alb, RBP, TTrans no change
Merritt et al. 1980	16 (10M 6F) 12.9 years OW% 80 ± 6	PSMF 1.4–3 g P/(kg day)	4 wk	N balance	Total nitrogen loss by 4th week: 28.8 g Main loss during first 3 wk: 29.5 g
Merritt et al. 1983	8 (6M 2F) 11–15 years OW% 91.8 ± 20.3	PSMF 2–3 g P/(kg day) (a) P + Fat (400 kcal) (b) P + C (400 kcal)	3 wk	N balance	(a) No reduction (b) Stable

Study	Subjects	Diet	Duration	Methods	Results
Pencharz et al. 1980	5 (2M 3F) 18.6 ± 1.4 years OW% 96 ± 25.5	PSMF 1.5 g P/(kg day)	4 wk	1. N balance 2. Whole-body N turnover	1. No change 2. No change
Pencharz et al. 1988	16 (M3 F13) 14.4 ± 0.9 years OW% 49 ± 11	PSMF 2.5 g P/(kg day)	18 d	1. N balance 2. P turnover by labelled amino-nitrogen	1. No change 2. Adaptive changes in urea – end products evident after first week. Change in ammonia – end product evident until 18th day
Schwingshandl & Borkenstein 1995	41 (19M 22F) 11.6 ± 1.7 years OW% 51 ± 20	500–1000 kcal/day P 20% Fat 30% C 50%	3 wk	BIA	Very heterogeneous LBM change: 19 subjects increased LBM 22 subjects decreased LBM
Stallings et al. 1988	17 (4M 13F) 15 ± 1.4 years OW% 58 ± 16.3	PSMF 2–2.5 g P/(kg day)	3 mo.	1. 4 Skinfolds Durnin or Brook formula 2. TB^{40}K 3. TB N (prompt γ-ray analysis)	1. 8.7% reduction in FFM at 3 mo. no change in FFM at 1 year 2. 19% reduction at 3 mo. 13% reduction at 12 mo. 3. 14.3% reduction only at 12 mo.
Stallings & Pencharz 1992	7 (2M 5F) 13.8 ± 1.3 years OW% 66 ± 13	PSMF 2–2.5 g P/(kg day)	8 wk	1. Skinfolds 2. TB^{40}K 3. TBW (^{18}O) 4. ECW (by bromide space)	1. 9% reduction in FFM 2. No change 3. No change 4. No change
Wabitsch et al. 1996	146 (NR) 12.7 ± 3 years BMI 28.8 ± 4.8	1033 ± 125 kcal day P 26% Fat 18% C 56%	40 d	BIA	5.7% reduction in LBM
Widhalm & Zwiauer 1987	8 (3M 5F) 12 ± 2.5 years OW% 78.5 ± 23	VLCD P 55% Fat 3% C 42% Modifast formula®	3 wk	N balance	Positive N balance at 3rd week, except one patient. High interindividual variability

PSMF: Protein Sparing Modified Fast; LBM: Lean Body Mass; TB^{40}K: Total body ^{40}K; TB N: Total Body Nitrogen; Alb: Albumin; Som C: Somatomedin C; TTrans: Total Transferrin; RBP: Retinol Binding Protein; FFM: Fat Free Mass; BIA: Bioimpedence Analysis; TBW: Total Body Water; ECW: Extracellular Water; OW: overweight; P: protein; C: carbohydrate; M: male; F: female.

Table 14.5. Studies of protein nutrition and lean body mass in children on VLCDs and BLCDs

Authors		Subjects		Diet	Time	Method		Results
Caroli et al. 1991	(A)	10 (3M, 7F) age 14.2 ± 2.2 years OW% 37.7 ± 12.7	(A)	BLCD 1.000 kcal/day	9 wk	Serum protein	(A)	No change in Alb, TTrans Reduction in C3
	(B)	13 (4M, 9F) age 14.8 ± 1.8 years OW% 46.35 ± 17.4	(B)	VLCD 600 kcal/day	9 wk		(B)	No change in Alb, TTrans or C3
Di Toro et al. 1997	(A)	33 (15M, 18F) age 8.8 ± 3.2 years OW% 60 ± 20	(A)	BLCD 60% RDA	13 wk	1. Skinfolds + Frisancho formula 2. Serum protein 3. Serum Fe, Zn and Cu	(A)	Reduction in C3 No change in Fe, Zn or Cu
	(B)	22 (13M, 9F) age 12.6 ± 2.6years OW% 64 ± 22	(B)	PSMF 25% RDA	10 wk		(B)	Reduction in C3 and LBM No change in Fe, Zn or Cu
Figueroa-Colon et al. 1993	(A)	9 (4M, 5F) age 11.3 ± 3.30 years OW%78.3 ± 19.6	(A)	BLCD 1000 kcal/day	10 wk	1. Skinfolds + Harsa formula	(A, B)	No change in LBM Visceral protein serum level in normal range
	(B)	10 (4M, 6F) age 11.5 ± 2 years OW% 82.2 ± 25.6	(B)	PSMF 1.8–2.5 g P/(kg day)	10 wk	2. Serum protein		

BLCD: balanced low-calorie diet; VLCD: very-low-calorie diet; PSMF: protein sparing modified fast; Alb: albumin; TTrans: total transferrin; LBM: lean body mass; OW: overweight; M: male; F: female.

of glycogen. Glycogen is the first energy source depleted in the early phases of any diet. Thus K loss at the beginning of any diet, but particularly a VLCD, includes the loss of glycogen-bound K. Thus, K loss estimations can distort estimates of body composition during dieting. For example, a loss of 200 g of glycogen results in about 90 mmoles of K loss; since each kilogram of LBM is associated with about 60 mmol K. This could be misinterpreted as a loss of at least 1.5 kg LBM (Kreitzman, 1992).

Obesity is associated with increased LBM for height, age and sex. The LBM loss occurring with VLCDs seems to be within the 'safe' range, since 'safe weight loss' is deemed a loss of no more than 25% total weight loss as LBM. A reduction of LBM at this level can be viewed as loss of excess lean tissue or regression towards the mean (Archibald et al., 1983; Stallings et al., 1988), rather than as a disadvantage of the diet. Further, since the lower LBM and PNS do not fall below the mean for age, sex and height, weight loss seems to lead to the development of a new steady PNS. This new equilibrium is set at a lower level than in the obese state, but remains within the normal range.

Reduced linear-growth velocity

Obesity is considered by some as the main cause for growth acceleration in early childhood and for the early onset of puberty (Vignolo et al., 1988; Vanderschueren-Lodeweyckx, 1993). The majority of obese prepubertal children are not only above average weight but also above average height for age. Height seems less advanced in obese children around puberty.

Reduced growth velocity during dietary management of obese children was described in early studies (Brook et al., 1974) and, although not observed in all studies, has been a major concern in the management of obese children.

Reduced growth velocity and lowering of predicted adult height have been reported with both very modest dietary restrictions (Dietz & Hartung., 1985; Amador et al., 1990) and with VLCDs (Archibald et al., 1983). However, some studies show that VLCDs (Brown et al., 1983; Caroli et al., 1992; Figueroa-Colon et al., 1993) and BLCDs (Figueroa-Colon et al., 1993) do not necessarily have a negative effect on the growth of prepubertal children in the short and medium term. Long-term growth was not impaired in children treated for about a year with a traffic-light diet (Epstein et al., 1993). Considering the variation in growth of obese children and their final height even if they are not treated, any observed growth velocity reductions probably represent regression to the mean rather than the negative effects of a diet. Moreover, if slow growth rates are associated with longevity (Stini, 1978) and lower risk for developing cancer (Staszewsky, 1971) and autoimmune diseases (Blom et al., 1992) there might even be some beneficial effects from slowed growth rates.

Anorexia and binge-eating disorders

In theory, anorexia and binge-eating disorders are long-term complications of obesity treatment even if, as some believe, they are not the precipitating problems (Chapter 8). Appetite disorders are thought to follow VLCDs more frequently than other forms of dieting.

Binge-eating behaviour is quite common amongst obese individuals (Marcus et al., 1985). However, the obese show as many personality types and traits in eating behaviour as in other behaviours, and as much variation in eating behaviour as in any normal population. Obese people differ from each other as much as they differ from normal-weight people. Differences between those seeking treatment and those not seeking treatment for example must always be considered (O'Neil & Jarrell, 1992). Thus, it becomes difficult with such a wide variety of psychopathological traits to make specific conclusions about how much dieting predisposes to the development of eating behaviour disorders.

Raised serum uric acid

Elevated serum uric acid has been found in several, but not all, studies using VLCD treatment in obesity (Merritt, 1978; Brown et al., 1983). There are no data on serum uric acid levels with BLCDs. Serum uric acid returns to normal levels when children treated with VLCDs move on to BLCDs. The metabolic explanation for the elevated uric acid may be that the urinary excretion of ketones interferes with excretion of uric acid. When ketonuria declines as energy intakes increase following return to more normal diets, the ability to excrete uric acid improves and serum values return to normal. There are no reports of clinical problems related to transitory hyperuricaemia in dieting obese.

Gallstones

The incidence of cholelithiasis in the obese adult population ranges from 10% to 33%, increasing with age and severity of obesity (Fiedman et al., 1966; Wattehow et al., 1983). The sole report on gallstone incidence in children and adolescents (Palasciano et al., 1989) found the overall prevalence of gallstones in a population aged 6–19 years was 0.13%, when the overall prevalence of obesity was 25%. These data confirm a very low prevalence of gallstone disease in subjects younger than 20 years, whether or not they are obese.

An increased incidence of cholelithiasis in adult obese subjects being treated with VLCDs (Liddle et al., 1989) has been reported. However, the increased incidence was only described in severely obese adults taking liquid formula VLCDs, not in patients receiving BLCDs or VLCDs composed of natural foods (Kamrath et al., 1992). There are no reports of cholelithiasis in obese children or adolescents treated with BLCDs or with VLCDs.

In conclusion, the negative effects of weight loss in obese children such as hyperuricacidaemia and LBM loss should not discourage dieting when this is indicated. Some so-called negative effects, such as slowed growth velocity, may reflect the return to normal rather than a disadvantage to the child. However, reliable short- and long-term paediatric data on some hypothesized consequences of dieting (gallstones and anorexia/binge eating) are needed to determine how much, if at all, these problems do occur following dietetic treatment.

14.6 Guidelines for weight goals and dietetic treatments

Providing useful dietary advice to obese children and their families is neither simple nor straightforward. Obesity is a multifactorial disease and diet is only one of many tools used in its management. For each obese child or adolescent, different factors are of significance in the development of his or her obesity. Moreover, obesity presents with different degrees of severity. All these issues influence management. As a consequence, treatment needs to be tailored to the needs of each child. We have dealt with first-line approaches to home management of obese children and adolescents in Chapter 13. We discuss dietary treatment in more detail here.

Table 14.6 presents guidelines for specific dietary approaches which relate to the child's age, the severity of, and the presence or not of complications to the obesity.

The schedule indicates dieting strategies which are implemented step by step in discussion with children and adolescents, their families and their carers and with the support of the clinical team – paediatricians, nutritionists, dieticians and all other professionals involved (Chapters 19 & 20).

We have really presented three strategies, all in association with nutritional counselling. Appropriate nutritional counselling can also be given with benefit to children who are not overweight to try to prevent overweight. Of course counselling needs tailoring to each child's condition and must be given by someone trained in paediatric nutrition and dietetics.

Weight maintenance. This should interfere least with the normal child's diet and provided the child is eating a balanced diet should present least risk of either secondary problems to dieting or negative responses from child and family. However, the goal of keeping a child's weight the same over months or years whilst the child grows 'into the weight' is only practical for young children who are not many kilograms overweight and who are still growing rapidly, or for children who are only marginally overweight. Occasional obese adolescent boys beginning their growth acceleration manage to maintain weight and grow into their weight, particularly if they can make the lifestyle changes that increase energy expenditure. The growth spurt in girls is shorter than in boys and this, together with the

Table 14.6. Guidelines for dietetic treatments and weight goals in different degrees of obesity

BMI centile	Age				
	0–2 years	2–6 years	6–10 years	10–14 years	14–18 years
90–97 no complications	Nutritional counselling weight maintenance	Nutritional counselling weight maintenance	Nutritional counselling weight maintenance	Nutritional counselling weight maintenance/ weight loss	BLCD weight loss
90–97 with complications	Nutritional counselling weight maintenance	BLCD weight loss	BLCD weight loss	BLCD weight loss	BLCD weight loss
> 97 no complications	Nutritional counselling weight maintenance	Nutritional counselling/BLCD weight maintenance/ weight loss	BLCD/VLCD weight loss	BLCD/VLCD weight loss	BLCD weight loss
> 97 with complications	Nutritional counselling weight loss	BLCD weight loss	BLCD/VLCD weight loss	BLCD/VLCD weight loss	BLCD/VLCD weight loss

BLCD: balanced low-calorie diet; VLCD: very-low-calorie diet.

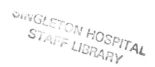
physiological tendency of pubertal girls to put on fat rather than lose it, makes weight maintenance a less hopeful prospect in adolescent girls.

Moderate versus severe obesity. We have tended to divide children according to the severity of their obesity as well as according to their age, since severity affects the risk of complications. Evidence of complications makes the need for fat loss urgent. Chapter 1 presents the current consensus view of body mass index (BMI) cut-off points for defining overweight and obesity in childhood – although other clinical features, as mentioned, need to be taken into account before selecting the most appropriate therapeutic strategies. In some cases, long-term inpatient treatments will be indicated (Chapter 20) but, whatever the obese individual's specific needs, a nutrition plan has to be developed and discussed. Diets remain, even so, only one part, albeit an important part, of the overall management plan.

Compliance. Whilst it would seem wise to prescribe more restrictive diets for children who are most severely affected by obesity, there remains little point in doing this if the child and the family are not prepared to comply with the advice. This raises the point we stressed earlier: diets must be tailored to each child's circumstances. A little fat loss is better than no loss and can improve well-being and enhance self-esteem. The positive effects of even slight weight loss should encourage further pursuit of restrictive diets and further weight loss.

Positive feedback does, of course, come from the diets – provided those diets are followed in the first place. In adolescence, however, it is our opinion that only those obese adolescents with BMI above the 97th centile and who are already affected by complications of obesity, should be treated with VLCDs rather than BLCDs. The limited use of VLCDs in this age-group is due to the risk of causing the illusion of a rapid and easy weight control in obese adolescents, since VLCDs produce rapid and remarkable weight loss. It is thought this can lead later to a 'yo-yo' syndrome of weight loss and weight gain. No controlled data are available to support this view.

14.7 Conclusions

Prescribing diets for obese children and adolescents requires evaluation of the children's nutritional status, possibly with metabolic assessment as well. Personal, family, socioeconomic and environmental factors also need evaluation. In this chapter, the long-term effects of dieting per se have not been considered since they are only one tool in the armamentarium of tools for management of obesity, both in children and in adults. Dieting is unlikely to have much effect without other long-term lifestyle changes: increased physical activity (Chapter 15); psychological help (Chapter 16); and the supportive effects provided by interdisciplinary management (Chapters 19 & 20).

It is not reasonable to expect that diet per se, whether a BLCD for 6 months or a VLCD for 2 months or modest changes in food consumption, will show positive effects 5, 10 or even 20 years later. However, dieting can begin the slimming process and initiate changes which encourage sustainable lifestyle changes for maintaining healthy weight into and throughout adult life. Related to overall guidelines for healthy nutrition, these recommendations contribute to prevention policies, even in children and adolescents, targeting not only cardiovascular diseases and cancer but social and psychological issues as well.

14.8 REFERENCES

Amador, M., Ramos, L., Morono, M. & Hermelo, M. (1990). Growth rate reduction during energy restriction in obese adolescents. *Experimental Clinical Endocrinology*, **96**, 73–82.

Archibald, E., Harrison, J. & Pencharz, P. (1983). Effect of a weight-reducing high-protein diet on the body composition of obese adolescents. *American Journal of Diseases in Childhood*, **137**, 658–62.

Becque, D., Katch, V., Rocchini, A., Marks, C. & Moorehead, C. (1988). Coronary risk incidence of obese adolescents: reduction by exercise plus diet intervention. *Pediatrics*, **81**, 605–12.

Blom, L., Persson L.A. & Dahlquist G. (1992). A high linear growth is associated with increased risk of childhood diabetes mellitus. *Diabetologia*, **35**, 528–33.

Brook, C.G.D. & Lloyd, J.K. (1973). Adipose cell size and glucose tolerance in obese children and effect of diet. *Archives of Disease in Childhood*, **48**, 301–4.

Brook, C.G.D., Lloyd, J.K. & Wolff, O.H. (1974). Rapid weight loss in children. *British Medical Journal*, **2**, 44–5.

Brown, M., Klish, W., Hollander, J., Campbell, M.A. & Forbes, G. (1983). A high protein, low calorie liquid diet in the treatment of very obese adolescents: long-term effect on lean body mass. *American Journal of Clinical Nutrition*, **38**, 20–31.

Brownell, K., Kelman, J. & Stunkard, A. (1983). Treatment of obese children with and without their mothers: changes in weight and blood pressure. *Pediatrics*, **71**, 515–23.

Burniat, W. & Van Aelst C. (1993). Therapeutic approach to childhood obesity. *Nutrition Research*, **13** (S1), 117–32.

Burns, T.L., Moll, P.P. & Lauer, R.M. (1989). The relationship between ponderosity and coronary risk factors in children and their relatives: the Muscatine Ponderosity Family Study. *American Journal of Epidemiology*, **129**, 973–87.

Caprio, S., Hyman, L.D., Limb, C., McCarthy, S., Lange, R., Sherwin, R.S., Shulman, G. & Tamborlane, W.V. (1995). Central adiposity and its metabolic correlates in obese adolescent girls. *American Journal of Physiology*, **269**, E118–26.

Caprio, S., Hyman, L.D., McCarthy, S., Lange, R., Bronson, M. & Tamborlane, W.V. (1996). Fat distribution and cardiovascular risk factors in obese adolescent girls: importance of the intraabdominal fat depot. *American Journal of Clinical Nutrition*, **64**, 12–17.

Caroli, M., Chiarappa, S., Borrelli, R., Martinelli, R. & Bratta, P. (1991). Weight loss and protein nutritional status in obese adolescents on balanced hypocaloric diet: comparison between 600 calorie diet vs. 1000 calorie diet. *International Journal of Obesity*, **15S**, P44.

Caroli, M., Chiarappa, S., Borrelli, R. & Martinelli, R. (1992). Efficiency and safety of using protein sparing modified fast in pediatric and adolescent obesity treatment. *Nutrition Research*, **12**, 1325–34.

Caroli, M., Chiarappa, S., Di Toro, A. & Pisconti, C. (1994). Variazioni dello stato di nutrizione proteica in bambini ed adolescenti obesi in corso di trattamento con protein sparing modified fast. *Bambini e Nutrizione*, **1**, 50–4.

Caroli, M., Chiarappa, S., Kutty, K.M. & Chandra, R.K. (1998). Changes in lean body mass in obese children and adolescents treated with protein sparing modified fast. *Nutrition Research*, **18**, 191–9.

Chiumello, G., Del Guercio, M.J., Carnelutti, M. & Bidone, G. (1969). Relationship between obesity, chemical diabetes and beta pancreatic function in children. *Diabetes*, **18**, 238–43.

Deschamps, I., Desjeux, F., Machinot, S., Rolland, F. & Lestradet, H. (1978). Effects of diet and weight loss on plasma glucose, insulin, and free fatty acids in obese children. *Pediatric Research*, **12**, 757–60.

Dietz, W. & Hartung, R. (1985). Changes in height velocity of obese preadolescents during weight reduction. *American Journal of Diseases in Childhood*, **139**, 705–7.

Dietz, W. & Schoeller, D. (1982). Optimal dietary therapy for obese adolescents: Comparison of protein plus glucose and protein plus fat. *Journal of Pediatrics*, **100**, 638–44.

Di Toro, A., Marotta, A., Todisco, N., Ponticiello, E., Collini, R., Di Lascio, R. & Perrone, L. (1997). Unchanged iron and copper and increased zinc in the blood of obese children after two hypocaloric diets. *Biological Trace Element Research*, **57**, 97–104.

Duffy, G. & Spence, S.H. (1993). The effectiveness of cognitive self-management as an adjunct to behavioural intervention for childhood obesity: a research note. *Journal of Childhood Psychology and Psychiatry*, **34**, 1034–50.

Endo, H., Tagaki, Y., Nouze, T., Kuwahata, K., Uemasu, F. & Kobayashi, A. (1992). Beneficial effects of dietary intervention on serum lipid and apolipoprotein levels in obese children. *American Journal of Diseases in Childhood*, **146**, 303–5.

Epstein, L., Wing, R.R., Penner, B.G. & Kress, M.J. (1985). Effects of diet and controlled exercise on weight loss in obese children. *Journal of Pediatrics*, **107**, 358–61.

Epstein, L., Kuller, L.H., Wing, R.R., Valoski, A. & McCurley, J. (1989). The effect of weight control on lipid changes in obese children. *American Journal of Diseases in Childhood*, **143**, 454–7.

Epstein, L., Valoski, A. & McCurley, J. (1993). Effect of weight loss by obese children on long-term growth. *American Journal of Diseases in Childhood*, **146**, 1076–80.

Fiedman, G.D., Kamel, W.B. & Dawber, J.R. (1966). The epidemiology of gall-bladder disease: observations in the Framingham study. *Journal of Chronic Diseases*, **19**, 273–92.

Figueroa-Colon, R., von Almen, K., Franklin, F., Schuftan, C. & Suskind, R. (1993). Comparison of two hypocaloric diets in obese children. *American Journal of Diseases in Childhood*, **147**, 160–6.

Flatt, J.P. & Blackburn, G. (1974). The metabolic fuel regulatory system: implications for protein-sparing therapies during caloric deprivation and disease. *American Journal of Clinical Nutrition*, **27**, 175–87.

Flodmark, C.E., Sveger, T. & Nilsson-Ehle, P. (1994). Waist measurement correlates to a potentially atherogenic lipoprotein profile in obese 12–14-year-old children. *Acta Paediatrica Scandinavica*, **83**, 941–5.

Garrow, J. (1989). Very low calorie diets should not be used. *International Journal of Obesity*, **13** (S2), 145–7.

Ginsberg-Fellner, F. & Knittle, J.L. (1981). Weight reduction in young obese children. I. Effect on adipose tissue cellularity and metabolism. *Pediatric Research*, **15**, 1381–9.

Graves, T., Meyers, A.W. & Clark, L. (1988). An evaluation of problem-solving training in the behavioural treatment of childhood obesity. *Journal of Consultant Clinical Psychology*, **56**, 246–50.

Hall, J.E. (1997). Mechanisms of abnormal renal sodium handling in obesity hypertension. *American Journal of Hypertension*, **10**, 49S–55S.

Heyden, S. & De Marsa W. (1973). Weight reduction in adolescents. *Nutrition and Metabolism*, **15**, 295.

Hills, A. & Parker, A. (1988). Obesity management via diet and exercise intervention. *Child Care, Health and Development*, **14**, 409–16.

Hoffman R.H. (1957). Obesity in childhood and adolescence. *American Journal of Clinical Nutrition*, **5**, 1–10.

Hoffman, R., Stumbo, P., Janz, K. & Nielsen, D. (1995). Altered insulin resistance is associated with increased dietary weight loss in obese children. *Hormone Research*, **44**, 17–22.

Horswill, C. & Zipf, W. (1991). Elevated blood pressure in obese children: influence of gender, age, weight, and serum insulin levels. *International Journal of Obesity*, **15**, 453–9.

Kamrath, R., Plummer, L., Sadur, C., Adler, M., Strader, W., Young, R. & Weinstein, R. (1992). Cholelithiasis in patients treated with a very-low-calorie diet. *American Journal of Clinical Nutrition*, **56**, 255–7S.

Knip, M. & Nuutinen, O. (1993). Long-term effects of weight reduction on serum lipids and plasma insulin in obese children. *American Journal of Clinical Nutrition*, **57**, 490–3.

Knip, M., Lautala, P. & Puukka, R. (1988). Reduced insulin removal and erythrocyte insulin binding in obese children. *European Journal of Pediatrics*, **148**, 233–7.

Kreitzman, S.N. (1992). Factors influencing body composition during very low calorie diets. *American Journal of Clinical Nutrition*, **56**, 217–23S.

Lauer, R., Burns, T., Clarke, W. & Mahoney, L. (1991). Childhood predictors of future blood pressure. *Hypertension*, **18** (S I), I-74–I-81.

Liddle, R.A., Goldstein, R.B. & Saxton, J. (1989). Gallstone formation during weight-reduction dieting. *Archives of International Medicine*, **149**, 1750–3.

Marcus, M.D., Wing, R.R. & Lamparasky, D.M. (1985). Binge eating and dietary restraint in obese patients. *Addictive Behaviour*, **10**, 163–8.

Martin, M.M. & Martin, A.L.A. (1973). Obesity, hyperinsulinism, and diabetes mellitus in childhood. *Journal of Pediatrics*, **82**, 192–201.

Merritt, R. (1978). Treatment of pediatric and adolescent obesity. *International Journal of Obesity*, **2**, 207–14.

Merritt, R., Bistrian, B., Blackburn, G. & Suskind, R. (1980). Consequences of modified fasting in obese pediatric and adolescent patients. I. Protein-sparing modified fast. *Journal of*

Pediatrics, **96**, 13–19.

Merritt, R., Blackburn, G., Bistrian, B., Batrus & C., Suskind, R. (1983). Consequences of modified fasting in obese pediatric and adolescent patients. *Nutrition Research*, **3**, 33–41.

O'Neil, P.M. & Jarrell, M.P. (1992). Psychological aspects of obesity and very low calorie diets. *American Journal of Clinical Nutrition*, **56**, 185–9S.

Palasciano, G., Portincasa, P., Vinciguerra, V., Velardi, A., Tardi, A., Baldassarre, G. & Albano, O. (1989). Gallstones prevalence and gallbladder volume in children and adolescents: an epidemiological ultrasonographic survey and relationship to body mass index. *American Journal of Gastroenterology*, **84**, 1378–82.

Pencharz, P., Motil, K., Parsons, H. & Duffy, B. (1980). The effect of an energy-restricted diet on the protein metabolism of obese adolescents: nitrogen-balance and whole-body nitrogen turnover. *Clinical Science*, **59**, 13–18.

Pencharz, P., Clarke, R., Archibald, H. & Vaisman, N. (1988). The effect of a weight-reducing diet on the nitrogen metabolism of obese adolescents. *Canadian Journal of Physiology and Pharmacology*, **66**, 1469–74.

Perosa, N., Aingorn, H., Metelskaya, V., Dorofoeva, T. & Belokonj, N. (1988). Plasma lipid and apolipoprotein levels in children hereditarily predisposed to coronary heart disease. *Acta Paediatrica Scandinavica*, **77**, 559–62.

Rocchini, A.P., Katch, V., Anderson, J., Hinderliter, J., Becque, D., Martin, M. & Marks, C. (1988). Blood pressure in obese adolescents: effect of weight loss. *Pediatrics*, **82**, 16–23.

Rocchini, A.P., Key, J., Bondie, D., Chico, R., Moorehead, C., Katch, V. & Martin, M. (1989). The effect of weight loss on the sensitivity of blood pressure to sodium in obese adolescents. *New England Journal of Medicine*, **321**, 580–5.

Schwingshandl, J. & Borkenstein, M. (1995). Changes in the lean body mass in obese children during a weight reduction program: effect on short term and long term outcome. *International Journal of Obesity*, **19**, 752–5.

Stallings, V., Archibald, E., Pencharz, P., Harrison, J. & Bell, L. (1988). One-year follow-up of weight, total body potassium, and total body nitrogen in obese adolescents treated with the protein-sparing modified fast. *American Journal of Clinical Nutrition*, **48**, 91–4.

Stallings, V. & Pencharz, P. (1992). The effect of a high protein-low calorie diet on the energy expenditure of obese adolescents. *European Journal of Clinical Nutrition*, **46**, 897–902.

Senediak, C. & Spence, S.H. (1985). Rapid versus gradual scheduling of therapeutic contact in a family based behavioural weight control programme for children. *Behavioral Psychotherapy*, **13**, 265–87.

Staszewsky, J. (1971). Age of menarche and breast cancer. *Journal of National Cancer Institute*, **47**, 935–40.

Stini, W.A. (1978). Early nutrition, growth, disease and human longevity. *Nutrition and Cancer*, **1**, 31–9.

Valverde, M.A., Patin, R.V., Oliveira, F.L.C., Lopez, F.A. & Vitolo, M.R. (1998). Outcomes of obese children and adolescents enrolled in a multidisciplinary health program. *International Journal of Obesity*, **22**, 513–19.

Vanderschueren-Lodeweyckx, M. (1993). The effect of simple obesity on growth and growth hormones. *Hormone Research*, **40**, 23–30.

Vignolo, M., Naselli, A., Di Battista, E., Mostert, M. & Aicardi, G. (1988). Growth and development in simple obesity. *European Journal of Pediatrics*, **147**, 242–4.

Wabitsch, M., Hauner, H., Böckman, A., Parthon, W., Mayer, H. & Teller, W. (1992). The relationship between body fat distribution and weight loss in obese and adolescents girls. *International Journal of Obesity*, **17**, 905–11.

Wabitsch, M., Hauner, H., Heize, E., Muche, R., Bockmann, A., Parthon, W., Mayer, H. & Teller, W. (1994). Body-fat distribution and changes in the atherogenic risk-factor profile in obese adolescent girls during weight reduction. *American Journal of Clinical Nutrition*, **60**, 54–60.

Wadden, T.A., Stunkard, A.J. & Brownell, K.D. (1983). Very low calorie diets: their efficacy, safety, and future. *Annals of Internal Medicine*, **99**, 675–84.

Wattehow, D.A., Hall, J.C., Whiting, M.J., Bradley, B., Iannes, J. & Watts, J.M. (1983). Prevalence and treatment of gallstones after gastric bypass surgery for morbid obesity. *British Medical Journal*, **286**, 763.

Widhalm, K. & Zwiauer, K. (1987). Metabolic effects of a very low calorie diet in obese children and adolescents with special reference to nitrogen balance. *Journal of American College of Nutrition*, **6**, 467–74.

Zwiauer, K., Kerbl, B. & Widhalm K. (1988). No reduction of high density lipoprotein-2 during weight reduction in obese children and adolescents. *European Journal of Pediatrics*, **149**, 192–3.

Management through activity

Jana Parizkova,[1] Claudio Maffeis[2] and Elizabeth M.E. Poskitt[3]

[1]Centre for the Management of Obesity, Prague. [2]Department of Paediatrics, University Hospital, Verona.
[3]International Nutrition Group, London School of Hygiene and Tropical Medicine

15.1 Introduction

Physical activity is usually included in treatment programmes for obesity and can be considered a cornerstone in management. Yet, what do we mean by physical activity? Too often physical activity is equated with formal exercise, since these two terms, physical activity and exercise, tend to be interchangeable although they refer to different constructs. For the purposes of this chapter and in conformity with the definitions used by others in this book, we have adopted the following definitions of physical activity, exercise and physical fitness (Caspersen et al., 1985):

- *Physical activity:* any bodily movement produced by skeletal muscles which results in increased energy expenditure.
- *Exercise:* a subcategory of physical activity which is repetitive, structured and purposive in the sense that improved maintenance of physical fitness is an objective.
- *Physical fitness:* the ability to carry out daily tasks with vigour and alertness without undue fatigue and with ample energy to enjoy leisure-time pursuits and to meet unforeseen circumstances.

Physical activity programmes should be part of all multifaceted programmes for the treatment of childhood obesity. Skeletal muscle is the site of most fat oxidation in the body. Physical activity affects total fat oxidation and fat balance through promotion of more favourable body composition (loss of fat, especially of visceral fat; preservation of lean body mass). Moreover, increased fat oxidation rates help maintain glycogen stores, thus influencing the regulation of food intake and energy balance (Flatt, 1987a).

Thus, physical activity benefits obese children by:

- Increasing lean body mass;
- Increasing energy expenditure;

- Improving the metabolic profile;
- Improving psychological well-being (Brown, 1990; Knip & Nuutinen, 1993).

Independent of any effect on excess weight, these changes justify the promotion of physical activity in children. Moreover, increased levels of skeletal muscle work to improve long-term prognosis in terms of both morbidity and mortality (Paffenbarger et al., 1986). Nevertheless, despite these potential benefits, the process of increasing physical activity, and maintaining the increase, has many problems.

The aim of this chapter is to provide an overview of programmes of physical activity for obese children. We discuss the positive and negative side effects of these programmes and propose strategies for intervention and future research.

15.2 Aims of the programmes

The US Surgeon General's report (Surgeon General, 1996) stated that 30–60 min of purposeful walking almost every day substantially increases energy expenditure, thus reducing body weight and fat in adults. Even the most common physical activities can be helpful in reducing the health risks of obesity, especially hypertension, dyslipoproteinaemia and impaired glucose tolerance (Blair et al., 1992). Walking, climbing stairs, domestic activities in house and garden – provided they occupy at least 30–40 min per day – have been shown to be efficient health promoters (Epstein, 1995; Epstein et al., 1995). Although specific physical activity guidelines are not available for children, it seems reasonable to encourage spontaneous activities such as walking to school (at least part of the way), walking and playing outdoors with peers, using stairs rather than lifts and escalators in buildings. These activities increase energy output and, however slightly, help improve energy balance. Evidence for the disadvantage of doing otherwise is that low levels of physical activity during childhood/adolescence have been associated (independent of other factors) with morbidity and mortality in adulthood (Paffenbarger et al., 1986). Reduced time spent in sedentary activities per se promoted greater weight loss after 1 year of study than exercise programmes (Epstein et al., 1995).

Plans for successful physical-activity programmes have to incorporate several factors (Table 15.1). Physical activity is the only discretionary component of total daily energy expenditure (TEE), so increased energy expenditure due to muscle work should increase TEE (Ravussin et al., 1986). In terms of energy, the higher the intensity of exercise, the higher the energy expenditure (Maffeis et al., 1993). However, fatigue and training affect this relationship. Theoretically, postexercise resting may compensate for some of the cost of exercise (Brehm & Gutin, 1986). A controlled training programme (cycling at 60% of $VO_{2\,max}$ for 45 minutes, five

Table 15.1. Factors influencing outcome of physical activity programmes

Intensity
Duration
Type of activity: aerobic or anaerobic
Training level
Fatigue induced by activity
Extent of compensatory rest following activity
Effect of activity on food intake
Risk of injury or trauma from activity

times a week, for 4 weeks) with a group of nonobese boys showed the children had higher energy expenditures during the training period than before (Blaak et al., 1992). Even so, the energy expenditure in the exercise programme only explained 50% of the increased TEE in these children suggesting that exercise training stimulated physical activity and not the contrary. Although compensatory falls in activity have not been documented in nonobese children following physical exercise programmes, lack of data means we can draw no definite conclusions about the possible effects of activity in obese subjects.

Training improves children's individual energetic efficiency when performing exercise thus reducing the final energy costs of the exercise itself (Astrand & Rodahl, 1986). Exercise intensity also has consequences on postexercise food intake and could influence children's overall compliance. Exercise at intensities above anaerobic threshold (corresponding to the level of VO_2 consumption (ml/min) at which the metabolism becomes mainly anaerobic) promotes a higher carbohydrate to fat oxidation ratio (Astrand & Rodahl, 1986). Exhaustion of glycogen stores may favour higher postexercise food intakes – as seems to happen in both animals and humans (Flatt, 1978, 1987a,b) – since glycogen depletion is one of the factors that stimulates appetite (Flatt, 1987a,b). Different types of exercise, performed at different intensities, may have different impacts on glycogen depletion and variable effects on appetite. Moderate intensity aerobic exercise, which uses a high proportion of fatty acids as substrate, may affect appetite proportionally less than anaerobic exercise (i.e. heavy exercise), which uses glucose as the principal substrate, and thereby depletes glycogen stores (Flatt, 1987a,b). The individual variation in ability to increase fat oxidation in response to exercise may also affect the rate of glycogen depletion, thereby determining the carbohydrate deficit and the postexercise carbohydrate and energy intake (Flatt, 1987a,b). Thus, one of the goals of activity in obesity should be to favour activities which promote low carbohydrate/fat oxidation ratio, that is aerobic activities, because relatively high fat oxidation stimulates appetite less than high carbohydrate oxidation.

Children's food preferences, the availability of food, and the composition of foods ingested can play important roles in compensating for the energy costs of exercise. In adults, highly palatable foods consumed after exercise may exceed the energy deficit created by the exercise thus promoting fat gain (Blundell et al., 1993; Rolls et al., 1994). Although studies of children's postexercise food consumption are needed to clarify this issue, it seems advisable to limit the availability of energy-dense food after exercise.

Weight loss during the treatment of obesity is usually due to loss of both fat and lean mass (Parizkova, 1977, 1979; Dore et al., 1982; Maffeis et al., 1992). Reduced lean body mass (LBM) – the metabolically active tissue – leads to reduced basal energy expenditure, which is determined by LBM (Maffeis et al., 1992). Reduced basal metabolic rate (BMR) thus presents a risk factor for further weight gain if energy intakes are not balanced to the new energy requirements.

The possible traumatic side effects of exercise have to be carefully considered when designing individual physical activity programmes. High-intensity exercises cause discomfort in obese children independent of their risk for injury. If obese individuals are to adhere to a physical activity programme, any proposed exercise should relate to their physical characteristics – and should be both safe and enjoyable.

Thus an 'ideal' physical activity programme should be designed so as:
- to preserve LBM;
- to avoid promotion of compensatory food intake;
- to be tailored on the basis of the preferences of the child;
- to be aerobic (walking, cycling, swimming, etc.);
- to be realistic in intensity and duration;
- to avoid psychological discomfort;
- to develop a level of activity which can be maintained after the programme has ended.

15.3 Efficacy of exercise in lowering fat mass

The quantity of energy expended during a bout of exercise is generally modest in comparison to the deficit that can be achieved by diet. For example, in a 9-year-old moderately obese girl (body weight 46 kg, 32% body fat), the energy expenditure during brisk walking at a speed of 5 km/h is about five times greater than her basal energy expenditure (BEE 3.5 kJ/min or 0.84 kcal/min) (Ainsworth et al., 1993). Walking for 1 hour, the girl expends about 1050 kJ (60 min × 5 × 3.5 kJ/min)

Table 15.2. Examples of relative energy costs for adults of sports and activities

Activity	Multiples of BMR
Walking, 3 km/h, no slope	2.5
Walking, 5 km/h, no slope	4
Walking, 5 km/h, uphill	6
Walking and running	6
Jogging	7
Running, 8 km/h	9
Cycling, no slope, < 15 km/h	4
Cycling, no slope, 15–20 km/h	6–7
Cycling, no slope, > 20 km/h	> 10
Volleyball (noncompetitive)	3
Basketball (noncompetitive)	6
Football (noncompetitive)	8
Tennis	7
Skateboarding	5
Roller skating	7
Judo, karate	10
Health club exercises (nonspecific)	5.5
Aerobic dancing	6
Swimming	6–12
Skiing	7–16.5

Modified from Sasaki et al., 1987.

(Table 15.2) (World Health Organization, 1985; Ainsworth et al., 1993). The energy expenditure during resting activity (sitting, standing quietly) for 1 hour is approximately 273 kJ (60 min × 1.3 × 3.5 kJ/min, where 1.3 is the mean multiple of the BEE for the resting activities considered) (WHO, 1985; Ainsworth et al., 1993). Net extra energy expenditure attributable to 60 minutes of exercise instead of sedentary activity is approximately 777 kJ (186 kcal). Assuming all the other components of energy expenditure and energy intake remain constant, walking daily for 1 hour at a speed of 5 km/h should theoretically create an energy deficit equivalent to the loss of 1 kg of adipose tissue in approximately 5 weeks. This seems a relatively modest result but, over the course of 6 months, this quantity of exercise could induce the reduction of approximately one-third of this girl's adipose mass.

Increased postexercise oxygen consumption is directly proportional to duration and intensity of exercise, although a workload greater than 50% of maximal aerobic capacity ($VO_{2\,max}$) appears necessary to induce a detectable effect (Brehm & Gutin, 1986). Postexercise glycogen-store replenishment, increased protein turnover, lactic-acid clearance, increased fatty-acid mobilization, oxidation and cycling, and other factors consequent to exercise such as increased core temperature, increased heart and breathing rates, and β-adrenergic stimulation, contribute to this phenomenon (Ekblom, 1992). However, after most low intensity activities, the postexercise energy debt is usually small ($< 100\,kJ$ or $25\,kcal$) and of short duration (<60 minutes from the end of the exercise). Its contribution to weight loss is thus negligible.

High-intensity exercise increases BEE for more than 24 hours in adults (Poehlman, 1989). However, the increase in BEE disappears after short-term interruptions in training (Tremblay et al., 1988). A prolonged postexercise debt seems the most reasonable explanation for this phenomenon.

Sustained training, in particular weight training, increases muscle mass (Faulkner & White, 1990). Because BEE is directly related to fat-free mass (FFM), increased FFM due to exercise should increase BEE. However, in obese subjects, the potential increase of muscle mass following training may be counterbalanced by the reduction of FFM that accompanies weight loss, especially with severely hypocaloric diets (Donnelly et al., 1993). The use of exercise with less-restrictive diets may reduce this FFM loss thus reducing the fall in BEE (Belko et al., 1986; Nieman et al., 1988). Maintenance of BEE should enhance rates of weight loss since, if energy spent on physical activity remains constant, energy deficit will not change as weight loss progresses.

Several studies in adults designed to evaluate the effects of exercise on weight loss show that exercise per se can induce weight loss but weight lost is modest (Ballor & Keesey, 1991). The use of exercise alone in the treatment of childhood obesity seems more effective. Running 20 minutes per day, 7 days a week, for 2 years, reduced overweight by about 50% in a group of male and female Japanese children (Sasaki et al., 1987). Increasing total energy expenditure by 240–500 kcal/day through either programmed exercise or altered 'lifestyle' activity with obese children produced losses averaging 15% overweight after 8 weeks (Epstein et al., 1982). Follow-up 15 months later demonstrated further 10% and 19% reduction of overweight in the two ('programmed exercise' and 'altered lifestyle activity') groups (Epstein et al., 1982). Additional exercise for 4–12 months also increased the weight losses induced by hypocaloric diets in children (Epstein et al., 1985a; Reybrouck et al., 1990) conforming with similar findings in obese adults (King & Tribble, 1991). Changes in lifestyle activity combined with dieting were more effective in maintaining long-term weight loss than programmed exercise combined with dieting amongst groups of obese children (Epstein et al., 1985b).

In adults, endurance training appears to mobilize abdominal fat more readily in males than in females (Wing et al., 1992), and in older than in younger subjects (Schwartz et al., 1991). Because upper-body fat is particularly associated with the morbid consequences of obesity (Björntorp, 1992), reductions in visceral fat have clinical interest. However, the association of fat distribution and morbidity, and the effect of exercise on fat distribution have not been studied in detail in childhood.

15.4 General principles

Subjects adapted to dynamic, weight-bearing aerobic exercise usually have high ratios of lean to fat mass, high levels of aerobic power (characterized by high maximal oxygen uptake per kilogram of total and/or lean body weight) and a characteristic profile of enzymatic activities in skeletal muscles. Significantly negative correlations were found between hydroxyacyl-coenzyme-A activity (HOAD) in the vastus lateralis muscles and relative adiposity (fat mass per cent) in skiers, runners and other dynamic adult athletes (Parizkova et al., 1987).

In obesity-prone adults, the activity of fat-oxidizing enzymes in the vastus lateralis muscle is decreased (Raben et al., 1997). Smaller areas of type 1 and type 2B muscle fibres were found in postobese compared with nonobese individuals, in spite of the lower energy and fat intakes amongst the former (Raben et al., 1997). Resting metabolic rates and respiratory exchange ratios were similar in both groups, but $VO_{2\,max}$ tended to be lower in postobese individuals than in controls: 28.0 (SE 1.9) vs. 34.2 (SE 2.3) ml/(kg min), $p = 0.06$. The results of this study suggest that reduced HOAD activity (a key enzyme in β-oxidation of fatty acids) along with reduced citrate-synthetase activity (a rate-limiting enzyme in the Krebs cycle) could explain lower fatty acid oxidation rates (Raben et al., 1997) in these subjects. Theoretically, these enzymatic changes, which are significantly related to lower levels of aerobic power in hypokinetic subjects, could be responsible for increased fat deposition. This might apply even more during growth and development, when levels of spontaneous physical activity may be higher than during adult life. An individual adapted to a higher level of dynamic, aerobic motor activity during growth may develop not only greater aerobic power, but also greater activity in specific enzymes which metabolize and utilize fatty acids and other fat metabolites as sources of energy for regular muscle work. All this fits in with the characteristic body composition of the aerobic athlete: that is, low deposition of fat, and high absolute and relative values of LBM. At present there are no biopsy data on the effects of exercise on enzymatic activity in the skeletal muscles of children.

15.5 Physical activity and exercise programmes

Obesity is characterized by great interindividual variability. Obese children and adolescents may have different levels of adiposity, fat distribution, duration of obesity, complications and comorbidities. Previous levels of physical activity, fitness and functional capacity vary not only with age and gender, but also with other factors in children's environments and previous health. Some overweight children are quite skilled, especially in techniques involving small muscle groups, or have considerable muscular strength. It should be standard practice to individualize all components of movement therapy.

No evidence-based guidelines exist from which to design exercise programmes for obese children. Aerobic exercise with intensity lower than 60% of maximum heart rate (HR) (or $VO_{2\,max}$) and duration of at least 30 minutes repeated with a frequency of 3 days/week should avoid stimulating appetite or inducing conflicting postexercise rest. The higher free fatty acid (FFA)/glucose oxidation ratio during moderate exercise will promote depletion of fat stores. The type of exercise chosen is relatively unimportant, although walking is easy and costs nothing. The energy expenditure of brisk walking is comparable to that of other exercises such as basketball, aerobic dancing, leisure swimming, 'keep fit' and cycling at 15 km/h (Table 15.2) (Ainsworth et al., 1993). Exercise programmes should be slowly progressive, preceded and followed by gradual warm-up and cool-down periods, respectively. Symptoms (pain, fatigue, weakness, dizziness) or the inability to sustain a conversation should halt the exercise. Fun, enthusiastic leadership, group activities, and parental support and participation are strong motivating factors in children (Jopling, 1988). Incentives and outdoor activities may improve adherence (Jopling, 1988).

Programmed exercise is difficult to enforce, except under strictly controlled conditions, for example on a residential basis. Summer holidays can also be used for this purpose. Special camps with training programmes suitable for obese children and youth have been used since the 1950s in some countries (Parizkova, 1972) and are becoming more widespread (Vamberova et al., 1971).

15.5.1 Leisure time

Video games and television programmes predominate as leisure-time activities for too many children and youths. The time spent with these programmes has been increasing during recent decades, helping to promote physically inactive behaviours. This creates serious problems, not only for obese individuals, but also for normal-weight adolescents, as such programmes are likely to be more attractive than exercise. This applies especially for those who have not been adapted to higher levels of activity since early childhood, and for whom movement and

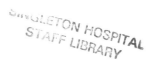

Table 15.3. Individual components of a physical activity and exercise regime

Warm-up exercises
Stretching exercises
Exercises directed at specific parts of the body and specific muscle groups: supervised by physical education teachers and individually designed for each child
Exercises aimed at preparing the child for participation in team sports, gymnastics, track and field events: again organized and supervised by qualified teachers
Walking ⇒ alternating walking and running ⇒ jogging
Dancing

exercise have become demanding and strenuous. The only recipe for a healthy and active lifestyle is to encourage participation in interesting physical activities and adequate work loads as young as possible.

Individual exercises and sports events must be chosen carefully so as to avoid obese children becoming disheartened over their difficulties and discomforts. Supervised activities are likely to be preferred by parents who are afraid of allowing their children to play freely in streets or parks. Formal supervised activities can be expensive, in which case parents may need persuading about the far-reaching health effects of physical activity and exercise regimes. It is unrealistic for children and families to dream of obese subjects growing into sustainable and acceptable adult body weight, body mass index (BMI) and fatness, if they continue to follow, unchanged, the typical lifestyle of the majority in westernized countries today.

15.5.2 The choice of exercise for the obese child

It is impossible to prescribe specific exercise programmes to cover growing children of different age, gender, degree and duration of obesity and from different environments and with different health histories. Recommendations already available on the kind, duration and intensity of exercise that should be practised are mostly very general. However, some principles can be outlined (Table 15.3).

Many obese children have orthopaedic problems such as bad posture, mild, or even severe, scoliosis, kyphosis, genu valgum, uneven shoulders and slack, weak abdominal musculature leading to characteristic slouching silhouettes. These problems have to be taken into account when designing training programmes for obese children. In the more serious cases, it may be necessary to consider whether the children should take part in school physical education classes with their peers who may not act very sensitively or constructively. The same question can apply to leisure-time physical education and sports. In some countries special physical education classes for children with some health problems already exist. Usually there are no classes specifically for obese children. Where they do exist, such classes are mostly organized by outpatient services for obese children attached to some paediatric hospitals, special sports clubs, or other groups with reasons for special concern with the obese.

It is necessary to develop obese children's interest in increased movement and exercise. The influence of environmental factors and the role of the family are very significant. The personality of the physical education instructor and the ambience of gym, sports hall or sport grounds need to be friendly and attractive. The educator should be kind, patient and cheerful, drawing attention to errors sensitively and praising any success, however small. Attractive sportswear can also add to the pleasure of organized exercise. The psychological aspects of the approach to weight reduction in childhood obesity are given in greater detail in Chapter 16.

As mentioned above, reducing excess fat is best achieved by dynamic, aerobic exercise, which is rarely practical for obese subjects at the beginning of a slimming regimen. For this reason, it can be ideal to begin exercise programmes in swimming pools, since these make movement easier for those who are extremely obese. Later, after some weight reduction and adaptation to increased physical activity, children become more able to exercise from lying down or sitting positions, and even to use cycle ergometers for short periods of time (Table 15.4).

Our recommendations for a programme of physical activity and exercises would include:
- morning exercise 10–15 min;
- afternoon and/or evening (ideally both) warm-up and exercise 15–20 min;
- at least 2 hours per day devoted to walking (running) in the open air, games, sport activities, and exercises;
- twice a week, normal (if possible) physical education classes at school, and/or special physical education classes suitable for obese subjects;
- at least 5–6 hours of physical activity, games, exercise and sport at weekends – when possible away from large urban agglomerations;
- ideally, all muscle groups should be exercised every day, even though some muscle groups (e.g. abdominal wall, hips) may require more specific attention.

Parents and other members of the family should be encouraged to take part in the programmes. Activities need to be lively, attractive and entertaining. Children should be supervised so as to perform exercises effectively with practice after a preliminary period of adaptation and practice.

At the beginning, movements and exercises need to be performed slowly, efficiently, purposefully and, if possible, also rhythmically. This approach reduces the disharmony of movement often observed in obese individuals, develops and maintains correct body posture and achieves symmetric and stable gait. (Even those of normal body weight may benefit from this.)

Exercises aimed at correcting posture belong to the most important compo-

Table 15.4. Outlines of exercise programmes for different degrees of obesity

Morbid/severe obesity

Aim at successive use of different muscle groups in different parts of the body

   Exercises in water: swimming

   Exercises lying down

   Exercises in sitting position

Moderate obesity

Begin with exercises as with severe obesity then:

   Exercises in standing position

   Cycle ergometer for 10–15 minutes at a time

   Walking

   Exercises preparatory to participation in team games etc.

   Dancing

   Stretching

Mild obesity

Begin as with moderate obesity and then:

   Exercises in all positions using all parts of the body and all muscle groups

   Participation in team games and sports as appropriate

   Walking and running for increasing distances and increasing duration

Body weight maintenance after fat loss

   All of the above and aerobics and endurance running

nents of movement therapy. Older children and adolescents can be encouraged to learn these exercises by looking at themselves in mirrors at the gym. The exercises should develop the skill, speed, endurance, strength and general physical fitness of obese children but will require specific, although different, approaches to make them individually suitable. Obese children cannot usually cope with long walks when first introduced to exercise programmes, so short runs, or alternating run–walk exercises along shorter distances are used. Intermittent jumping, obstacle courses and other natural movements are recommended.

In older children, exercises aimed towards participation in team games such as football, basketball, badminton, volleyball and so on, and seasonal individual sports (swimming, skiing, tennis etc.) should be included in the programme. Basic preparations for track-and-field are also recommended. It is important that obese children master some basic movement stereotypes which enable them to participate later in these sports in the company of their nonobese peers.

Dancing is a good motivator of exercise, especially amongst groups of obese children, for example during special summer camps where children often lose the inhibitions they show in the company of normal-weight children. Dancing can increase energy expenditure significantly although the fashion and style of dancing must be energy demanding. Generally, children enjoy participation in dancing activity even when they refuse other motor activities and exercise because they are 'too tired'.

We have already recommended swimming. The benefits of swimming need little explanation. Archimedes' principle facilitates lifting one's own body weight. Swimming involves almost all muscle groups in the body, that is, it is an all-round exercise suitable for growing subjects. It is also an activity which teaches a useful skill. Cycling – at a normal rate – is also helpful, although it does not encourage the development of chest muscles.

Skating is not a good choice of exercise for obese subjects. Genu valgum is a common problem for obese children and may be made worse by skating. Skiing should, preferably, only be introduced after some weight reduction and adaptation to exercise have taken place, and then as careful cross-country skiing.

Aerobics, stretching (callisthenics) and yoga have become fashionable not only among young adults, but also amongst adolescents. At the onset of exercise, stretching, which helps muscle tone, can be helpful to obese individuals, especially if accompanied by other suitable exercises. However, its energy expenditure is relatively low. Aerobics is best reserved for weight maintenance after marked reduction of weight.

15.5.3 Details of some progressive postural exercises

Body posture

The head is drawn up, the chin and the neck are held at a right angle. Shoulders are spread and drawn down, arms hang along the trunk, elbows are rotated aside so thumbs are directed forwards and inwards. Abdomen musculature is pulled in and buttock muscles are contracted. The pelvis is thus supported and inclined forwards. Mild rotation of the thighs also rotates knees and feet. When standing, the feet are oriented in such a way that body weight is concentrated on the insteps. Increased lordosis of the neck which is common in obese children can be improved by contraction of the muscles between scapulae and vertebral column ('pull your shoulders back and stand up straight!'), especially between 6–9th vertebrae. The sternum is lifted at the same time and shoulders are drawn to the sides and down. Thus the chest is better positioned for adequate breathing.

Breathing exercises

Breathing exercises should not be carried out until children have adopted correct body posture. During all exercises children should be aware of unobstructed flow of air in and out of the lungs. Most children breathe superficially, automatically, and unconsciously.

Conscious breathing is best done in a lying position. Attention should be concentrated on expiration. Various rhythms are used. During these exercises the abdomen should be drawn in, and small of the back should be pressed towards the ground. Expiration should always last longer than inspiration since it has been shown that inspiration is more efficient after full expiration. It is also important that the children do not hyperventilate. These exercises can exercise the costal muscles. Adoption of more effective respiration can also improve body posture.

As regards other exercises, it is best for obese children to start from a low supported position, such as lying on the back or abdomen, sitting, kneeling, and so on. It is important to have a slow start or gradual 'warm-up' with some simple exercise, for which the procedures, benefits, and disadvantages if practised incorrectly, have been fully explained. Rhythmic co-ordination of exercise and breathing is essential. Relaxation after a period of exercise involving prolonged muscle contraction is indispensable. Exercises are initially performed four to six times on each occasion but later on can be performed as many as eight to ten times. A kindly encouraging approach helps to gain the confidence of children, creates a pleasant ambience and makes it easier to overcome children's physical and psychological restraints.

All exercises can be executed correctly or incorrectly. Incorrect techniques not only limit their effect but can cause harm. Only experienced teachers should exercise obese children. The consequences of not using the correct procedures for exercise or of practising exercises in unsupervised environments are potentially serious in unfit obese individuals.

Exercising individual parts of the body

To exercise the spine, the abdominal wall muscles need strengthening, the contracted shoulder and back muscles need to relax – as do the hip joints – and, simultaneously, muscles around joints need strengthening. Initially, children should be helped when performing exercises, for example assisted to get up from lying to sitting by pulling them up by their arms. During all exercises breathing should be relaxed, with no holding of breath but concentration on expiration. There are a number of exercises for the vertebral column with the subject lying on the back or sides, with various movements of the legs and arms. Other sets of exercises can be executed in kneeling, sitting or standing positions. Each exercise must be followed by a period of relaxation.

When exercising lower extremities, we stress the strengthening of the thighs. In spite of their large circumference, thigh muscles are often weak and flaccid. For this purpose it is helpful to trot on the spot, lifting knees up high, or exercise with a skipping rope. Such exercises should be limited in number at the beginning of a programme of activity, but can be gradually increased. Skipping should be low and relaxed. These exercises can be supplemented by intermittent squatting, at the same time as maintaining good truncal posture and regular breathing.

Movements of the upper extremities should involve the active support of other parts of the body and can be carried out from standing, sitting, kneeling and lying positions. Shoulder joints, as well as all other joints, should be relaxed. These exercises can be used for preclass warm-ups. They should prepare children for the main activity and need to be varied and attractive.

Obese children with orthopaedic complications can be given exercises modified specifically to meet their needs. For example, children with lordosis or kyphos-coliosis need to strengthen their back and interscapular and abdominal muscles. Chest muscles must be relaxed and lengthened. Children with winging of the scapulae have slack and feeble muscles especially down their backs. These children need advice on how to achieve better chest posture by drawing their shoulders back and practising keeping their scapulae flat against their backs.

Special exercises for the correction of scoliosis can also help to rectify simple rounded back and winged scapulae. There are as many exercises for this purpose as there are for the correction of pathological flat feet and genu valgum. The detailed descriptions of such exercises, especially those developed for obese children with or without additional health and orthopaedic problems, are available in handbooks prepared by specialized physical educators.

15.6 How to improve compliance

Usually, obese children have poor compliance with exercise programmes (Epstein et al., 1983). Longitudinal measurements in obese children show that the majority of children regain body weight and any fat lost when obesity treatment stops. This happens even after successful periods of inpatient and/or outpatient treatment, during which the children have significantly improved their morphological, functional and biochemical status. In our clinical experience, the main reason given for noncompliance or drop-out is that exercise is time consuming, tiring, costly, boring and causes injuries. Programmes must appeal to children's preferences. A return to the lifestyle and environmental conditions which induced obesity reverses many of the positive changes promoted by therapy. However, if we follow children long enough, we can show improved fitness in spite of fluctuations in weight, fatness and functional capacity. After attending summer camps over 4 years, mean values for BMI, LBM, depot fat and functional capacity in a group of adolescent obese boys were closer to the mean for normal-weight boys of the same age than before attending the camps (Parizkova, 1998). Some of the boys even achieved normal anthropometry.

Recognizing some of the concepts which underlie the programmes can increase obese children's adherence to exercise. For example:

- The importance of increased fitness without necessarily decreased fatness. There is always some benefit in terms of fitness even after short periods of exercise, provided that the exercises are executed properly and regularly. There may be no change in total body weight due to simultaneous growth in height. BMI might reduce slightly but, in the absence of that, reduction in skinfold thickness, at least in some parts of body surface, could be present. Children must be encouraged to recognize that there are positive results from their efforts even if not demonstrated in loss of weight.

- The recognition that only permanent adherence to programmes of activity can bring lasting reductions to weight and fatness and improved functional capacity and physical performance. Physical activity needs to be seen in a positive light. It may be helpful to find role models, with public profiles, who have slimmed or who are known to be involved in physical-activity programmes. As mentioned above, exercise must be enjoyable and amusing. The personality of the trainer/physical educator, the environment, the overall ambience have to be friendly and kind and the sportswear attractive and comfortable. These all help keep children interested and participating.

- Appreciation of the positive value of the programme for other members of the family and for peers. This should encourage children to continue with the programme – and even encourage peers to participate too.

- The sense of well-being and achievement resulting from the activity, supported by the congratulation of others, creates very positive feelings towards the regime. Good results will encourage permanent commitment to organized forms of physical education as well as increasing the levels of spontaneous physical activity and exercise at home and during leisure time.

- Activity programmes which do not appear to be having much effect should not dwell on weight and fat loss but try to find other positive output, such as evidence for improved performance of some physical tasks, improved silhouette and so on (Parizkova, 1995; Parizkova & Hill 2000; Strakova & Simsova, unpublished data).

15.7 The role of the family

Family members are usually those closest to obese children. Their emotional and psychological support are essential for successful slimming programmes. Ideally, regimes should be adhered to, at least in part, by all members of obese children's families. It is an absolute requirement that they do not eat sweets and energy-dense, tempting foodstuffs in the presence of the obese children. Family members are unlikely to be harmed and may benefit from following the exercise regimen with their children, particularly if there is familial overweight. The same applies to physical activity regimes. It is difficult to persuade children to adopt greater workloads when they are constantly seeing their overweight parents move only when absolutely necessary. Joining in physical activities as a family should be seen as an essential adjunct to treatment of the obese. Walking and some games should be part of family outings – and should not be less frequent than twice a month. Holidays can be spent together as a family, with excursions and exercises in the open air.

When caring parents have one or more obese children, the support required from the family is easy to see. The greatest problems arise when only one child in the family is obese. Then family arrangements to meet the obese child's dietary and physical activity needs may appear to interfere with normal lifestyle.

Encouragement from family members, sensitive support and appreciation of what they are achieving enhance children's willingness to continue exercise to improve their physical and functional status and to maintain active lifestyles in the future.

15.8 Conclusions

Exercise produces significant effects on body weight and/or fat mass, provided that it is intense enough. Reduction of inactivity, promotion of a more active lifestyle and the development of an exercise programme can increase the success of obesity therapy. Even when exercise does not reduce obesity, it may independently reduce morbidity. Organized physical activity regimes and increased exercise have to be accompanied by controlled energy intakes, so that increased energy outputs are not paralleled by increased energy intakes, especially of undesirable food items. Aerobic exercise increases cardiorespiratory capacity. The increased enzymatic activity of skeletal muscles facilitates the utilization of fat metabolites during muscle work. This in itself results in reduced adiposity and changes fat distribution. Therefore, aerobic exercise is the most suitable form of exercise for obese children.

In spite of the need for further research, some principles for planning exercise programmes can be tentatively proposed. Each programme should be individualized and adapted to the needs of the particular child. Supportive help from family, peers, physical educators and teachers can combine to guarantee lasting positive effects of physical activity therapy until adulthood. High rates of drop-out can be reduced by programmes which are cheap, which involve group aerobic activities, and which are of low intensity but of more than 30 minutes duration.

15.9 REFERENCES

Ainsworth, B.E., Haskell, W.L., Leon, A.S., Jacobs, D.R., Montoye, H.J., Sallis, J.F. & Paffenbarger, R.S. (1993). Compendium of physical activities: classification of exercise costs of human physical activities. *Medicine and Science in Sports and Exercise*, **25**, 71–80.

Astrand, P.O. & Rodahl, K. (1986). *Textbook of Work Physiology*. 3rd edn. New York: MacGraw-Hill.

Ballor, D.L. & Keesey R.E. (1991). A meta-analysis of the factors affecting exercise-induced changes in body mass, fat-mass and fat-free mass in males and females. *International Journal of Obesity*, **15**, 717–26.

Belko, A.Z., Van Loan, M., Barbieri, T.F. & Mayclin, P.P.P. (1986). Diet, weight loss, and energy expenditure in moderately overweight women. *International Journal of Obesity*, **11**, 93–104.

Björntorp, P. (1992). Abdominal fat distribution and disease: an overview of epidemiological data. *Annals of Medicine*, **24**, 15–18.

Blaak, E.E., Westerterp, K.S., Bar-Or, O., Wouters, L.J.M. & Saris, W.H.M. (1992). Total energy expenditure and spontaneous activity in relation to training in obese boys. *American Journal of Clinical Nutrition*, **55**, 777–82.

Blair, S.N., Kohl, H.V., Gordon, N.F. & Paffenbarger, R.S. (1992), How much physical activity is good for health? *Annual Review of Public Health*, **13**, 99–126.

Blundell, J., Burley, V.J. & Lawton, C.L. (1993). Dietary fat and the control of energy intake: evaluating the effects of fat on meal size and postmeal satiety. *American Journal of Clinical Nutrition*, **57** (suppl.), 772–8S.

Brehm, B. & Gutin, B. (1986). Recovery energy expenditure for steady state exercise in runners and nonexercisers. *Medicine and Science in Sports and Exercise*, **18**, 205–10.

Brown, D.R. (1990). Exercise, fitness, and mental health. In *Exercise, Fitness, and Health.* eds. C. Bouchard, R.J. Shepard, T. Stephens, J.R. Sutton & B.D. McPherson, pp. 607–26. Champaign, IL: Human Kinetics Books.

Caspersen, C.J., Powell, K.E. & Christensen, G.M. (1985). Physical activity fitness: definitions and distinctions for health-related research. *Public Health Reports*, **100**, 126–31.

Ceesay, S.M., Prentice, A.M., Day, K.C., Murgatroyd, P.R., Goldberg, G.R., Scott, W. & Spurr, G.B. (1989). The use of heart-rate monitoring in the estimation of energy expenditure using whole body calorimetry: a validation study. *British Journal of Nutrition*, **61**, 175–86.

Donnelly, J.E., Sharp, T., Houmard, J., Carlson, M.G., Hill, J.O., Whatley, J.E. & Israel, R.G. (1993). Muscle hypertrophy with large-scale weight loss and resistance training. *American Journal of Clinical Nutrition*, **58**, 561–5.

Dore, C., Hesp, R., Wilkins, D. & Garrow, J.S. (1982). Prediction of energy requirements of obese patients after massive weight loss. *Human Nutrition: Clinical Nutrition*, **36C**, 41–8.

Ekblom, B. (1992). Energy expenditure during exercise in obesity. In *Obesity*, eds. P. Björntorp, B.N. & J.B. Brodoff, pp. 136–44. Philadelphia, PA: Lippincott Co.

Epstein, L.H. (1995). Exercise in the treatment of childhood obesity. *International Journal of Obesity and Related Metabolic Disorders*, **19** (suppl. 4), 117–21.

Epstein, L.H., Wing, R.R., Koeske, R., Ossip, D. & Beck, S. (1982). A comparison of lifestyle change and programmed aerobic exercise on weight and fitness changes in obese children. *Behaviour Therapy*, **13**, 651–65.

Epstein, L.H., Koeske, R. & Wing, R.R. (1983). Adherence to exercise in obese children. *Journal of Cardiac Rehabilitation*, **4**, 185–9.

Epstein, L.H., Wing, R.R., Penner, B.C. & Kress, M.J. (1985a). Effect of diet and controlled exercise on weight loss in obese children. *Journal of Pediatrics*, **107**, 358–61.

Epstein, L.H., Wing, R.R., Koeske, R. & Valoski, A. (1985b). A comparison of lifestyle exercise, aerobic exercise, and calisthenics on weight loss in obese children. *Behaviour Therapy*, **16**, 345–56.

Epstein, L.H., Valoski A.M., Vara, L.S., McCurley, J., Wisniewski, L., Kalarchian, M.A., et al. (1995). Effects of decreasing sedentary behaviour and increasing activity on weight change in obese children. *Health Psychology*, **14**, 109–15.

Faulkner, J.A. & White, T.P. (1990). Adaptation of skeletal muscle to physical activity. In *Exercise, Fitness, and Health*, eds. C. Bouchard, R.J. Shepard, T. Stephens, J.R. Sutton & B.D. McPherson, pp. 265–279. Champaign, IL: Human Kinetics Books.

Flatt, J.P. (1978). The biochemistry of energy expenditure. In *Recent Advances in Obesity Research*, vol. II, ed. G.A. Bray, pp. 211–19. London: Newman Publishing.

Flatt, J.P. (1987a). Dietary fat, carbohydrate balance, and weight maintenance: effect of exercise. *American Journal of Clinical Nutrition*, **45**, 296–306.

Flatt, J.P. (1987b). The difference in the storage capacities for carbohydrate and for fat, and its implications in the regulation of body weight. *Annals of the New York Academy of Sciences*, **499**, 104–23.

Jopling, R.J. (1988). Health-related fitness as preventive medicine. *Pediatric Review*, **10**, 141–8.

King, A.C. & Tribble, D.L. (1991). The role of exercise in weight regulation in nonathletes. *Sports Medicine*, **11**, 331–49.

Knip, P. & Nuutinen, O. (1993). Long-term effects of weight reduction on serum lipids and plasma insulin in obese children. *American Journal of Clinical Nutrition*, **57**, 490–3.

Maffeis, C., Pinelli, L. & Schutz, Y. (1992). Effect of weight loss on resting energy expenditure in obese prepubertal children. *International Journal of Obesity*, **16**, 41–7.

Maffeis, C., Schutz, Y., Schena, F., Zaffanello, M. & Pinelli, L. (1993). Energy expenditure during walking and running in obese and nonobese prepubertal children. *Journal of Pediatrics*, **123**, 193–9.

Nieman, D.C., Haig J.L., DeGula, E.D., Dizon, G.P. & Registed, U.D. (1988). Reducing diet and exercise training effects on resting metabolic rate in mildly obese women. *Journal of Sports Medicine*, **28**, 79–88.

Paffenbarger, R.S., Hyde, R.T., Wing, A.L. & Hsieh, C.C. (1986). Physical activity, all-cause mortality, and longevity of college alumni. *New England Journal of Medicine*, **314**, 605–13.

Parizkova, J. (1972). Obesity and physical activity. In *Proceedings of the Nutricia Symposium 'Nutritional Aspects of Physical Performance'*, pp. 146–60 Papendal, The Netherlands, 1971. The Hague: Mouton & Company.

Parizkova, J. (1977). *Body fat and physical fitness. Body composition and lipid metabolism in different regimes of physical activity*. The Hague: Martinus Nijhoff B.V. Medical Division.

Parizkova J. (1979). Activity, obesity and growth. *Monographs of the Society for the Research in Child Development*, **35**, 28–32.

Parizkova, J. (1995). Obesity and physical fitness: an age-dependent functional and social handicap. In *Social Aspects of Obesity*, eds. I. DeGarine & N.J. Pollock, pp. 163–75. Australia: Gordon & Breach.

Parizkova, J. (1998). Treatment and prevention of obesity by exercise in Czech children. Physical fitness and nutrition during growth. In *Studies in Children and Youth in Different Environments*. ed. J. Parizkova & A.P. Hill, pp. 145–54. Basel: S. Karger.

Parizkova, J. & Hill, A. P. (2000). *Childhood Obesity: Prevention and Treatment*. Boca Raton, London: CRC Press.

Parizkova, J., Bunc, V., Sprynarova, S., Mackova, E. & Heller, J. (1987). Body composition, aerobic power, ventilatory threshold, and food intake in different sports. *Annals of Sports Medicine*, **3**, 171–7.

Poehlman, E.T. (1989). A review: exercise and its influence on resting energy expenditure in man. *Medicine and Science in Sports and Exercise*, **21**, 515–25.

Raben, A., Mygind, E., Saltin, B. & Astrup, A. (1997). Decreased activity of fat-oxidizing enzymes in muscle of obesity-prone subjects. *International Journal of Obesity*, **21** (Suppl. 2), S43.

Ravussin, E., Lillioja, S., Anderson, T.E., et al. (1986). Determinants of 24-hour energy expenditure in man: methods and results using a respiration chamber. *Journal of Clinical Investigation*, **78**, 568–78.

Reybrouck, T., Vinckx, J., Van den Berghe, G. & Vanderschueren-Lodeweyckx, M. (1990). Exercise therapy and hypocaloric diet in the treatment of obese children and adolescents. *Acta Paediatrica Scandinavica*, **79**, 84–9.

Rolls, B.J., Kim-Harris, S., Fischman, M.W., et al. (1994). Satiety after preloads with different amounts of fat and carbohydrate: implications for obesity. *American Journal of Clinical Nutrition*, **60**, 476–87.

Sasaki, J., Shindo, M., Tanaka, H., Ando, M. & Arakawa, K. (1987). A long-term aerobic exercise program decreased the obesity index and increased the high density lipoprotein cholesterol concentration in obese children. *International Journal of Obesity*, **11**, 339–45.

Schwartz, R.S., Shurman, W.P., Larson, V., Cain, K.C., Fellingham, G.W., Beard, J.C., Kahn, S.E., Stratton, J.R., Cerqueira, M.D. & Abrass, I.B. (1991). The effect of intensive endurance exercise training on body fat distribution in young and older men. *Metabolism*, **40**, 545–51.

Surgeon General (1996). *Physical activity and health: a report of the surgeon general*. Washington, DC: US Department of Health and Human Services.

Tremblay, A., Nadeau, A., Fournier, G. & Bouchard, C. (1988). Effect of a three-day interruption of exercise-training on resting metabolic rate and glucose-induced thermogenesis in trained individuals. *International Journal of Obesity*, **12**, 163–8.

Vamberova, M., Parizkova, J. & Vaneckova, M. (1971). Vegetative reactions to optimal work load as related to body weight and composition in adolescent boys and girls. *Physiologica Bohemoslovaca*, **20**, 415.

WHO (1985). Energy and protein requirements: *report of a joint FAO/WHO/UNU expert consultation*. Geneva, World Health Organization, p. 189.

Wing, R.R., Jeffery, R.W., Burton, L.R., Thorson, C., Kuller, L.H. & Folsom, A.R. (1992). Change in waist-hip ratio with weight loss and its association with change in cardiovascular risk factors. *American Journal of Clinical Nutrition*, **55**, 1086–92.

16

Psychotherapy

Carl-Erik Flodmark[1] and Inge Lissau[2]

[1]Department of Paediatrics, University Hospital in Malmö. [2]National Institute of Public Health, Copenhagen

16.1 Obesity – a disease put into perspective

Obesity itself is not usually regarded as an eating disorder, although sometimes obesity and eating disorders (commonly binge eating) coexist. The prevalence of eating disorders in association with obesity used to be thought as high as 20–50% of those seeking help for their obesity, but recent studies of adolescents enrolled into an obesity programme suggest a prevalence of around 7% of obese (Decaluwé et al., 2000). The reason for this difference is that diagnostic interviews do not confirm the findings of earlier questionnaires (Stunkard et al., 1996; Ricca et al., 2000). Further, amongst obese children in the general population and not seeking help for their obesity, the prevalence of eating disorders may be even lower. However, we do not propose to discuss the use of psychotherapy in the treatment of eating disorders here. This chapter is concerned with how psychotherapy can be used more generally for the understanding and treatment of obesity.

Psychotherapy is one tool for achieving the lifestyle changes necessary to counteract strong genetic influences on the development of obesity. The multifactorial causes of obesity demand lifestyle changes which can only be achieved through a combined approach using many different treatment components, for example combining advice on exercise and diet, training in social skills, even drug treatment in the most severe cases.

16.1.1 Psychosocial aspects of society

Psychosocial factors are certainly important in childhood obesity, although the extent to which they are relevant varies with the population selected and the differences in environmental support provided by family and peers.

There are conflicting results regarding the self-esteem of obese children (Braet et al., 1997a; Kimm et al., 1997; Stradmeijer et al., 2000; Strauss, 2000). Most obese children in a population-based sample seem to have normal self-esteem (Rumpel

& Harris, 1994; Renman et al., 1999; Strauss, 2000) although Braet et al. (1997a) disagree. However, in a more recent study, weight status rather than self-esteem was most closely linked to dietary restraint (Braet & Wydhooge, 2000).

Whatever the prevalence or extent of specific psychosocial problems in childhood obesity, the strong association of obesity with some psychosocial factors indicates that this area needs more attention. For further discussion, see Chapter 6.

16.2 The treatment of obesity

16.2.1 Why do we need new treatments?

Many different kinds of treatment for obesity have been investigated, including diet, exercise, surgery and medication. None is totally effective as sole treatment.

Treatment needs to be affirmative and long lasting. Single physical treatments or short periods of treatment are insufficient because they fail to take into account lifelong genetic influences and/or societal pressures promoting obesity. However, increased understanding of genetics means that the need for the long-term management of childhood obesity is more widely recognized. Many children probably have some inherited susceptibility for the development of obesity. Management thus needs to be lifelong and not merely a short period of diet and exercise. With these latter children, after successful periods of fat reduction, obesity would be considered 'cured' and affected individuals would return to their earlier but only marginally improved lifestyles without being thought at risk of redeveloping obesity. If they gained weight again, it was thought that their lifestyles were less healthy than those of normal-weight persons. Now, better understanding of gene–environmental interaction gives room for other interpretations.

For those who have inherited a predisposition to obesity, it is not sufficient to follow the average lifestyle regarding exercise and diet – a healthier lifestyle is needed. Many studies show that obese people eat less than the nonobese. This is usually explained by the belief that obese people under-report their eating behaviours (Epstein, 1993). However, metabolic adjustments may return body fat to base-line levels if energy intakes are constrained to hold fat stores constantly above or below the base-line levels (Leibel et al., 1995). Thus, it is difficult to deviate from a set point for body fat and body weight. This may explain why obese individuals may eat small amounts of food and still remain obese.

Healthy lifestyles could be followed early in life and thus counterbalance the genetic inheritance. In such cases individuals might not notice the effects of the genetic influence and thus not see themselves as having a disease, that is being obese. However, if lifestyles change due to external factors, such as through diseases affecting the motor system, these individuals might then develop obesity.

Below, we describe a choice of strategies which can be used to manage child-hood obesity. For those who are not genetically susceptible to obesity, it should be easy to reduce weight. They should just live like those of normal weight! However, for those who appear to have the genes for obesity, lifestyles need special care. And for those at high risk of adult obesity – the most obese children – health and lifestyle programmes for the whole population (see Section 16.2.5) may help, but specific, personalized management is also necessary.

16.2.2 Psychodynamic therapy – an early perspective

Psychodynamic therapy is used less for the management of obesity than for eating disorders. Bruch's early clinical observations on obesity included subjects' families in the management programme (Bruch, 1964, 1970, 1974). The obese child was described as living in a dysfunctional family, with disturbed communication between parents and child. The child had difficulties discriminating between emotions and other bodily sensations, such as hunger. Eating was then used as a substitute for emotional needs. This abnormal response developed early in the mother–child interaction if the child's needs for love, warmth, food and so on were not adequately met.

All this work remains relevant since there are no recently published studies regarding psychodynamic therapy in obesity (Porter, 1980).

16.2.3 Behavioural and cognitive therapies – a traditional and a new approach

Behavioural therapy has been used in obesity management since it was first developed (Stuart, 1967). Programmes were based on the belief that obesity was a 'learned disease' and potentially amenable to cure by 'relearning'. However, long-term successes were not achieved (Brownell & Wadden, 1991). Nevertheless, booster sessions over a 4-year period did create lasting effects for adults in one 10-year follow-up. This study showed the difficulties of achieving a good response and the need for long-term treatment (Björvell & Rössner, 1992).

Behavioural therapy for obesity is centred on the concept of bad eating habits in which insufficient control of external stimuli to eat, or rewarding behaviours, result in increased food intakes. Bad eating habits can be broken down into small sequences: the frequency of chewing; the frequency of meals and so on. Parents may be seen as reinforcing children's eating habits. For example, children may be encouraged to diet by rewarding weight reduction with money (Epstein et al., 1980).

In 1983, Brownell and coworkers evaluated a programme consisting of behaviour modification, social support, nutrition and exercise (Brownell et al., 1983). They noted that groups in which obese children and their mothers met the group therapist separately gave better results than those in which children were seen alone or children were seen together with their mothers.

Other strategies may be more efficient. Epstein et al. (1990) studied the effects of parent interaction, using three groups: a child and parent group where parent and child behavioural change and weight losses were reinforced by behavioural techniques; a children-only group where child behavioural change and weight loss were reinforced; and a nonspecific control group where families were reinforced only for attendance. The best response came from the parent and child behavioural change group.

Recently, cognitive therapy has been combined with behavioural therapy in the treatment of obesity. The presumption is that, through practice and reward, changes in key areas of children's cognitive processing lead to behavioural changes. However, the causal connections between the attempt to influence children's cognition and the observed behaviour changes were not subjected to stringent research design (Kendall & Lochman, 1994).

There are few studies evaluating cognitive and behavioural therapy. In one such study, 27 children aged 7–13 years were randomized to either cognitive therapy or behavioural therapy. No differences between the groups were found after 3 and 6 months follow-up. Therapies were equally effective (Duffy & Spence, 1993) but the follow-up period was short.

In another study, behavioural treatment was combined with either cognitive therapy or nutrition education (Kalodner & DeLucia, 1991). The different treatments induced different ways of controlling weight. For example, in the cognitive group the weight-related cognitions were more adaptive than in the other groups. However, although there were significant differences in obesity status over time, there was none between treatments. Another study with 3 months follow-up also showed that the addition of cognitive therapy to a behavioural programme was no better than behavioural therapy alone (DeLucia & Kalodner, 1990).

However, cognitive therapy can be effective in treating childhood obesity (Braet, 1999; Braet & Van Winckel, 2000; Braet et al., 1997b). In these studies, cognitive behavioural therapy was given for 6 months in different settings and subjects were followed up for 6 months after treatment stopped. Individual treatment was compared with group treatment given both as an outpatient programme and during a summer camp. 'Advice in one session' was given to those who could not participate in the full programme. All groups were compared with the control group. The camp group had significantly better results initially: 8.2% weight loss vs. 3.3–5.7% in other groups at 3 months and 15.6% vs. 8.3–8.4% at 6 months. However, at 1 year the differences were no longer significant, although the effect of treatment overall was significant using analysis of covariance. At 1 year the camp approach showed a weight reduction of 14.7%, the group treatment 13.1%, the individual treatment 9.8% and the 'advice in one session' approach 6.8%. The control group increased in weight by 2.5%. The best results were in moderately overweight children ($<55\%$ excess weight) aged less than 14 years.

After 5 years, 80% of the original sample were followed up again (Braet & Van Winckel, 2000). Seventy-two subjects (72%) showed no increase in percentage overweight, 18% were no longer obese and 29% were moderately obese. Overweight fell by 11%, although mean overweight was still 42%. Important to remember is that the goals of treatment in obese adolescents have to be different from those used in adults as the child is growing, making both body mass index (BMI) and body fat age-dependent. In this study, using the Eating Disorder Inventory (Garner et al., 1983), five adolescents in a subgroup ($n = 53$), that is 9%, had an 'at-risk' score on the bulimia subscale. This shows that the risk of developing eating disorders is lower than previously thought using this type of treatment.

Treatment was based on cognitive strategies, behavioural strategies, education and motivation. Self-regulation techniques were introduced according to a 12-session manual aiming at self-instruction, self-observation, self-evaluation and self-reward. Modelling, behavioural rehearsal and homework were used to train these skills. The emphasis was on developing a healthy lifestyle so as to avoid the presumed psychologically negative effects of strict dieting. The treatment was combined with family discussions although specific family therapy was not given. Epstein et al. (1990) have shown the importance of involving families in the treatment process.

Although emerging from a different therapeutic background this programme has many similarities with programmes based on family therapy (Flodmark et al., 1993). Similarities are seen in the behavioural strategies, educational components and work needed to increase motivation. Both programmes develop weight stabilizing rather than weight reducing strategies. Prescribed diets involve moderate calorie restriction. However, there are differences in the emphasis placed on families in family-therapy programmes and in the fewer visits necessary (six family-therapy sessions in 18 months) with cognitive behavioural programmes. The explanation of why fewer visits still lead to significant effects may relate to the home supervision of children by their families but induced by the therapists. In the family therapy programme, exercise at home was encouraged and no exercise was performed using supervision.

These two studies show that combined programmes are effective using a careful selection of different approaches.

16.2.4 Group therapy – more research is needed

Many different types of therapy can be utilized within the context of a group, and there have been some studies of this approach. For example, with adolescents, a peer-group behaviour-modification programme gave better results than individual contact (Zakus et al., 1979). Although the development of group cohesion was tenuous and temporary, the girls who were functioning most independently achieved the greatest weight loss. However, the study was not randomized and the patient group was small. In another study, individual dietetic counselling, group dietetic counselling, and group dietetic counselling with behaviour modification were compared (Long et al., 1983). The first and third treatment programmes were equally effective at 1-year follow-up and better than group dietetic counselling alone. The general impression is that group therapy has no decisive advantage when compared with individual therapy (Aimez, 1976). Exceptions may be shown by those groups for whom there has been very careful selection for strong homogeneity regarding, for example, gender, age and social background.

It is probably easier to get preschool children to accept groups formed by adults than older children, who need to create their own groups. Further, group activities may be more successful in preschool than older children. Our experience is that during puberty, acceptance of these group activities is low. Only 10% of 14-year-old children identified after screening, accepted group therapy as an alternative to individual treatment (unpublished data). Braet et al. (1997a) give more information on how to use groups in cognitive behavioural therapy but more research is still needed on its use in childhood obesity.

16.2.5 School-based treatments – the basic approach

Behavioural therapy has also been used in schools (Brownell & Kaye, 1982). Programmes comprised behaviour modification, nutrition education and physical activity. Parents and school personnel were involved. Sixty (95%) of 63 children (5–12 years) in one 10-week programme lost weight, compared to only three (21%) of 14 control children. Programme children showed a mean decrease of 15.4% in their percentage overweight, and lost an average of 4.4 kg.

Providing treatment in the wider context of schools and promoting a good lifestyle, not only to obese children but to *all* children, may be fruitful approaches to childhood obesity. However, long-term follow-up is difficult in such studies with so many individuals being treated and so many potential variables. A review of school-based treatments found no single programme significantly better than the others. No recommendations could be made (Ward & Bar-Or, 1986). Most programmes were not directed at obese children specifically but instead at groups of children of all nutritional states.

This area needs more research and should be seen more as health education rather than psychotherapy.

16.2.6 Early treatment – the treatment of choice

Early treatment, that is beginning before the peak incidence of childhood obesity around 10 years old, has shown best results with preschool children (Davis & Christoffel, 1994). The treatment is similar to school-based treatment in that it also uses groups of children but is specifically directed at obese children (see above). Treatment of children seems more effective than treatment of adults (Epstein et al., 1995a) and 50–75% of adults in excess of 160% of ideal body weight were also obese as children (Dietz, 1983). Thus, early treatment should prevent many of the most severe cases of obesity in adults.

16.2.7 Family therapy – a new view on treatment

The family is basic to a child's psychological development and is a major factor influencing the child's quality of life. Family therapy has been widely used for children with behavioural and/or emotional disturbances, and for children with chronic diseases.

Several reviews (Gurman & Kniskern, 1981; Hazelrigg et al., 1987; Lask, 1987; Dare, 1992) show that family therapy is effective in asthma, diabetes, anorexia nervosa, bereavement and adult schizophrenia. It has also been possible to develop family-based diagnostic tests for those families where a child is showing other symptoms (Hansson, 1989).

Psychoeducational family therapy has been used in schizophrenia. Orhagen (1992) and coworkers have studied whether the educational or the therapeutic part of the programme was most effective and have shown that both are needed. Another Swedish study demonstrated that family therapy was a cost-effective treatment for childhood asthma (Gustafsson, 1987).

Not surprisingly, therefore, it has also been suggested that family therapy might be helpful for treating obesity (Ganley, 1986). Several studies by Epstein's group have highlighted the importance of obese children's interaction with their parents (Epstein et al., 1980, 1990). Flodmark et al. (1993) demonstrated that family therapy is more effective than conventional treatment with obese children screened at school at the age of 10 years when children are compared 4 years later. These families were selected from a population-based sample and three treatment groups were compared: conventional treatment, that is regular visits to physician and dietician; six sessions of family therapy; and no treatment. The duration of treatment was 14–18 months for both treatment groups.

At follow-up 1 year after the end of treatment, BMI was significantly lower in the family therapy group than in the untreated control group. Furthermore, physical fitness was significantly higher and fat mass (measured by skinfold thickness) significantly lower in the family therapy group than in the conventionally treated group. There was no difference in mean BMI between the family therapy group and the conventionally treated group, perhaps because better physical fitness in combination with reduced fat mass led to greater muscle mass and thus an unchanged BMI.

The diets used in the study described above contained 1500–1700 kcal/day with 30% total energy from fat. Such diets have been used in other programmes (Epstein et al., 1990) and give sufficient calorie restriction whilst not impeding normal pubertal growth (Epstein, 1993). However, the energy content of diets does need adjusting upwards for factors such as physical activity. Diets of lower energy content are rarely needed. It is often more effective to discuss general strategies for changing lifestyle than the technicalities of diets.

Children are naturally active. It is not usually necessary to prescribe exercise programmes for those under 10 years old, since they are spontaneously active. However, they do need support from their families for time and space to move, and particularly the freedom to play out of doors.

In adolescence, a sedentary lifestyle becomes habitual, making it important that teenagers are encouraged to maintain high levels of physical activity. A combined approach which encourages both formal exercise and a more active lifestyle has been investigated in other studies (Epstein et al., 1995b). The best results were in those groups which focused only on lifestyle changes, not in the groups targeting exercise and a less sedentary lifestyle. Routine or lifestyle activities such as fidgeting may account for more expenditure than once thought (Dietz, 1991). Encouraging lifestyle changes within the context of mixed programmes which include dietary changes could have significant impact on childhood obesity.

During family therapy sessions, families were encouraged to be physically active at home (Flodmark et al., 1993). Those receiving family therapy had better physical fitness than the control group who had received similar advice to the family therapy group regarding physical activity. This emphasizes that the psychological aspects of changing lifestyle are more important than the precise exercise adopted. In the past, when treating obesity, too much emphasis has been placed on techniques rather than on global approaches to changing lifestyles (Flodmark, 1997).

What sort of psychotherapy was offered? A combination of Minuchin's structural model (Minuchin et al., 1975, 1978; Minuchin & Fishman, 1981) and de Shazer's brief therapy model (de Shazer, 1982, 1985, 1988, 1991) was used.

The therapist used a structural model as the basis of therapy but within this, the solution-based model could be influential. Usually families wanted to discuss the difficulties they or their children experienced following prescribed diets or recommended exercise regimens, rather than the recommendations per se. Adequate information during therapy was essential for success in finding solutions. Families were asked to discuss different solutions at home between sessions. The beliefs and thoughts of the obese children were essential to this whole process.

To summarize, the following goals were found to be useful; to:

- provide families with low intensity, nonconfrontational, contact;
- identify and acknowledge family resources;
- show respect for the family and use noncondemning interventions;
- involve other significant individuals;
- try to identify the whole system and relate it to its context;
- accept individual's definitions of problems;
- rephrase comments in positive contexts;
- emphasize positive solutions;
- start with small simple solutions. Give appreciation;
- discuss realistic and appropriate lowest weights;
- advise families about the length of time needed to achieve goals for fat loss;
- convey the message that controlling overweight is hard work.

Finally, it should be acknowledged that the experiences of those providing family therapy and studies of obese children and their families recognize that families with obese children show no differences in communication with, or support of, their children when compared with families of normal-weight children (Valtolina & Marta, 1998).

16.2.8 The questions are the answers

Below are some examples of how to use different types of questions in the treatment of obesity in children and adolescents.

You are interviewing a 15-year-old boy with his parents. The setting is perhaps a doctor in his or her office or a family therapist in a research setting (Fig. 16.1).

Linear questions

Dr: How are things going with John's obesity?
Mother: He is trying to eat less but I don't know what he is doing when he comes home from school.
Dr: Did you follow the lists I gave you, John?
John: I have tried to but I don't know where they are.
Dr: When did you see them last?
John: I don't remember.
Father: My wife says he is always trying to escape his responsibilities!
Dr: Do you remember anything from my lists, John?
John: No, I don't. Didn't I tell you that one minute ago? I want to go home now.

Although unintentional, these linear questions can lead to a scapegoating process. John is being blamed for not being able to follow the diet. This process began with the initial complaint of the mother. The doctor then used linear questions without any intention to attribute blame but this was counterbalanced

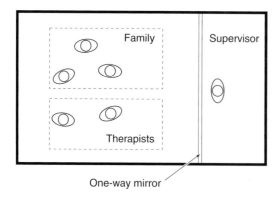

Figure 16.1 A supervisor is needed to train therapists. Behind a one-way mirror the supervisor can give support and instructions to the therapists either by phone or during gaps in the therapy. The session may also be video-taped.

as mother's view was supported by father saying that he really did not know what was going on at home.

Circular questions

Dr: How are things going with John's obesity?
Mother: He is trying to eat less but I don't know what he does when he comes home from school.

Now you know that the mother is worried. Instead you use circular questions to investigate the problem.

Dr: Who would know that?
Father: My wife says he is always trying to escape his responsibilities!

Now you know the father is worried but that he also does not know what is happening.

Dr: Who is most worried about your obesity John? Your father or your mother?
John: It is my mother.
Dr: How do you know that?
John: She is always nagging me about what I eat when I get home from school.
Dr: Is there any difference in how your mother or your father reminds you about what you are eating?
John: Yes, my father reminds me but my mother nags me all the time.
Dr to mother and father: What can you do to help each other to remind John about his late afternoon snack?

These questions are more neutral but still need care. Although using circular questions, mother may need more support.

Strategic questions

Now let us continue the conversation with something more powerful!

These questions are used by lawyers and journalists and are not recommended in obesity. They could be useful in certain psychiatric conditions and an example is given below. The doctor wants to increase the involvement of the father.

Father answers: I don't know.
Dr to father: Can't you see that you disappoint your wife by not helping her?
Father: I have too much to do at work.
Dr to father: How can you abandon your family totally?
Father: I am really trying, you know.
Dr to father: How long do you think your wife will let you choose between your job and your family?

After this you might never see the family again. Of course, these questions may be efficient so far as probing the problem, but they are too powerful. Instead reflexive questions are recommended.

Reflexive questions

Father answers: I don't know.
Dr to father: If you thought about it, what could you do to help?
Father: I might call John at home when I have my coffee break and remind him about what he is going to eat.
Dr to mother: If this was done regularly do you think this would help John lose weight?
Mother: Of course it would. I would be so happy if I didn't have to take responsibility for John's eating all the time.

Reflexive questions create the possibility of envisaging new solutions and testing them even if, at first, they seem impossible due to external circumstances. Thus, 'if you don't know what to do, what would be your best guess?' Many reflexive questions start with 'if . . .'. This gives more space for patients to test whether new solutions are possible. The external factors which need to be changed to make this possible or who could be of help in this process are other areas for discussion.

16.2.9 Perspective on different psychotherapies

Family therapy or, more correctly, family systems therapy could be defined as follows: improving a family member's health by observing and analysing interactions between family members and between families and therapists, as well as by improving a family's ability to use its own resources.

Cognitive therapy, by contrast, aims at changing the cognitive process through a system of practice and reward (key elements in behavioural therapy). The changes in the cognitive process are supposed to lead to behavioural changes.

Psychodynamic therapy is not widely used with obesity but management does have a tradition of discussing transference and countertransference – something not widely used in other psychotherapies.

As stated earlier, behavioural therapy is based on the belief that obesity is a 'learned disease', amenable to cure by 'relearning'. However, the focus today is more often on finding the most efficient therapeutic technique for the treatment of obesity. If there are many efficient techniques which benefit from being used in combination, behavioural therapy may be one which is more efficient if used in conjunction with other treatments.

Finally, environmental therapy can be used in day-care programmes, institutions or child guidance clinics to teach individuals how to interact using, for example, training meals where the personnel all participate in patient-to-patient, and patient-to-staff, interactions.

We suggest combining the best aspects of different programmes into a general management programme for childhood obesity. The most important aspect must be to use scientific tools to identify the most effective features in each major treatment programme.

Table 16.1 outlines a suggestion for the use of different types of psychotherapeutic programmes in the management of childhood obesity. Treatments could be offered in several contexts such as schools, specialized environments (day-care programmes, boarding schools) and hospitals. Social and educational support could be offered together with traditional psychiatric therapy.

Obesity type A

In the preschool setting, educational methods might be used for groups of children as they are more cost effective than direct therapy to individual patients. At this young age, children are taught many different skills and the addition of teaching about healthy lifestyles regarding food and exercise could be beneficial. Obese children would not have to be identified. Education for a healthy lifestyle for all could be justified merely from a public-health perspective. The exact methods used need more research but Braet's treatment programmes mentioned earlier may be good examples (Braet et al., 1997b; Braet, 1999; Braet & Van Winckel, 2000).

We do not use family-therapy-based programmes in Malmö, Sweden for children less than 4 years old. From 4 to 10 years of age, the emphasis is on education to develop healthy lifestyles for all children within the preschool day-care centres and the schools. Children with BMI above the 95th centile are given basic instructions by the child health-care nurse or the school nurse. In some cases a primary-health-care dietician gives basic guidance which aims to reduce the fat content of the diet to 30% of total energy and total energy to 1500 kcal/day.

Table 16.1. Outline of treatment progress related to age

Type of obesity	Recommended treatment	Next step
(A) Childhood obesity 4–10 years of age	Education in preschool settings and in schools giving dietary advice and physical activity in groups	Cognitive behavioural therapy Family therapy
(B) Adolescent obesity 10–18 years of age	Obesity treated at school health centre Severe obesity treated with family therapy and social support or cognitive behavioural therapy	Day-care programme Specialized school environments (boarding schools)
(C) Eating disorders in adolescent obesity over 15 years of age	Child guidance clinic Family therapy Cognitive behavioural therapy Individual therapy	Day-care programme Hospital treatment using environmental therapy
(D) Syndromes and impaired cognitive function, e.g. Prader–Willi syndrome	Family therapy Social and educational specialized support at home	Day-care programme Hospital treatment using environmental therapy

Family therapy is rarely given at a paediatric outpatient clinic and then only at very low intensity. This means that families receive basic guidelines only at one or two sessions and are then reviewed every 6 months. Alternatively, they receive only one session and are invited to return when the standard treatment programmes start at the age of 10 years amongst children with BMI above the 99th centile and one or both parents with BMI greater than 30.

US recommendations suggest interventions as early as 3 years (Barlow & Dietz, 1998). The greatest risk for developing adult obesity is during adolescence, but the period between 3 and 5 years is also a high risk period if both parents are obese (Whitaker et al., 1997). This seems to encourage early intervention. Braet et al. (1997b) used cognitive behavioural therapy in early interventions and showed that treatment of preschool children was promising and that single-session interventions were useful although less effective.

Obesity type B

Our programme in Malmö starts with screening at school between 10 and 11 years. At this age most childhood obesity has become manifest (Rolland-Cachera et al., 1984). Children with BMI above the 95th centile are given basic instruction by the school nurse and those with BMI above the 99th centile are referred to paediatricians trained in family therapy or supported by child guidance teams.

Family therapy is useful and effective when offered to children with BMI above the 98th centile (we choose this BMI cut-off because of lack of health-care resources).

When treatment does not give acceptable weight control, day-care programmes or, for older children, education in specialized school environments can be added. However, outpatient-based treatment involves most children since obesity is such a common disease. Thus, when treatment is ineffective, special inpatient units or specially trained personnel sent to patients' homes to help parents in their daily family management can be used. These approaches are already practised in Sweden with children suffering from other severe disabilities. Our programmes need to focus on obesity treatment and the personnel need special training. The decision whether to opt for outpatient or inpatient treatment is always difficult. It may be argued that inpatient treatment is needed to give children initial encouraging weight loss. Rapid weight loss at an early phase of treatment may make further weight loss easier. However, there is little support for this view since it has been shown that the addition of very-low-calorie diet (VLCD) (usually a guarantee of rapid weight loss) to behavioural therapy in adults produces long-term outcomes which are no better than behavioural treatment alone (Wadden et al., 1989).

Obesity type C

The management of eating disorders in older teenagers requires all the resources of clinical child psychiatry. These cases are rare, but effective treatment is available and the diagnosis is an important one to make.

Obesity type D

For conditions such as Prader–Willi syndrome and others where the child has impaired cognitive function, treatment is much more difficult. In many cases family therapy is useful in providing families with extra support at home. Without this, day-care programmes are probably needed (Chapter 9).

16.3 Conclusions

Different types of psychotherapy have been used in the treatment of childhood obesity. The major programmes for children aim to produce lifestyle changes based on psychotherapy – family therapy or cognitive behavioural therapy. We suggest the best parts of different programmes should be introduced into general programmes for the treatment of childhood obesity.

Age is a major factor influencing choice of strategies for helping obese children control their weight. With preschool children, group teaching is more important than individual treatment. With preschool children, it is easy to get children to accept groups formed by adults. Older children need to create their own groups.

Thus, group activities may be more successful with preschool groups than with older children.

Later on, the treatment of individuals becomes more and more necessary. In early childhood the family of origin is critically important for management but, with older teenagers and young adults (16–25 years), new homes and social groupings are more important. Then, later still, families, but new and self-chosen, become important again. Thus, family therapy can also be helpful with adults. The treatment of childhood obesity is important. We have the impression that the change to a healthy lifestyle – one which includes appropriate eating patterns and exercise – is more easily incorporated into adult life if learned in childhood than if attempted later.

New possibilities provided by ongoing research in the field of genetics, and indications of more effective prevention of obesity in childhood, offer hope for better controls of the ongoing 'weight explosion'. However, management of the problem must involve all stakeholders if it is to be effective. We need to listen to what the long-suffering obese subjects and their families say: 'Diets don't work'! All obese individuals, but particularly children, need help to develop lifestyles for maintenance of normal, healthy weight.

16.4 REFERENCES

Aimez, P. (1976). [Modification of pathogenic dietary behaviour. Group technics]. *Annales de Nutrition et d'Alimentation*, **30**, 289–99.

Barlow, E. & Dietz, W. (1998). Obesity evaluation and treatment: Expert Committee Recommendations. *Pediatrics*, **102**, E29.

Björvell, H. & Rössner, S. (1992). A ten-year follow-up of weight change in severely obese subjects treated in a combined behavioural modification programme. *International Journal of Obesity*, **16**, 623–5.

Braet, C. (1999). Treatment of obese children: A new rationale. *Clinical Child Psychology and Psychiatry*, **4**, 579–91.

Braet, C. & Van Winckel, M. (2000). Long-term follow-up of a cognitive behavioral treatment program for obese children. *Behavior Therapy*, **31**, 55–74.

Braet, C. & Wydhooge, K. (2000). Dietary restraint in normal weight and overweight children. A cross-sectional study. *International Journal of Obesity*, **24**, 314–18.

Braet, C., Mervielde, I. & Vandereycken, W. (1997a). Psychological aspects of childhood obesity: a controlled study in a clinical and nonclinical sample. *Journal of Pediatric Psychology*, **22**, 59–71.

Braet, C., Van Winckel, M. & Van Leeuwen, K. (1997b). Follow-up results of different treatment programs for obese children. *Acta Paediatrica*, **86**, 397–402.

Brownell, K.D. & Kaye, F.S. (1982). A school-based behavior modification, nutrition education, and physical activity program for obese children. *American Journal of Clinical Nutrition*, **35**,

277–83.

Brownell, K.D. & Wadden, T.A. (1991). The heterogeneity of obesity. *Behavior Therapy*, **22**, 153–77.

Brownell, K.D., Kelman, J.H. & Stunkard, A.J. (1983). Treatment of obese children with and without their mothers: changes in weight and blood pressure. *Pediatrics*, **71**, 515–23.

Bruch, H. (1964). Psychological aspects of overeating and obesity. *Psychosomatics*, **5**, 269–74.

Bruch, H. (1970). Eating disorders in adolescence. *Proceedings of the Annual Meeting of the American Psychopathological Association*, **59**, 181–202.

Bruch, H. (1974). The family as background to obesity. In *The International Book of Family Therapy*, ed. F.W. Kaslow. p. 229–43. New York: Bruner

Dare, C. (1992). Change the family, change the child? *Archives of Disease in Childhood*, **67**, 643–8.

Davis, K. & Christoffel, K.K. (1994). Obesity in pre-school and school-age children. Treatment early and often may be best. *Archives of Pediatric and Adolescent Medicine*, **148**, 1257–61.

Decaluwé, V., Braet, C. & Fairburn, C. (2000). Binge eating in obese children and adolescents. *International Journal of Obesity*, **24** (suppl. 1), S162.

DeLucia, J.L. & Kalodner, C.R. (1990). An individualized cognitive intervention: does it increase the efficacy of behavioral interventions for obesity? *Addictive Behaviors*, **15**, 473–9.

de Shazer, S. (1982). *Patterns of Brief Family Therapy*. New York: Guilford.

de Shazer, S. (1985). *Keys to Solution in Brief Therapy*. New York: Norton.

de Shazer, S. (1988). *Clues: Investigating Solutions in Brief Therapy*. New York: Norton.

de Shazer, S. (1991). *Putting Difference to Work*, 1st edn. New York: W.W. Norton & Company, Inc.

Dietz, W.H. (1983). Childhood obesity: susceptibility, cause and management. *Journal of Pediatrics*, **103**, 676–86.

Dietz, W. (1991). Physical activity and childhood obesity. *Nutrition*, **7**, 295–6.

Duffy, G. & Spence, S.H. (1993). The effectiveness of cognitive self-management as an adjunct to a behavioural intervention for childhood obesity: a research note. *Journal of Child Psychology and Psychiatry*, **34**, 1043–50.

Epstein, L.H. (1993). New developments in childhood obesity. In: *Obesity. Theory and Therapy*. Second edition, eds. A.J. Stunkard & T.A. Wadden. New York: Raven Press.

Epstein, L.H., Wing, R.R., Steranchak, L., Dickson, B. & Michelson, J. (1980). Comparison of family based behavior modification and nutrition education for childhood obesity. *Journal of Pediatric Psychology*, **5**, 25–36.

Epstein, L.H., Valoski, A., Wing, R.R. & McCurley, J. (1990). Ten-year follow-up of behavioral, family-based treatment for obese children. *JAMA*, **264**, 2519–23.

Epstein, L.H., Valoski, A. & McCurley, J. (1993). Effect of weight loss by obese children on long-term growth. *American Journal of Diseases in Children*, **147**, 1076–80.

Epstein, L.H., Valoski, A.M., Kalarchian, M.A. & McCurley, J. (1995a). Do children lose and maintain weight easier than adults: a comparison of child and parent weight changes from six months to ten years. *Obesity Research*, **3**, 411–17.

Epstein, L.H., Valoski, A.M., Vara, L.S., McCurley, J., Wisniewski, L., Kalarchian, M.A., et al. (1995b). Effects of decreasing sedentary behavior and increasing activity on weight change in obese children. *Health Psychology*, **14**, 109–15.

Flodmark, C.E. (1997). Childhood Obesity. *Clinical Child Psychology and Psychiatry*, **2**, 283–95.

Flodmark, C.E., Ohlsson, T., Ryden, O. & Sveger, T. (1993). Prevention of progression to severe obesity in a group of obese schoolchildren treated with family therapy. *Pediatrics*, **91**, 880–4.

Ganley, R.M. (1986). Epistemology, family patterns, and psychosomatics: the case of obesity. *Family Process*, **25**, 437–51.

Garner, D.M., Olmsted, M.P. & Polivy, J. (1983). Development and validation of a multidimensional eating disorder inventory for anorexia nervosa. *International Journal of Eating Disorder*, **2**, 15–34.

Gurman, A. & Kniskern, D. (1981). Family therapy outcome research: knowns and unknowns. In *Handbook of Family Therapy*, pp. 742–75. New York: Branner/Mazel.

Gustafsson, P.A. (1987). Family interaction and family therapy in childhood psychosomatic disease. Doctoral Dissertation. Linköping.

Hansson, K. (1989). Familjediagnostik. Doctoral Dissertation. Lund University.

Hazelrigg, M., Cooper, H. & Bourdin, C. (1987). Evaluating the effectiveness of family therapy: an integrative review and analysis. *Psychological Bulletin*, **101**, 428–42.

Kalodner, C.R. & DeLucia, J.L. (1991). The individual and combined effects of cognitive therapy and nutrition education as additions to a behavior modification program for weight loss. *Addictive Behaviors*, **16**, 255–63.

Kendall, P. & Lochman, J. (1994). Cognitive-behavioural therapies. In *Child and Adolescent Psychiatry*, eds. M. Rutter, E. Taylor & L. Hersov, pp. 844–57. London: Blackwell Science.

Kimm, S., Barton, B., Berhane, K., Ross, J., Payne, G. & Schreiber, G. (1997). Self-esteem and adiposity in black and white girls: the NHLBI Growth and Health Study. *Annals of Epidemiology*, **7**, 550–60.

Lask, B. (1987). Family therapy. *British Medical Journal*, **294**, 203–4.

Leibel, R., Rosenbaum, M. & Hirsch, J. (1995). Changes in energy expenditure resulting from altered body weight. *New England Journal of Medicine*, **332**, 621–8.

Long, C.G., Simpson, C.M. & Allott, E.A. (1983). Psychological and dietetic counselling combined in the treatment of obesity: a comparative study in a hospital outpatient clinic. *Human Nutrition Applied Nutrition*, **37**, 94–102.

Minuchin, S. & Fishman, C. (1981). *Family Therapy Techniques*. 1st edn. Cambridge MA: Harvard University Press.

Minuchin, S., Baker, L., Rosman, B.L., Liedman, R., Milman, L. & Todd, T.C. (1975). A conceptual model of psychosomatic illness in children: family organisation and family therapy. *Archives of General Psychiatry*, **32**, 1031–8.

Minuchin, S., Rosman, B. & Baker, L. (1978). *Psychosomatic Families*. 1st edn. Cambridge MA: Harvard University Press.

Orhagen, T. (1992). Working with families in schizophrenic disorders: the practice of psychoeducational intervention. Doctoral dissertation. Linköping.

Porter, K. (1980). Combined individual and group psychotherapy: a review of the literature 1965–1978. *International Journal of Group Psychotherapy*, **30**, 107–14.

Renman, C., Engström, I., Silfverdal, S. & Aman, J. (1999). Mental health and psychosocial characteristics in adolescent obesity: a population-based case-control study. *Acta Paediatrica*,

88, 998–1003.

Ricca, V., Mannucci, E., Moretti, S., Di Bernardo, M., Zucchi, T., Cabras, P.L., et al. (2000). Screening for binge eating disorder in obese outpatients. *Comprehensive Psychiatry*, **41**, 111–15.

Rolland-Cachera, M.F., Deheeger, M., Bellisle, F., Sempe, M., Guilloud, B.M. & Patois, E. (1984). Adiposity rebound in children: a simple indicator for predicting obesity. *American Journal of Clinical Nutrition*, **39**, 129–35.

Rumpel, C. & Harris, T.B. (1994). The influence of weight on adolescent self-esteem. *Journal of Psychosomatic Research*, **38**, 547–56.

Stradmeijer, M., Bosch, J., Koops, W. & Seidell, J. (2000). Family functioning and psychosocial adjustment in overweight youngsters. *International Journal of Eating Disorders*, **27**, 110–14.

Strauss, R. (2000). Childhood obesity and self-esteem. *Pediatrics*, **105**, e15.

Stuart, R.B. (1967). Behavioral control of overeating. *Behaviour Research and Therapy*, **5**, 357–65.

Stunkard, A., Berkowitz, R., Wadden, T., Tanrikut, C., Reiss, E. & Young, L. (1996). Binge eating disorder and the night-eating syndrome. *International Journal of Obesity*, **20**, 1–6.

Valtolina, G. & Marta, E. (1998). Family relations and psychosocial risk in families with an obese adolescent. *Psychological Reports*, **83**, 251–60.

Wadden, T.A., Sternberg, J.A., Letizia, K.A., Stunkard, A.J. & Foster, G.D. (1989). Treatment of obesity by very low calorie diet, behavior therapy, and their combination: a five-year perspective. *International Journal of Obesity*, **2**, 39–46.

Ward, D. & Bar-Or, E. (1986). Role of the physician and physical education teacher in the treatment of obesity at school. *Pediatrician*, **13**, 44–51.

Whitaker, R.C., Wright, J.A., Pepe, M.S., Seidel, K.D. & Dietz, W.H. (1997). Predicting obesity in young adulthood from childhood and parental obesity. *New England Journal of Medicine*, **337**, 869–73.

Zakus, G., Chin, M.L., Keown, M., Hebert, F. & Held, M. (1979). A group behavior modification approach to adolescent obesity. *Adolescence*, **14**, 481–90.

17

Drug therapy

Dénes Molnár[1] and Ewa Malecka-Tendera[2]

[1]Department of Paediatrics, University of Pečs. [2]Department of Pathophysiology, Silesian School of Medicine, Katowice, Poland

The present chapter focuses on the current pharmacotherapy of obesity and agents under development. It is intended to update clinical practitioners especially paediatricians in this rapidly progressing field and to give indications for eventual drug support in childhood obesity. It should be noted, though, that few treatments are currently recognized and licensed for use in children.

The medical history of obesity dates back to the Stone Age (Bray, 1990). The first drug for the management of obesity, thyroid hormone, was introduced in 1893. It was believed to be therapeutic because overweight patients were thought to have a reduced metabolic rate. Dinitrophenol, a drug that was noted to increase metabolic rate due to the uncoupling of oxidative phosphorylation and to produce weight loss, was soon abandoned because of severe side effects. The development and synthesis of amphetamines initiated a new area of pharmaceutical therapy for obesity. Drugs used for the management of obesity are usually classified according to the mechanism of their action (Table 17.1).

17.1 Appetite suppressants

These drugs are commonly divided into centrally acting noradrenergic agents (benzphetamine, phendimetrazine, diethylpropion, mazindol, phenyl-propanolamine, phentermine) and serotoninergic agents (i.e. fenfluramine, dex-fenfluramine).

17.1.1 Noradrenergic agents

The discovery of ephedrine from the Chinese plant *Ephedra sinica* led to the synthesis of the amphetamines in 1933. Amphetamine, metamphetamine and phenmetrazine are no longer recommended for obesity treatment because of their addictive potential (Bray, 1995a). However, chemical manipulation of the side chains and ring structure of amphetamine have led to the development of several

Table 17.1. Classification of antiobesity agents by main mode of action

Mechanism	Category	Drug
Appetite suppressants	noradrenergic	Benzphetamine
		Phendimetrazine
		Diethylpropion
		Mazindol
		Phenylpropanolamine
		Phentermine
	serotoninergic	Fenfluramine[a]
		Dexfenfluramine[a]
		Fluoxetine
	adrenergic/serotoninergic	Sibutramine
Thermogenic agents	adrenergic	Ephedrine, Caffeine
	β₃-agonists	*BRL 26830A*
		BRL 35135
		RO 402148
Digestive inhibitors	lipase inhibitor	Orlistat®
	fat substitutes	Olestra®
Hormonal effects	*leptin analogues*	
	neuropeptide Y antagonists	
	cholecystokinin promoters	

Drugs in *italics* are investigational.
[a]Withdrawn from the market in 1997.

β-phenetylamines with reduced risk for central nervous system stimulation and abuse. With the exception of phentermine these agents are infrequently used in clinical practice (Bray, 1993; National Task Force on the Prevention and Treatment of Obesity, 1996).

Phentermine

Phentermine modulates noradrenergic neurotransmission to decrease appetite. However, it has little effect on the dopaminergic system and, thus, there is little risk of abuse. The use of phentermine as a single agent is limited by intolerance to its stimulatory activity. Previously, phentermine was used in combination with fenfluramine, which counteracted the undesirable effects of phentermine. This combination has been demonstrated to be more effective, in terms of weight loss, than either agent used alone (Goldstein & Potvin, 1994). The most common adverse effects of phentermine are headache, insomnia, nervousness, irritability, palpitation, tachycardia and elevation of blood pressure. Safety has not been established and phentermine is not recommended for children.

17.1.2 Serotoninergic agents

While amphetamines release dopamine and noradrenaline within the lateral hypothalamus, serotoninergic drugs release serotonin and/or inhibit its reuptake in presynaptic neurones terminating within the paraventricular nucleus of the hypothalamus. Serotonin anorexia differs from that caused by amphetamines. It is characterized by decreased rate of eating and early termination of meals, rather than by inhibition of eating (Blundell et al., 1979). These anorectic effects of serotonin are mediated by 5-hydroxytryptamine (5-HT)$_{1B/D}$ and 5-HT$_{2C}$ receptors. Currently seven types of 5-HT receptors and further subfamilies are known (Baez et al., 1995). Studies suggest that serotoninergic drugs reduce carbohydrate craving (Wurtman & Wurtman, 1995) and increase basal metabolic rate by 100 calories per day thus promoting further weight reduction (Scalfi et al., 1993).

Fenfluramine

Fenfluramine was synthesized in the 1960s. It is a mixture of two racemic compounds, L-fenfluramine and D-fenfluramine, which are metabolized to active but pharmacologically distinct products. Among patients who remain in the trials, fenfluramine is clearly more effective than placebo in producing and maintaining weight loss. In a double blind, randomized trial, fenfluramine combined with phentermine has been shown to improve the magnitude of weight loss in obese subjects when compared to placebo (Weintraub et al., 1992). The side effects were generally transient and mild. However, increased risk of primary pulmonary hypertension was reported in patients exposed to derivatives of fenfluramine (Abenhaim et al., 1996). Valvular heart disease was identified in 24 women who were treated with the phentermine–fenfluramine combination for a mean of 11 (SD ± 6.9) months (Connolly et al., 1997) and presented with cardiovascular symptoms. Cardiac surgical intervention was necessary in five patients. Further echocardiographic investigations revealed that in 291 asymptomatic patients receiving phentermine–fenfluramine or phentermine–dexfenfluramine combination, 92 had abnormal valve findings. Subsequently, both fenfluramine and dexfenfluramine were withdrawn from the market.

Dexfenfluramine

Dexfenfluramine, the dextrorotary stereoisomer of fenfluramine was developed during the 1970s. It was found to be more effective in reducing food intake in rats and to have greater specificity for serotonin release and reuptake inhibition (Campbell, 1991).

The International Dexfenfluramine Study (Guy-Grand et al., 1989) including 822 patients from 24 centres in nine European countries showed a continued efficacy for up to 1 year. In 1997, valvular disease was observed after long-term therapy and the drug was withdrawn from the market.

Other serotonin agonist drugs including the selective serotonin reuptake inhibitors such as fluoxetine, fluvoxamine and sertraline have been evaluated as anti-obesity agents (Goldstein et al., 1995; National Task Force on the Prevention and Treatment of Obesity, 1996), but are not approved by Food and Drug Administration (FDA) and not recommended for the treatment of obesity.

Noradrenergic/serotoninergic agent (sibutramine)

FDA has recently approved this drug. It is a serotonin and noradrenaline reuptake inhibitor. Devoid of antidepressant effect, it decreases food intake through its action on β_1 and 5-$HT_{2A/2C}$ receptors, and is thought to enhance metabolic activity through the stimulation of peripheral β_3 receptors (Ryan et al., 1995; Finer, 1997). Placebo-controlled studies (Ryan et al., 1995; Bray et al., 1996) reported significant effects of this drug on weight loss.

Although the incidence of adverse effects was not reported in these studies, the most common adverse events associated with sibutramine treatment were constipation, dry mouth and insomnia. The studies showed slight elevations in blood pressure and heart rate (Ryan et al., 1995; Bray et al., 1996). There are no reports of the use of sibutramine in children.

17.2 Thermogenic agents

Interventions that increase exercise and activity are valuable components of any weight-reduction programme. It is, however, often difficult for severely obese patients to be physically active. Consequently, there has been a concerted search for drugs that might safely increase metabolic rate and dissipate excessive energy stores as heat. The ideal thermogenic drug should increase thermogenesis without any effect on heart rate, cardiac output, myocardial oxygen consumption or blood pressure. Such an agent still awaits discovery.

The first thermogenic drug, dinitrophenol, was abandoned because of multisystem side effects. Thyroid hormones are also not used in clinical practice for the treatment of obesity since they cause tachycardia, dysrhythmias and myocardial infarction, and are associated with accelerated protein loss.

17.2.1 Ephedrine and xanthines

Ephedrine decreases body fat in obese subjects by a dual action: suppression of appetite and stimulation of energy covered by fat oxidation (Astrup et al., 1992b, 1995). Adenosine antagonists such as caffeine potentiate the thermogenic and clinical effects of ephedrine. Ephedrine is both an indirect sympathomimetic causing the release of noradrenaline from the sympathetic nerve endings and a direct agonist on β-adrenergic receptors (β-AR$_{1,2}$, but mainly β-AR$_3$) (Astrup et al., 1995). A combination of ephedrine and caffeine (20 mg ephedrine and 200 mg caffeine three times a day) has been shown to be effective for the treatment of obesity. After 24 weeks the ephedrine/caffeine group lost 3.4 kg more than the placebo group (Astrup et al., 1992a). Tachyphylaxis developed for the cardiovascular, but not for the weight-loss-producing effects of the ephedrine/caffeine mixture. In a double blind comparison of ephedrine/caffeine and dexfenfluramine, the former therapy seemed to be more effective in younger and more severely obese subjects. The latter therapy was preferable in middle-aged and elderly patients and in hypertensive obese subjects (Breum et al., 1995). Experience with ephedrine/caffeine combinations in obese children and adolescents is insufficient to allow proper evaluation.

17.2.2 Atypical β-adrenoreceptor agonists

The finding of atypical β-adrenoreceptor agonists in 1983 (Arch & Ainsworth, 1983), soon led to the discovery of atypical receptors (β_3 receptor) that mediate the thermogenic effects of sympathomimetic drugs, but not the β_1 effects of heart-rate stimulation, or β_2 effects on smooth muscle contraction and tremor. The existence of a novel receptor involved in energy expenditure stimulated the development of new thermogenic drugs. In animal models, the principal mechanism of the β_3 receptor seems to be enhanced thermogenesis in brown adipose tissue. The β_3 receptor agonists stimulated metabolic rate and led to weight loss in rodents, but the findings were inconsistent in humans and the thermogenic effect could not be separated from heat produced by troublesome skeletal muscle tremor (Chapman et al., 1988; Connacher et al., 1990). The human β_3 receptor has recently been cloned and is known to differ from the rodent receptor. Existing compounds appear to have only poor affinity and specificity to human receptors. More specific compounds are being developed, but they are still a long way from clinical use.

17.3 Digestive inhibitors

17.3.1 Lipase inhibitor

Orlistat is a potent and irreversible inhibitor of gastric, pancreatic, and pancreatic carboxylester lipases (Guerciolini, 1997), thus decreasing the hydrolysis of the ingested triglycerides. It produces a dose-dependent reduction in dietary fat absorption, which is nearly maximal at a dose of 120 mg thrice daily. Short-term (12 weeks) and long-term (1 year) human studies demonstrated that together with a low-fat diet, orlistat induced a significantly higher weight loss as compared to the placebo group (Drent et al., 1995; James et al., 1997). Adverse effects of orlistat are predominantly related to fat malabsorption (loose stools, faecal urgency, fat-soluble vitamin deficiency). The FDA has recently approved the drug. Absolutely no experience is available in obese children concerning the effects and side effects of orlistat.

17.3.2 Fat substitutes

Olestra is a noncaloric fat substitute that is a mixture of hexa-, hepta- and octa-esters formed from the reaction of sucrose with long-chain fatty acids. Three studies evaluated the effect of olestra on weight loss with equivocal results (Glueck et al., 1982, 1983; Mellies et al., 1985). The main problems concerning the use of olestra are the gastrointestinal adverse effects (diarrhoea, bloating, flatulence, anal leakage, reduction of fat-soluble vitamins). Currently there are no contraindications to the use of olestra. The manufacturer does not recommend it for children younger than 2 years of age. Perhaps it is prudent to say that those at risk of fat-soluble vitamin deficiencies, that is paediatric and elderly population's should avoid the use of olestra.

17.4 Hormone analogues and antagonists

Hormonal control of appetite is a complex system affected by several peptides found in the gastrointestinal tract and central nervous system. This system is currently the focus of widespread investigation. Many of these hormones, their agonists and antagonists are in the early stages of development (Bray, 1995b). In healthy subjects, cholecystokinin (CCK), serotonin and insulin decrease food intake. The role of serotonin-receptor stimulation as a potential antiobesity drug has already been discussed. CCK is a physiologic satiety factor which reduces meal size, whether administered peripherally or centrally. Peripheral CCK-A receptors, when stimulated, inhibit feeding by slowing gastric emptying and sending information about feeding to the hypothalamus through the vagus nerve. A number of CCK-A promoters and an inhibitor of the enzyme metabolizing CCK (butabindide) are subject to ongoing research (Levine & Billington, 1996).

Neuropeptide Y (NPY) is the most potent stimulator of food intake, and also increases energy expenditure. Data suggest that leptin, in part, exerts its actions by modulating hypothalamic NPY (Smith et al., 1996). A number of pharmaceutical companies have developed NPY inhibitors, but it is not clear how peripherally administered polypeptides cross the blood–brain barrier.

A comprehensive review of leptin has recently been published (Caro et al., 1996), and Chapters 3, 7, 8 and 10 of this book also discuss the possible role of leptin in the development and treatment of human obesity. Most obese people have high leptin in the plasma levels, however, a subset of patients with low serum leptin concentrations may benefit from leptin administration.

The new developments in obesity research, at least in adults, have resulted in paradigm shifts concerning obesity treatment: (a) obesity is now recognized as a chronic disease that requires long-term treatment; (b) loss of only 10% or even 5% of body weight is now considered sufficient to improve the health-risk factors such as insulin resistance, hypertension and hyperlipidaemia; (c) because exercise, diet and behavioural modification alone are usually not sufficient to maintain long-term weight loss, there has been renewed interest in drug therapy; (d) the weight regain after cessation of drug therapy has been ascribed to failure of drug treatment. However, the latest conclusion is that medications do not work if not taken.

In adults, it seems to be justified to use drugs for long-term treatment of 'medically important' obesity. Unfortunately, most drugs previously used in obesity have had to be withdrawn from the market because of serious side effects. New drugs are still in the experimental stage of development. The only two new drugs recommended for the treatment of adult obesity are sibutramine and orlistat. The old ephedrine/caffeine combination does not have serious adverse effects and is effective in certain cases but marketed only in Denmark.

In childhood there is only very limited experience with antiobesity drugs. The thermogenic effects of ephedrine and aminophylline were investigated in obese children (Molnár, 1993). Both drugs caused a significant increase of resting metabolic rate in obese adolescents. However, the number of nonresponders was high. Supplementation of a low-calorie diet with ephedrine led to a greater weight loss in children than diet alone (Malecka-Tendera, 1993). The side effects were mild and transient. The results of the first double-blind, placebo-controlled study in obese adolescents treated with caffeine/ephedrine mixture were encouraging (Molnár et al., 2000).

A double-blind, placebo-controlled study could not demonstrate any advantage of dexfenfluramine treatment over diet in obese children (Grugni et al., 1995). Two other studies (Madeiros-Neto, 1993; Malecka-Tendera et al., 1996) found dexfenfluramine treatment effective in obese children.

In Prader–Willi syndrome the effects of fenfluramine and naloxone (an opiate antagonist) have been investigated in double-blind, placebo-controlled trials with equivocal results (Kyriakides et al., 1980; Selikowitz et al., 1990). With the ready availability of biosynthetic growth hormone, there is pressure on clinicians to treat Prader–Willi patients with growth hormone. The most recent study (Davies et al., 1998) demonstrated significant and beneficial changes in body composition of Prader–Willi patients after 6 months of treatment with growth hormone. However, the results are contradictory (Hauffa, 1997) and further, more prolonged trials are needed before growth hormone treatment can be recommended for this subset of obese children.

The newly introduced antiobesity drugs, orlistat and sibutramine, have not been studied in childhood, so we cannot recommend any antiobesity agent for use in children. However, the problem of acceptable treatment for the extremely obese adolescent remains. A rationale needs to be developed for well-designed trials of pharmacological treatment in these children.

17.5 REFERENCES

Abenhaim, L., Moride, Y., Brenot, F., Rich, S., Benichou, J., Kurz, X., Higenbottam, T., Oakley, C., Wouters, E., Aubier, M., Simonneau, G. & Begaud, B. (1996). Appetite-suppressant drugs and the risk of primary pulmonary hypertension. *New England Journal of Medicine*, **335**, 609–15.

Arch, J.R.S. & Ainsworth, A.T. (1983). Thermogenic and antiobesity activity of a novel β-adrenoreceptor agonist (BRL 26830A) in mice and rats. *American Journal of Clinical Nutrition*, **38**, 549–58.

Astrup, A., Breum, L., Toubro, S., Hein, P. & Quaade, F. (1992a). The effect and safety of an ephedrine/caffeine compound compared to ephedrine, caffeine and placebo in obese subjects on an energy restricted diet. A double blind trial. *International Journal of Obesity*, **16**, 269–77.

Astrup, A., Toubro, S., Christensen, N.J. & Quaade, F. (1992b). Pharmacology of thermogenic drugs. *American Journal of Clinical Nutrition*, **55** (Suppl.), 246–8.

Astrup, A., Breum, L. & Toubro S. (1995). Pharmacological and clinical studies of ephedrine and other thermogenic agonists. *Obesity Research*, **3** (Suppl. 4), 537–40.

Baez, M., Kursur, J.D., Helton, L.A., Wainscott, D.B. & Nelson, D.L.G. (1995). Molecular biology of serotonin receptors. *Obesity Research*, **3** (Suppl. 4), 441–7.

Blundell, J.E., Latham, C.J., Moniz, E., McArthur, R.A. & Rogers, P.J. (1979). Structural analysis of the actions of amphetamine and fenfluramine on food intake and feeding behaviour in animals and man. *Current Medical Research Opinion*, **6** (Suppl. 1), 34–54.

Bray, G.A. (1990). Obesity: historical development of scientific and cultural ideas. *International Journal of Obesity*, **14**, 909–26.

Bray, G.A. (1993). Use and abuse of appetite-suppressant drugs in the treatment of obesity. *Annals of Internal Medicine*, **119**, 707–13.

Bray, G.A. (1995a). Evaluation of drugs for treating obesity. *Obesity Research*, **3** (Suppl. 4), 425–34.

Bray, G.A. (1995b). Peptides and food intake. Nutrient intake is modulated by peripheral peptide administration. *Obesity Research*, **3** (Suppl. 4), 569–72.

Bray, G.A., Ryan, D.H., Gordon, D., Heidingsfelder, S., Cerise, F. & Wilson, K. (1996). A double blind randomized placebo controlled trial of sibutramine. *Obesity Research*, **4**, 263–70.

Breum, L., Frimodt-Moller, J., Ahlstrom, F. & Pedersen, J.K. (1995). Age, but not BMI and gender predicts weight loss during treatment with serotonergic or sympathomimetic drugs. *Obesity Research*, **3** (Suppl. 4), 627.

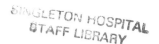

Campbell, D.B. (1991). Dexfenfluramine: an overview of its mechanisms of action. *Review of Contemporary Pharmacotherapy*, **2**, 93–113.

Caro, J.F., Sinha, M.K., Kolaczynski, J.W., Zhang, P.L. & Considine, R.V. (1996). Leptin: the tale of an obesity gene. *Diabetes*, **45**, 1455–62.

Chapman, B.J., Farquahar, D.L., Galloway, S.M., Simpson, G.K. & Munro, J.F. (1988). The effects of a new β-adrenoreceptor agonist BRL 26830A in refractory obesity. *International Journal of Obesity*, **12**, 119–23.

Connacher, A.A., Lakie, M., Powers, N., Elton, R.A., Walsh, E.G. & Jung, R.T. (1990). Tremor and the antiobesity drug BRL 26830A. *British Journal of Clinical Pharmacology*, **30**, 613–15.

Connolly, H.M., Crary, J.L., McGoon, M.D., Hensrud, D.D., Edwards, B.S., Edwards W.D. & Schaff, H.V. (1997). Valvular heart disease associated with fenfluramine–phentermine. *New England Journal of Medicine*, **337**, 581–8.

Davies, P.S.W., Evans, S., Broomhead, S., Clough, H., Day, J.M.E., Laidlaw, A. & Barnes, N.D. (1998). Effect of growth hormone on height, weight, and body composition in Prader–Willi syndrome. *Archives of Disease in Children*, **78**, 474–6.

Drent, M.L., Larsson, I., William-Olsson, T., Quaade, F., Czubayko, F., von Bergmann, K., Strobel, W., Sjostrom, L. & van der Veen, E.A. (1995). Orlistat (Ro 18-0647), a lipase inhibitor, in the treatment of human obesity: a multiple dose study. *International Journal of Obesity*, **19**, 221–6.

Finer, N. (1997). Present and future pharmacologic approaches. *British Medical Bulletin*, **53**, 409–32.

Glueck, C.J., Hastings, M.M., Allen, C., Hogg, E., Baehler, L., Garside, P.S., Phillips, D., Jones, M., Hollenbach, E.J., Braun, B. & Anastasia, J.V. (1982). Sucrose polyester and covert caloric dilution. *American Journal of Clinical Nutrition*, **35**, 1352–9.

Glueck, C.J., Jandacek, R., Hogg, E., Allen, C., Baehler, L. & Tewksbury, M. (1983). Sucrose polyester: substitution for dietary fat in hypocaloric diets in the treatment of familial hypercholesterolemia. *American Journal of Clinical Nutrition*, **37**, 347–54.

Goldstein, D.J., Rampey, A.H., Roback, P.J., Wilson, M.G., Hamilton, S.H., Sayler, M.E. & Tollefson, G.D. (1995). Efficacy and safety of long-term fluoxetine treatment of obesity-maximizing success. *Obesity Research*, **3** (Suppl. 4), 481–90.

Goldstein, D. J. & Potvin, J. H. (1994). Long term weight loss: the effect of pharmacologic agents. *American Journal of Clinical Nutrition*, **60**, 647–57.

Grugni, G., Guzzaloni, G., Ardizzi, A., Moro, D. & Morabito, F. (1995). Dexfenfluramine in the treatment of prepubertal subjects with essential obesity. *Acta Medica Auxologica*, **27**, 69–78.

Guerciolini, R. (1997). Mode of action of orlistat. *International Journal of Obesity*, **21** (Suppl 3), 12–23.

Guy-Grand, B., Apfelbaum, M., Crepaldi, G., Gries, A., Lefebvre, P. & Turner, P. (1989). International trial of long term dexfenfluramine in obesity. *Lancet*, **2**, 1142–4.

Hauffa, B.P. (1997). One-year results of growth hormone treatment of short stature in Prader–Willi syndrome. *Acta Paediatrica*, **423** (Suppl.), 63–5.

James, W.P.T., Avenell, A., Broom, J. & Whitehead, J. (1997). A one-year trial to assess the value of orlistat in the management of obesity. *International Journal of Obesity*, **21** (Suppl. 3), 24–30.

Kyriakides, M., Silverstone, T., Jeffcoate, W. & Laurence, B. (1980). Effect of naloxone on hyperphagia in Prader–Willi syndrome. *Lancet*, **1**, 876–7.

Levine, A.S. & Billington, C.J. (1996). Peptides in the regulation of energy metabolism and body weight. In *Regulation of Body Weight: Biological and Behavioural Mechanisms*, eds. C. Bouchard & G.A. Bray, pp. 179–91. Chichester: John Wiley & Sons.

Madeiros-Neto, G.A. (1993). Should drugs be used for treating obese children? *International Journal of Obesity*, **17**, 363.

Malecka-Tendera, E. (1993). Postheparine lipoprotein lipase activity in obese children treated with hypocaloric diet supplemented with ephedrine or theophylline. (Abstract.) *International Journal of Obesity*, **17** (Suppl. 1), 80.

Malecka-Tendera, E., Kochler, B., Muchacka, M., Wazowski, R. & Trzciakowska, A. (1996). Efficacy and safety of dexfenfluramine treatment in obese adolescents. *Pediatria Polska*, **71**, 431–6.

Mellies, M.J., Vitale, C., Jandacek, R.J., Lamkin, G.E. & Glueck, C.J. (1985). The substitution of sucrose polyester for dietary fat in obese, hypercholesterolemic outpatients. *American Journal of Clinical Nutrition*, **41**, 1–12.

Molnár, D. (1993). Effects of ephedrine and aminophylline on resting energy expenditure in obese adolescents. *International Journal of Obesity*, **17** (Suppl. 1), 49–52.

Molnár, D., Török, K., Erhardt, E. & Jeges, A. (2000). Safety and efficacy of treatment with an ephedrine/caffeine mixture. The first double-blind, placebo-controlled study in adolescents. *International Journal of Obesity*, **24**, 1573–8.

National Task Force on the Prevention and Treatment of Obesity. (1996). Long-term pharmacotherapy in the management of obesity. *Journal of American Medical Association*, **276**, 1907–15.

Ryan, D.H., Kaiser, P. & Bray, G.A. (1995). Sibutramine: a novel new agent for obesity treatment. *Obesity Research*, **3** (Suppl. 4), 553–9.

Scalfi, L., D'Arrigo, E., Carradente, V., Coltori, A. & Contaldo, F. (1993). The acute effect of dexfenfluramine on resting metabolic rate and post prandial thermogenesis in obese subjects: a double blind placebo controlled study. *International Journal of Obesity*, **17**, 91–6.

Selikowitz, M., Sunman, J., Pendergast, A. & Wright, S. (1990). Fenfluramine in Prader–Willi syndrome: a double blind, placebo controlled trial. *Archives of Disease in Childhood*, **65**, 112–14.

Smith, F.J., Campfield, L.A., Moschera, J.A., Bailon, P.S. & Burn, P. (1996). Feeding inhibition by neuropeptide Y. *Nature*, **382**, 307.

Weintraub, M., Sundaresan, P.R., Madan, M., Schuster, B., Balder, A., Lasagna, L. & Cox, C. (1992). Long term weight control study I (weeks 0 to 34). The enhancement of behavior modification, caloric restriction, and exercise by fenfluramine plus phentermine versus placebo. *Clinical Pharmacology Therapy*, **51**, 586–94.

Wurtman, R.J. & Wurtman, J.J. (1995). Brain serotonin, eating behavior, and fat intake. *Obesity Research*, **3** (Suppl. 4), 477–80.

Surgical treatment

Alessandro Salvatoni,

Paediatric Department, University of Insubria, Varese

18.1 Introduction

Medical treatment for obesity and the prevention of obesity are, in most cases, discouraging and frustrating for subjects, doctors and dieticians. The surgical treatment of obesity ('bariatric surgery') was proposed 40 years ago after it was observed that those who had large portions of the stomach and/or small intestine removed during surgery for gastro-duodenal ulcers or cancer, tended to lose weight postoperatively.

The first operations attempted were intestinal by-pass operations which induced weight loss through gastrointestinal malabsorption. The problems were that intestinal by-pass also produced loss of essential nutrients. Side effects were thus unpredictable and sometimes fatal. As a result, the original intestinal by-pass operations are no longer used. Since these original operations, various other surgical techniques for treating obesity have been proposed and tested. These are predominantly of two kinds: *plastic surgery* and *gastrointestinal surgery*.

18.2 Surgical techniques and their complications

18.2.1 Plastic surgery in obesity

The two main techniques of aesthetic plastic surgery are liposuction and the surgical resection of fat tissue and redundant skin, particularly that around the abdomen (abdominoplasty) and around the breasts (mastoplasty). There is little comment on the use of these techniques in childhood and they are certainly rarely used in the young.

18.2.2 Gastrointestinal bariatric surgery in adults

Gastrointestinal bariatric surgery follows two different strategies: reducing food intake by gastrorestrictive operations (gastric banding: GB, with or without vertical gastroplasty: VGP) or reducing intestinal absorption by gastrointestinal by-pass (Roux-en-Y gastric by-pass: RYGB, or biliary–pancreatic diversion: BPD). In recent years, there has been considerable progress in the development of gastrorestrictive techniques which have become more and more popular. At present laparoscopic GB, using an adjustable silicon ring which is useful for optimizing gastric pouch size (15–25 ml) and minimizing vomit, is proposed as the first choice approach in bariatric surgery (Belachew et al., 1994; Belachew & Legrand, 1998). However, by-pass techniques may still be indicated in selected cases when the gastrorestrictive procedure is, for some reason, unsuccessful (Sugerman et al., 1996).

The medium- and long-term results of gastrointestinal bariatric surgery published over the last 10 years are encouraging, with consistent and persistent losses of 60–90% of excess weight and reversal of the main complications in severe or morbid obesity (Rand & Macgregor, 1994; Scopinaro et al., 1996). Fertility also increases after weight loss but pregnancy is not recommended in the first 18 months post-BPD (Marceau et al., 1998). However, there are several crucial points which relate to the surgical treatment of obesity. Patient selection is the most important. It is also important to inform and advise potential subjects of the likely psychological and psychosocial effects of postoperative changes in bowel habit (Adami et al.1994, 1995; Bonne et al., 1996).

18.2.3 Complications

Early and late anatomical complications and side effects must be considered before recommending bariatric surgery. Almost all bariatric surgery techniques have complications. Although liposuction is considered a relatively safe procedure and most new techniques tend to be safer than previous techniques, deaths and nonfatal serious complications such as sepsis, toxic-shock syndrome, thrombo-embolic disease, fat emboli, and adult respiratory-distress syndrome, have been reported (Palmieri et al., 1995; Samdal et al., 1995).

Gastrointestinal bariatric surgery has a perioperative mortality risk ranging from 0% to 0.7% (Mason et al., 1992; Desaive, 1995; Hell & Lang, 1996; Scopinaro et al., 1996). Preliminary results of the recent Swedish Obesity Study (SOS) reported a perioperative mortality rate of 2/1680 patients corresponding to 0.12% (Näslund, 1998). The short-term mortality rate for severe obesity is unknown so it is not possible to determine whether surgery reduces obesity-related mortality or not.

The main perioperative complications of bariatric surgery are cardiorespiratory impairment, infection, gastrointestinal leakage, deep venous thrombosis and, less frequently, wound dehiscence and renal complications. Three different types of long term complications exist:

- anatomical (incisional hernia, intestinal obstruction, gastro-oesophageal reflux, gastric ulcer, staple line disruption) (Scopinaro et al., 1996; Sugerman et al., 1996);
- nutritional (anaemia, protein malnutrition, electrolyte imbalance, vitamin deficiency) (Rhode et al., 1996; Seehra et al., 1996);
- psychological (binge eating, anorexia) (Adami et al., 1994; 1995; Bonne et al., 1996; Gandolfo et al., 1996; Hsu et al., 1996).

Laparoscopic GB has fewer complications (both early and late) than BPD and has other advantages, such as being less painful, causing little respiratory impairment, allowing earlier digestive recovery, carrying no risk of incisional hernia, and resulting in shorter hospital stay (Belachew et al., 1994; Lonroth et al., 1996; Belachew & Legrand, 1998). GB is also a reversible procedure. The band may be removed if intractable vomiting or gastro-oesophageal reflux occur and, when indicated, the intervention can be converted into BPD. Patients with GB must be advised about the risks of taking aspirin or other drugs which can cause gastric erosions. In a significant proportion (20–30%) of GB cases, banding has to be repositioned by laparoscopy or traditional open surgery. The risks of late complications indicate a need for lifelong medical surveillance for all subjects after bariatric surgery.

A National Institutes of Health (NIH) Conference (Anon, 1991) prepared a consensus statement which included criteria for the selection of candidates for bariatric surgery. These were: body mass index (BMI) above 40, or between 30 and 40 in the presence of associated diseases (hypertension, diabetes, sleep apnoea etc.); age between 18 and 50 years; obesity stable for more than 5 years; failure of dietary or drug therapy after at least a year; absence of endocrine pathology; good comprehension by the patient of issues relating to surgery and of the importance of compliance; no dependency on drugs or alcohol; and acceptable operative risks. However, the positive effects of long-term weight loss and the late complications of the different forms of banded gastroplasty reported in the past few years (Brolin, 1996) suggest the 1991 NIH Consensus Conference recommendations need reconsidering.

18.3 Bariatric surgery in adolescence

Morbid obesity in children and adolescents, arbitrarily defined as greater than 100% excess weight or BMI over $40 \, \mathrm{kg/m^2}$ is associated with major health complications (Drenick, 1981). Epidemiological surveys show recent dramatic increases in the prevalence of obesity in childhood and particularly of severe obesity (Troiano & Flegal, 1998). Obstructive sleep apnoea, mainly due to increased thickness of the lateral pharyngeal wall, is one of the most severe complications of obesity and is associated with high mortality even in childhood and adolescence (Riley et al., 1976), thus providing an indication for dramatic intervention. Even though the minimum recommended age for bariatric surgery has been placed at 18 years, a few cases have been reported where the severity of obesity and/or related complications were such that bariatric surgery was undertaken in younger subjects. Surveys of patients who underwent bariatric surgery report few cases of children under 18 years (Desaive, 1995; Scopinaro et al., 1996). The only report on the medium-term outcome of surgery for obese teenagers is that by Rand and Macgregor (1994). They reported a 6-year follow-up of 34 adolescents who underwent restrictive gastric surgery between the ages of 11 and 19 years. Average BMI before surgery was 47 kg/m². At follow-up the mean BMI was 32 kg/m².

Assessing the balance between the risks and benefits of bariatric surgery in childhood is hampered by the small number of paediatric patients reported in the literature. Results in the adult population cannot be applied directly to paediatric age-group. For example, recent preliminary results of the SOS showed positive results with bariatric surgery, mainly gastric banding or vertical gastroplasty, in patients with BMI lower than 40 kg/m². Therefore they proposed to lower the BMI limit for surgical treatment to 34 kg/m² in men and 38 kg/m² in women (Näslund, 1998). We have no evidence to suggest we should recommend these limits for the paediatric age-group at present.

18.4 Conclusions

Surgical treatment of obesity in childhood and adolescence is undesirable and, in general, should only be considered when all else has failed, when children have achieved adult height and when severe, potentially life-threatening complications of obesity are present. Certainly, bariatric surgery cannot, and never will, solve the problems of management for the vast majority of obese and morbidly obese children and adolescents.

18.5 REFERENCES

Adami, G.F., Gandolfo, P., Camostano, A., Bauer, B., Cocchi, F. & Scopinaro, N. (1994). Eating disorders inventory in the assessment of psychosocial status in the obese patients prior to and long-term following biliopancreatic diversion for obesity. *International Journal of Eating Disorders*, **15**, 265–74.

Adami, G.F., Gandolfo, P., Campostano, A., Cocchi, F., Bauer, B. & Scopinaro, N. (1995). Obese binge eaters: metabolic characteristics, energy expenditure and dieting. *Psychological Medicine*, **25**, 195–8.

Anon (1991). NIH conference. Gastrointestinal surgery for severe obesity. Consensus Development Conference Panel. *Annals of Internal Medicine*, **115**, 956–61.

Belachew, M. & Legrand, M. (1998) Update on laparoscopic surgery for morbid obesity. *International Journal of Obesity*, **22** (Suppl. 3), S51.

Belachew, M., Legrand, M.J., Defechereux, T.H., Burtheret, M.P. & Jacquet, N. (1994). Laparoscopic adjustable silicone gastric banding in the treatment of morbid obesity. *Surgical Endoscopy*, **8**, 1354–6.

Bonne, O.B., Bashi, R. & Berry, E.M. (1996). Anorexia nervosa following gastroplasty in the male: two cases. *International Journal of Eating Disorders*, **19**, 105–8.

Brolin, R.E. (1996). Update: NIH consensus conference. Gastrointestinal surgery for severe obesity. *Nutrition*, **12**, 403–4.

Desaive, C. (1995). A critical review of a personal series of 1000 gastroplasties. *International Journal of Obesity*, **19** (Suppl. 3), S55–60.

Drenick, E.J. (1981). Risk of obesity and surgical indications. *International Journal of Obesity*, **5**, 387–98.

Gandolfo, P., Gianetta, E., Meneghelli, A., Cuneo, S., Scopinaro, N. & Adami, G.F. (1996). Preoperative eating behaviour and weight loss after gastric banding for obesity. *Minerva Gastroenterological Dietological*, **42**, 7–10.

Hell, E. & Lang, B. (1996). 10 years experience with vertical banded gastroplasty for operative therapy of morbid obesity. *Zentralblatt fur Chirurgie*, **121**, 363–9.

Hsu, L.K., Betancourt, S. & Sullivan, S.P. (1996). Eating disturbances before and after vertical banded gastroplasty: a pilot study. *International Journal of Eating Disorders*, **19**, 23–34.

Lonroth, H., Dalenback, J., Haglind, E., Josefsson, K., Olbe, L., Fagevik Olsen, M. & Lundell, L. (1996). Vertical banded gastroplasty by laparoscopic technique in the treatment of morbid obesity. *Surgical Laparoscopy and Endoscopy*, **6**, 102–7.

Marceau, P., Simard, S., Hould, F.S. & Biron, S. (1998). Outcome of pregnancies after obesity surgery. *International Journal of Obesity*, **22** (Suppl. 3), S51.

Mason, E.E., Renquist K.E. & Jiang D. (1992). Perioperative risks of surgery for severe obesity. *American Journal of Clinical Nutrition*, **55** (Suppl. 2), 573–6S.

Näslund, I. (1998). Effects and side-effects of obesity surgery in patients with BMI below and above 40 in the SOS (Swedish Obese Subjects) study. *International Journal of Obesity*, **22** (Suppl. 3), S52.

Palmieri, B., Bosio, P., Catania N. & Gozzi, G. (1995). Ultrasonic suction lipectomy. A mini-invasive treatment of obesity. *Recenti Progressi in Medicina*, **86**, 220–5.

Rand, C.S. & Macgregor, A.M. (1994). Adolescents having obesity surgery: a 6-year follow-up. *Southern Medical Journal*, **87**, 1208–13.

Rhode, B.M., Arseneau, P., Cooper, B.A., Katz, M., Gilfix, B.M., MacLean, L.D. (1996). Vitamin B12 deficiency after gastric surgery for obesity. *American Journal of Clinical Nutrition*, **63**, 103–9.

Riley, D.J., Santiago, T.V. & Edelman, N.H. (1976). Complications of obesity- hypoventilation syndrome in childhood. *American Journal of Diseases of Children*, **139**, 671–4

Samdal, F., Aasen, A.O., Mollnes, T.E., Hogasen, K. & Amland, P.F. (1995). Effect of syringe liposuction on activation cascade system and circulating cells when using the superwet or tumescent technique. *Annals of Plastic Surgery*, **35**, 242–8.

Scopinaro, N., Gianetta, E., Adami, G.F., Friedman, D., Traverso, E., Marinari, G.M., Cuneo, S., Vitale, B., Ballari, F., Colombini, M., Baschieri, G. & Bachi V. (1996). Biliopancreatic diversion for obesity at eighteen years. *Surgery*, **119**, 261–8.

Seehra, H., MacDermott, N., Lascelles, R.G., Taylor, T.V. (1996). Wernicke's encephalopathy after vertical banded gastroplasty for morbid obesity. *British Medical Journal*, **312**, 434.

Sugerman, H.J., Kellum, J.M., DeMaria, E.J. & Reines, H.D. (1996). Conversion of failed or complicated vertical banded gastroplasty to gastric bypass in morbid obesity. *American Journal of Surgery*, **171**, 263–9.

Troiano, R.P. & Flegal, K.M. (1998). Overweight children and adolescents: description, epidemiology, and demographics. *Pediatrics*, **101** (Suppl. 3), 497–504.

19

Interdisciplinary outpatient management

Beatrice Bauer[1] and Claudio Maffeis[2]

[1]Centre for Eating Disorders (DIDASCO), Verona. [2]Department of Paediatrics, University of Verona

Social, biological and psychological factors interact in the development of obesity. Consequently, we believe an interdisciplinary team approach is necessary in order to cope with this multifactorial background. This enables varied technical expertise to create an integrated approach which can then develop into efficient and effective management of obesity in children.

The difference between the *multi*disciplinary approach and the *inter*disciplinary concept of treatment we present is a basic one. 'Multidisciplinary' suggests adding components to a process which then act in parallel upon a problem. 'Interdisciplinary' implies integration of different components to create a harmonious solution to a multifaceted problem. In this chapter, we present the various interventions, usually offered at outpatient treatment centres, then develop the possibilities and problems which arise from the need to integrate these interventions.

19.1 Goal and general philosophy

Enabling permanent change in a child's eating habits is one of the major aims in obesity management. The success of a treatment programme is measured in long-term maintenance rather than in short-term weight loss. This shifts the focus of treatment from kilograms and kilocalories, as the most relevant variables, to behavioural and attitudinal changes, as only these can lead to future maintenance of weight loss. However, eating behaviours and attitudes to food, body shape and health are influenced by a myriad of internal (metabolic, emotional, cognitive) and external (attractiveness and availability of food, educational practices) events. Research continues to expose complexity in the antecedents and consequences of eating behaviour. As a consequence, no satisfactory characterizations of obese children from which to specify treatment yet exist.

Behavioural changes can result from the development of an individual's self-control or through parents and/or the social environment exerting strong external controls on a child's behaviour. The difference between the forms of control is theoretical since, in practice, both forms of control are usually active in achieving any benefit. However, it is important to decide where to put most emphasis on a weight-control programme and when this should be followed consistently by all therapists during management. We explain self-control and external control in more detail.

In common speech, terms such as 'self-control' and 'will-power' are used interchangeably. They are behavioural qualities often considered as personality traits resulting from individuals' biological constitutions and from their experiences when learning to control actions and impulses. In behavioural approaches to treatment, individuals are encouraged to exert self-control whereby, without any immediate external constraints or urging, they engage in behaviours which would have seemed *less likely* than other more tempting behaviours, and which make the behaviours requiring control *less likely* to occur (Kanfer, 1971; Thorensen & Mahoney, 1974).

This does not mean that self-control is viewed as behaviour which unfolds during an individual's development, irrespective of environmental influences. On the contrary, its development is related to earlier training. Its success is related to outcomes in the social environment (Kanfer, 1980). Thus the decision to eat a salad instead of a cheeseburger when going to a 'fast-food' restaurant with friends after school can be heavily influenced by (a) the menu of the restaurant, (b) the decisions of other children (c) the information retained since the last treatment session for obesity and (d) the reward for weight loss expected by the child.

The Behaviour Modification Programme we present in this chapter stresses a self-control approach to the management of obese children. It aims to develop specific skills which gradually lead children to better self-control in varied environments. Success will only be achieved if professionals and parents reinforce even the smallest approximations to ideal behaviour and, in the process, learn how their external control can help their children. Through gradual changes, children develop the necessary abilities to deal with environmental, biological, cognitive and emotional cues which previously triggered dysfunctional behaviour. Any positive changes must be incorporated into family routines and ultimately maintained by the children themselves.

The traditional use of diets or exercise programmes aims to produce changes in behaviour, but changes which are too often perceived as 'all-or-none'. Children comply, if at all, for a short period of time only. It is commonly parents' belief that treatments delivered in highly controlled environments with strong authoritarian parent–child or therapist–child relationships bring results. Consequently, they tend to expect professionals to adopt strictly authoritarian attitudes so as to make children to submit to 'the rules'. Such management concepts are quite dangerous. Cohen et al. (1980) investigated these in a study on long-term maintenance of weight loss. Twenty-five children who had attended a children's weight-loss group 1–3 years earlier were classified as either regainers or maintainers. Seventeen normal-weight children also participated in the study. All subjects recorded their eating and exercise behaviours for 4 days. Their parents monitored these behaviours for 1 day. The results showed that maintainers reported more self-regulation of weight and more physical activity than either the regainers or the normal-weight subjects. The regainers reported more parental control than normal-weight subjects. (It might be argued that despair on seeing their children's failure to exercise self-control led the parents of the regainers to intervene more.)

It has been recognized that childhood obesity frequently progresses to adult obesity. Given the negative experiences of management regimens heavily based on external parental/professional control, it is not surprising that obese individuals who were obese as children seem particularly resistant to slimming interventions in adult life.

Our basic premise is that children should be involved in management of their own obesity. Treatment should be tailored to the motivation, drive and ability of each obese child. The aim of all parties involved in treatment should be to foster each child's autonomy rather than to stress adherence to rules. Most importantly, whatever behaviour or cognitive changes we want to stimulate in obese children need to be reinforced by success if they are to be maintained over time. Positive reinforcement can be produced using all sorts of external rewards but we cannot ensure behaviours will last beyond the reinforcement phase unless new behaviours are also intrinsically reinforcing for children and their families.

Obese children already have to carry a heavy burden due to social discrimination. Health professionals need to pay particular attention to enhancing children's self-esteem rather than lowering their already negative self-image even further by unsuitable attitudes and unsuccessful procedures.

As we shall see in the second part of the chapter, it is not enough to declare these principles as important. All professionals on the interdisciplinary team must show sensitivity to the more general philosophy behind the principles. This is not easily achieved.

For example, in academic departments, professionals dealing with obese children may be more interested in developing biological knowledge, such as body composition or energy expenditure research, than in reducing children's obesity. They may look at obese 'subjects' with intense *scientific* interest but be totally unaware of, or unable to develop, the interpersonal skills needed to work with children and influence their behaviour.

If different therapists work together as an interdisciplinary management team, they need to follow the same therapeutic guidelines, independent of their professional background. These guidelines include sharing:

- the same theoretical knowledge and research findings with regard to the aetiology and treatment of obesity;
- the same understanding of the principles concerning the teaching and learning procedures used in treatment;
- the same basic organizational knowledge on the functioning of an interdisciplinary team;
- the organizational behaviour which ensures successful team work.

19.2 Multifaceted treatment programmes

The majority of research studies published have involved multicomponent treatment programmes to which children are allocated in the hope that, with such a wide range of interventions, something will work for each participant. We propose to explore the literature and examine the contribution made by the various components of behavioural programmes.

19.2.1 Psychoeducation

Obese children and their families usually think they are well informed about nutrition, 'ideal weight' and weight loss. In reality, the general population is well read on these matters, but has often gained information from popular magazines or televisions advertisements, which offer 'what the public wants to buy' and which cannot be relied upon for good advice. As a starting point for any obesity management programme, it can be helpful to develop a short series of meetings or lectures during which parents with their children, or adolescents alone, have the opportunity to understand their obesity problem and how they might bring it under control.

Possible topics to be covered include the aetiology of obesity, environmental influences on eating behaviour, the risks associated with obesity, high-fat diets, the effects of television on children's food preferences, the importance of exercise and the goals of a management programme. Information helps parents and children change their attitudes and behaviours. What really matters, however, is the way this knowledge is offered. Adopting a collaborative educational approach during these initial encounters encourages children and their families to feel that they are active participants in the therapeutic process (Olmsted & Kaplan, 1995). Clinicians should offer expertise and support in ways which make children feel both that change is possible and that their pace in proceeding with the change process will be respected. Psychoeducation is the most basic aspect of management. It should act as the foundation for all other interventions. At the end of any psychoeducation group meeting, children and their families are usually better motivated to participate in treatment programmes or have, at least, acquired better understanding of their difficulties in initiating change. It is thus vital that the professional in charge of this part of the programme is well acquainted with motivational enhancement techniques and with the management of treatment resistance.

19.2.2 Diet

The majority of obesity management programmes base their intervention on some form of dietary regulation as the means of reducing energy intake (Epstein et al., 1998). Diet-based programmes, however, do not correspond with the need to acquire long-term healthy eating habits – the most important concern in managing obese children. Furthermore, it is important to consider the adverse effects which can result from dieting in childhood (Bryant-Waugh, 1993). Many children suffering from eating disorders claim their disorders began with dieting. Patton et al. (1990) have suggested that female adolescent dieters run eight times the risk of developing eating disorders compared to nondieters. Dieting is increasingly common amongst women and adolescent (or younger) girls (Hill et al., 1992). Rigid slimming diets should probably be avoided in the management of obese children and adolescents. The widely used food-exchange system is an alternative adopted in many dietary education programmes, such as in Epstein et al. (1981)'s 'traffic-light' diet. Children and parents learn how to develop nutritious and balanced meals keeping within 1000 to 1200 kcal per day. An even less prescriptive way to help children improve their eating habits is to use food sheets (or food diaries) on which children record all they have eaten. These are then discussed with children and their parents during nutritional counselling sessions. It is important to remember that low-calorie diets, as sole recommendation in obesity management, have only minimal success (Coates & Thorensen, 1978).

19.2.3 Exercise

Physical activity is, after basal metabolic rate (BMR), the second largest component of the total daily energy expenditure. The level of physical activity of an individual is influenced by the familial factors. In Pima Indians, approximately 55% of interindividual variance of spontaneous physical activity in a respiratory chamber can be explained by familial factors (Zurlo et al., 1992). However, other factors, like time spent out of doors, television viewing, peer-group activity overall and individual motivation, influence childhood physical activity (Maffeis, 1999). Education for a more active lifestyle and encouraging the pursuit of activity favour increased total daily energy expenditure and ultimately, fat loss (Maffeis & Tatò, 1998). Moreover, muscle work promotes fat oxidation and so contributes significantly to negative fat balance (Flatt, 1987). Research findings show that the addition of exercise programmes to dietary regimens (Epstein et al., 1985; Rey-brouch et al., 1990) leads to better maintenance of weight/fat loss over 1–3 years follow-up. (Cohen et al., 1980). As with obese adults, the problem is how to improve compliance. Compliance with exercise, as with other aspects of child-hood obesity management, is poor. One attempted solution is to start pro-grammes with supervised exercise (Martin & Dubbert, 1982). Any physical activity must be both enjoyable and rewarding for the children. Reinforcement of the benefits of exercise by both therapists and parents has an important role in increasing the likelihood that children will continue to take exercise of their own volition. New levels of activity will be maintained over time only if they are intrinsically reinforcing – that is if children feel physically fitter and/or develop a sense of achievement. Another way of creating natural reinforcement of exercise is to let children choose the kinds of activity they want to pursue from a list of lifestyle exercises. They are then taught how to monitor their own activity and this provides tangible reinforcement (Epstein et al., 1982). Determination to cycle, to walk instead of going by car, to go upstairs instead of using elevators and other everyday physical activity is strongly influenced by the behaviour of those around obese children. Friends and relatives can make differences. The changes children should follow must befit their environments if they are to continue for years. Again, as with bad eating habits, we need to consider who is responsible for children's bad exercise habits and direct our efforts into changing the attitudes of the carers also (Chapter 15).

19.2.4 Behaviour management

Self-monitoring is one of the most widely used procedures in the behavioural management of children. Information from self-monitoring can help diagnosis, functional analysis and evaluation of treatment outcomes. The information children and/or adults collect during self-monitoring varies from the sort of food eaten and the amount of food eaten to the situational and emotional antecedents and consequences of eating and to the use of special behaviours targeted during the different phases of treatment. We also ask children to report the frequency and duration of physical exercise, the number of snacks per day, social interaction with other children after school (as an alternative to watching television), how often children have refused food when it was offered, the number of servings of vegetables eaten, and so on. A thorough analysis of the information gleaned during self-monitoring can characterize various behaviours responsible for excess-ive eating or for lack of exercise. One or more behaviours can then be chosen as targets for change. Behaviours which we want to encourage as management proceeds are clearly defined and reported on specially prepared observation sheets which, ideally, the children prepare themselves.

When training children (and parents) in self-assessment procedures, the most important rule is to avoid collecting data on the frequency of negative, that is unwelcome, behaviour. Attention should always focus on learning to increase positive behaviour through positive comments and reinforcement. Punishment can be an easy way to avoid facing the difficulties of educating young people. At times, it is a powerful means of inducing change. Nevertheless, although punishment may account for (temporary) interruptions in dysfunctional behaviour (such as not eating junk food), it creates no positive learning experience such as becoming skilled in choosing the right food in difficult situations.

A second rule for working with obese children is always to create learning experiences which have a high probability of success. The generally low level of self-efficacy in obese children and the need to improve their self-esteem, makes success in any activity an important motivating factor.

There are problems in creating successful learning experiences which relate to definitions of 'success'. Parents, children's friends, the media and, sometimes, doctors, may define 'success' only in terms of the amount of weight lost by obese children and usually expect 'success' after a very short period of time. Recent changes in the diagnostic criteria of the *DSM-IV* (*Diagnostic and Statistical Manual of Mental Disorders*, American Psychiatric Association, 1994) recognize that linking individuals' sense of worth to their appearance, weight and shape is the psychopathology central to eating disorders in adult life (Garfinkel & Dorian, 1997). Thus, defining treatment goals in terms of positive behaviours with children and their parents and repeatedly explaining the folly of concentrating exclusively on weight, is *conditio sine qua non* for a constructive treatment approach.

The principles of behavioural change in the management of childhood obesity should be part of more general parent-training programmes which help adults understand child management procedures, such as reinforcement techniques and contracting methods (Senediak & Spence, 1985). These should also heighten awareness of how attitudes towards parents' own weight and that of their children are crucial to the development and management of eating disorders (Pike & Rodin, 1991).

19.2.5 Parent training

It is very important that parents are involved, at least in part, in any obesity-control programme. Ten-year follow-up studies have demonstrated that the inclusion of parents in habit change and weight loss (Epstein et al., 1994b) influences both children's weight and their exercise habits. The data indicate that the eating environment and support from family and friends are significant predictive variables. As a consequence the more parents become involved and change their own behaviour as part of the programmes, the greater the positive changes in children's nutritional environment and the greater the social support for their children.

This would all seem so self-evident that it should need no further discussion. However, developing appropriate involvement of children's parents is often the part of obesity management that leads to most controversy and conflict. It is too easy for the treatment team to underestimate the difficulties some parents have in accepting children's obesity and becoming active change agents. The concept that 'the child has a problem that needs solving' and the desire to have this 'solved' by health professionals rather than by themselves needs addressing before embarking on any management of the children (Barlow & Dietz, 1998). Premature drop-out from treatment programmes can be largely avoided if the issues of parental resistance and motivation are addressed in one or two motivation enhancement sessions. Motivation Enhancement Therapy, as this initial phase is generally called, helps parents accept direct involvement and become personally committed to changing their own lifestyles. This type of psychotherapy is effective in dealing with various health-related behaviours which are usually resistant to change (Miller & Rollnick, 1991).

Another important but unusual component of the parent-training programme is training in problem-solving abilities. In one such programme (Graves et al., 1988), children and parents participated in problem-solving group learning, through discussion, so as to identify and solve problems arising from attempts to control their children's weight. The positive results of this experiment supported the view that the addition of parental problem-solving training to behavioural weight-loss programmes could be beneficial. Children in the 'problem-solving' group demonstrated the greatest weight change at both post-treatment and 6-month follow-up when compared with the 'behavioural-treatment' and the 'instruction-only' groups.

19.2.6 Assertiveness training and social-skills training

The most common serious consequence for obese children in western countries is their poor psychosocial functioning (Hill & Silver, 1995).

Children who grow up with problems of overweight or obesity do not only have problems with food, eating and health. Because of their history of obesity, these children frequently develop emotional and interpersonal problems which need addressing as much as their physical symptoms.

For example, obese children may have learned to depend on strong environmental cues for initiating eating. They may come to rely on cues provided by their parents rather than those provided by their own physiological needs (Krasner & Ullmann, 1973). The cues for meal termination are no longer linked to internal satiety or other biological stimuli. The need to conform to parental rules in order to receive attention and affection can trigger the child's eating behaviour. Food may come to satisfy multiple emotional needs by being strongly and repeatedly associated with parental attention, comfort and affection. Through this association, food becomes a general way of coping with various emotional states or difficult social situations (Jordan & Levitz, 1975).

A second difficulty faced by obese children has been well described by Hilde Bruch (1975):

> Obese children are in danger of becoming the butt and laughing stock of their peers. While they look big, they rarely are good fighters or self-assertive in other ways. Quite often they are passive and fearful, incapable of defending themselves against their tormentors. It is not surprising that the insults which hit a fat child day-by-day make him or her miserable and reclusive.

Twenty years later the World Health Organization (WHO) Report for the prevention and management of obesity (WHO, 1997) lists the risk of obese children being socially isolated among the three 'Special considerations in the management of childhood obesity'.

Interpersonal behaviour plays an important role in an individual's acquisition of social and cultural reinforcers as well as in his or her acquisition of various social norms and roles. Children who do not possess effective and appropriate social skills experience isolation, rejection and overall diminished happiness. If interpersonal problems persist, as is often the case with obese children, they can interfere with school and peer experience and fuel a sense of failure, social isolation and friendlessness.

Assertiveness training and training in social skills help children learn specific, discrete verbal and nonverbal communication skills, behavioural repertoires and social skills for effective peer and adult interaction, self-assertion and problem solving in difficult situations and how to handle their own emotions and stress (McGinnis et al., 1984).

The group setting provides an ideal format for this kind of training. It is often the first real-life situation in which children can explore a better way of dealing with interpersonal problems and improve their self-esteem.

19.2.7 Psychiatric Intervention

Obesity, in childhood as in adolescence, is not a uniform condition. Some obese children hide severe emotional and personality disturbances behind their obesity. These may be the consequence of problems existing in their families or of traumas experienced outside the home (Bruch, 1975). There are few data on the prevalence of psychiatric problems in children with obesity but in a sample of obese children at the beginning of treatment Epstein et al. (1994a) found 29% of children met, or exceeded, the clinical criteria for psychological problems on the Child Behaviour Checklist (Achenbach, 1991).

A thorough psychological evaluation may help prevent worsening psycho-pathology due to inadequate or inappropriate management procedures. Weight reduction in significantly disturbed children can precipitate an even more serious illness. In severe cases, family therapy is the prerequisite for continuing to treat the eating behaviour. Play therapy is another form of intervention if the obese child is a victim of abuse and neglect (Mann & McDermot, 1973). The goal of play therapy is to help children master the multiple stresses of abuse and neglect and to correct or prevent deviations in future psychosocial development. Play is particularly useful, since most abused children express their innermost feelings and fantasies much more readily by action than by verbalization. If children are not too destructive or aggressive, group therapy may be possible (Kynissis & Halperin, 1996) but children are unlikely to profit from group therapy if they are unable to listen to, or interact with, others or if they are severely depressed and unable to feel at ease with their peers.

Given a recent increase in eating disorders amongst the mothers of very young children, therapists should understand possible relations between the pathological eating behaviour of the mothers and the obesity in their children.

19.3 Organizing team work

Every group of professionals involved in an obesity-management centre is confronted with the problem of organizing different treatments. A process of constant testing and reorganizing interventions as well as redefining the combinations and possible integration of professionals is necessary in order to find the 'ideal' therapeutic process.

To begin to realize an ideal vision requires the development of new ideas with only limited financial and professional resources. Programmes which were effective elsewhere need to be adapted to the local cultural and political environment. Willingness to innovate, to tolerate uncertainty, and, last but not least, to 'survive' internal and external power dynamics is essential.

19.3.1 Organizational aspects of the therapeutic process

The literature on the organizational aspects of interdisciplinary centres is still amazingly poor. Problems in this area involve everyone: patients, families, professionals, secretaries and administrative personnel.

There are many aspects we could analyse in order to understand the problems facing an interdisciplinary centre better and what makes it 'tick' as an organization. In our view the style of therapeutic approach is critical.

There are two main therapeutic approaches: the individually tailored approach and the standard approach.

The individually tailored approach: an illusion of interdisciplinary treatment?

The advantages of the traditional individualized approach are that interventions can be easily adapted to patients' needs. Usually, treatment is delivered by a paediatrician specialized in the management of obesity. Individualized treatment does not require extensive organizational effort in order to design a management programme. The individual caring for a child and family decides what is needed and tailors interventions to results. Changes in the approach to obesity occur almost imperceptibly over time, based on the experiences of the professionals in charge. Professionals working together in the same unit may develop quite different approaches to treatment, but the differences remain hidden behind the closed doors of offices unless unit management comes under discussion. The freedom experienced by professionals in decision making is one of the values of individualized treatment. The burden (real or imagined) of being simultaneously clinician, psychologist and dietician is the method's most serious limitation. Any interdisciplinarity, if it exists at all, is 'inside' the individual practitioner. Knowledge from different disciplines is integrated into a clinical approach but is confined to a 'one-man (or woman) conceptual framework'.

The standardized treatment: interdisciplinary management running through the programme

A standardized approach offers just one, preferably evidence-based, approach. The kind of intervention offered develops from the experience and 'best practice' perceptions of a group of professionals. Children and their families accept a predetermined management plan. The only variations in the programme relate to the speed at which the children cope with the phases of the programme.

The best way to guarantee that the treatment is sufficient or appropriate to particular children's needs is pretreatment screening. If it is clear that the programme does not suit a child, the child should be redirected to an obesity management programme more appropriate to his or her needs.

The standardized therapeutic model is used mainly in institutions which have only recently started working with obese children, or which have inexperienced or comparatively unqualified professionals. However, this approach can be used by organizations with highly qualified professionals, if personal and financial resources are insufficient to offer more complex interventions. The individual, or group of professionals, who design the programme decide the mix of medical, nutritional and psychological interventions. Coordination of the professionals involved in treatment is reduced to a minimum by using written guidelines or a treatment manual.

The limitations of the standardized approach are counterbalanced by the ease of organizing and managing a predefined programme. Beginners are usually reassured by manuals with precise instructions on conducting therapy, session by session. The anxieties and uncertainties which surround attempts to treat conditions as complex as obesity are controlled by guidelines. Any problems patients encounter with implementation of the programme tend to be dismissed as either 'not important' or as evidence of 'failure to collaborate'.

This is the treatment generally offered as group therapy – the most common treatment choice in western countries. Limited resources often determine health services' decisions to pursue standardized approaches. It is perhaps of interest that most professionals schooled in group interaction and group dynamics consider the positive effects of group therapy outweigh the extra efforts needed to learn the skills required to initiate treatment.

Adults, as well as children, benefit from learning in groups. Positive feelings and behaviours can be contagious. Group members act as role models and stimulate imitation of new behaviour by others. In difficult situations, group members help each other and offer precious support. Discussion amongst group members can help critical thinking and the acceptance of responsibility (Wilkinson, 1984).

Integrating the two approaches: interdisciplinarity embedded in the organization

Besides the standardized and individualized approaches, there is a third way to organize interdisciplinary work which respects the time and money resources of organizations and of their clients whilst guaranteeing an individualized approach to pathology (Fig. 19.1). This modality can be realized by arranging some basic therapy, such as psychoeducation and assertiveness training, in standardized groups. Clinicians can then devote their time to individual problems, knowing that the basic information for obesity control has been acquired in group sessions.

To personalize the programme there must be highly experienced therapists who can follow individuals' needs through initial assessments and then direct children and their families to appropriate management groups. The same therapists then assess the effects of group therapy, stimulate good practice in these sessions, and help patients optimize their session time. The frequency of individual meetings between group sessions depends on the extent of child–family difficulties and on professionals' availability.

This combined approach has numerous advantages. It reduces the costs of individual therapy. It guarantees high-quality group therapy. It gives the chance to adapt standardized therapies to individual needs. Nevertheless, it has important costs, mainly for the participating professionals. Most health-care professionals –

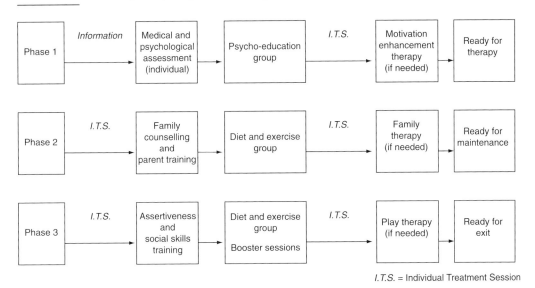

I.T.S. = Individual Treatment Session

Figure 19.1   Interdisciplinary approach to the treatment of childhood obesity.

physicians, dieticians, psychologists – are trained to work with patients on a personal basis. Their exclusive relationship with patients as individuals is an appealing element of their profession. The reciprocal interdependence among professionals required to work in an interdisciplinary organization is often perceived as a burden. No wonder therefore, that the most crucial aspect for perfect functioning in a matrix design is the motivation and management of professionals involved.

Organizational difficulties relate to the need for close collaboration with colleagues. Professionals who are strongly motivated to obtain good results are better able to cope with interpersonal conflicts amongst staff. However, people with strong desires to dominate their colleagues or, by contrast, who submit uncritically to more powerful colleagues are not useful members of the team.

Efficient briefings and quick, informal communications are also important if this approach is to succeed. Not all professionals involved in the programme can meet the criteria required for this form of teamwork and this can pose problems.

19.3.2 Collaboration problems

This dynamic vision of a fully integrated approach is unique in that success provides further impetus for cooperation. However, so often what prevails is a bureaucratic–normative vision of work organization, where specialization is important and where the separation of tasks, responsibilities and power remains. Specialization enables an individual to play one role well but without considering the whole process. It creates a tunnel vision of the outcome. Only the fraction of the outcome which concerns the specialist is seen – usually just a small part of the whole.

We perceive an interdisciplinary team as a complex solution to a complex problem. The management of childhood obesity will not succeed by ignoring the complexity of the problem. Lack of time and lack of resources are no excuse for the difficulties and problems experienced in managing the condition. We need to rethink the structure of relevant organizations. This may need time and money. However, the prime initiative in developing new solutions to the management of obesity must arise from dissatisfaction with present results.

To achieve an innovative and effective work organization, with strong goal orientation, is costly for both human and financial resources. Reciprocal interdependence requires widespread delegation of decisional powers whilst enabling all participants to share a global view of obese children's problems.

There are then the costs associated with conflicts, jealousy, incomprehension among people which stem from the fact that no one has taught us how to work together. On the contrary, the most important institutions in our life, from family to school, have competed to reward individual success, better if achieved with astuteness and at someone else's expenses. Our ambiguous relationship with authority doesn't help the openness to an interdisciplinary collaboration at all: power is a personal quality exhibited by the submissiveness of as many people as possible. The answer to this type of power is generally a formal and apparent servility, which hides cynicism, indifference, mistrust and a desire to do one's way. These characteristics, make whatever organization one is trying to build as whimsical and unreliable as a naughty child (Perrone, 1992).

19.4 Acknowledgements

We are indebted to Vincenzo Perrone, Professor of Organization at the Università L. Bocconi in Milan, Italy, for his help in the understanding of our organizational problems and the development of strategies to implement change.

19.5 REFERENCES

Achenbach, T.M. (1991). *Manual for the Child Behavior Checklist/4–18 and 1991 Profile*. Burlington, VT: University of Vermont Department of Psychiatry.

American Psychiatric Association (1994). Diagnostic and Statistical Manual of Mental Disorders. Fourth Edition. Washington DC: American Psychiatric Association.

Barlow, S.E. & Dietz, W.H. (1998). Obesity evaluation and treatment: expert committee recommendations. *Pediatrics*, **102**, e29.

Bruch, H. (1975). The importance of overweight. In *Childhood Obesity*, ed. P.J. Collip, Massachusetts: Publishing Science Group.

Bryant-Waugh, R. (1993). Epidemiology. In *Childhood Onset Anorexia Nervosa and Related Eating Disorders*, eds. B. Lask & R. Bryant-Waugh. Hove: Lawrence Erlbaum Ass. Publishers.

Coates, T. & Thorensen, C. (1978). Treating obesity in children and adolescents: a review. *American Journal of Public Health*, **68**, 143–9.

Cohen, E.A., Gelfand, D.M., Dodd, D.K., Jensen, J. & Turner, C. (1980). Self-control practices associated with weight loss maintenance in children and adolescents. *Behavior Therapy*, **11**, 26–37.

Epstein, L.H., Wing, R., Koeske, R., Androsik, F. & Ossip, D. (1981). Child and parent weight loss in family-based behaviour modification programs. *Journal of Consulting and Clinical Psychology*, **49**, 674–85.

Epstein, L., Wing, R.R., Koeske, R., Ossip, D. & Beck, S.A. (1982). Comparison of lifestyle change and programmed aerobic exercise on weight and fitness changes in obese children. *Behavior Therapy*, **13**, 651–65.

Epstein, L.H., Wing, R., Penner, B. & Kress, M.J., (1985). The effect of diet and controlled exercise on weight loss in obese children. *Journal of Pediatrics*, **107**, 358–61.

Epstein, L.H., Klein K.R. & Wisniewski, L. (1994a). Child and parent factors that influence psychological problems in obese children. *International Journal of Eating Disorders*, **15**, 151–7.

Epstein, L.H., Valovski, A., Wing, R.R. & McCurley J. (1994b). Ten-years outcomes of behavioral family-based treatment for childhood obesity. *Health Psychology*, **13**, 373–83.

Epstein, L.H., Myers, M.D., Raynor, H.A. & Saclens, B.E. (1998). Treatment of pediatric obesity. *Pediatrics*, **101**, 554–70.

Flatt, J.P. (1987). Dietary fat, carbohydrate balance, and weight maintenance: effect of exercise. *American Journal of Clinical Nutrition*, **45**, 296–306.

Garfinkel, P.E. & Dorian, B.J. (1997). Factors that may influence future approaches to the eating disorders. *Eating and Weight Disorders*, **2**, 1–16.

Graves, T., Meyers, A.W. & Clark, L. (1988). An evaluation of parental problem-solving training in the behavioral treatment of childhood obesity. *Journal of Consulting and Clinical Psychology*, **56**, 246–50.

Hill, A.J. & Silver, E.K. (1995). Fat, friendless and unhealthy: 9-year old children's perception of body shape stereotypes. *International Journal of Obesity*, **19**, 423–30.

Hill, A.J., Oliver, S. & Rogers, P. (1992). Eating in the adult world: The rise of dieting in childhood and adolescence. *British Journal of Clinical Psychology*, **31**, 95–105.

Jordan, H.A. & Levitz, L. (1975). Behavior modification in the treatment of childhood obesity. In *Childhood Obesity*, ed. M. Winick. New York: John Wiley.

Kanfer, F.H. (1971), The maintenance of behavior by self-regulated stimuli and reinforcement. In *The Psychology of Private Events*, eds. A. Jacobs & L.B. Sachs, New York: Academic Press.

Kanfer, F.H. (1980). Self-management methods. In *Helping People Change*, eds. F.H. Kanfer & A.P. Goldstein., Pergamon General Psychology Series, Volume 52.

Krasner, L. & Ullmann, L.P. (1973). *Behavior, Influence and Personality*. New York: Holt, Rinehart & Winston.

Kynissis, P. & Halperin, D.A. (1996). *Group Therapy with Children and Adolescence*, New York: American Psychyatric Press.

Maffeis, C. (1999). Role of energy metabolism in the pathophysiology of childhood obesity. In

Progress in Obesity Research, pp. 633–7. London: John Libbey.

Maffeis, C. & Tatò, L. (1998). Quel role jouent l'activité physique et la sedentarité dans le développement et le maintien de l'excès de poids chez les enfant? *Archives françaises de Pediatrie*, **5**, 1191–6.

Mann, E. & McDermot, J.F. (1973). Playtherapy for victims of child abuse and neglect. In *Handbook of Playtherapy*, eds. Schaefer, K.J. O'Connor. New York: John Wiley.

Martin, J.E. & Dubbert, P.M. (1982). Exercise applications and promotion in behavioral medicine: current status and future directions. *Journal of Consulting and Clinical Psychology*, **50**, 1004–17.

McGinnis, E., Goldstein, A.P., Sprafkin, R.P. & Gershaw, N.J. (1984). *Skillstreaming the Elementary School Child.* Champaign, IL: Research Press.

Miller, W. & Rollnick, S. (1991). *Motivational Interviewing: Preparing People to Change Addictive Behavior.* New York: Guilford Press.

Olmsted, M.P. & Kaplan, A.S. (1995). Psychoeducation in the treatment of eating disorders. In *Eating Disorders and Obesity*, eds. K.D. Brownell & C.G. Fairburn, New York: Guilford Press.

Patton, G.C., Johnson-Sabine, E., Wood, K., Mann A.H. & Wakeling, A. (1990). Abnormal eating attitudes in London schoolgirls – a prospective epidemiological study: outcome at twelve month follow-up. *Psychological Medicine*, **16**, 49–58.

Perrone, V. (1992). L'organizzazione interdisciplinare: solo costi o anche vantaggi? In *Oltre la dieta.* Verona: Atti del convegno ANDID.

Pike, K.M. & Rodin, J. (1991). Mothers, daughters and disordered eating. *Journal of Abnormal Psychology*, **100**, 198–204.

Reybrouch, T., Vinchk, J., Van de Berghe, G. & Vanderschueren-Lodeweychk, M. (1990). Exercise therapy and hypocaloric diet in the treatment of obese children and adolescents. *Acta Paediatrica Scandinavica*, **79**, 84–8.

Senediak, C. & Spence, S.H. (1985). Rapid versus gradual scheduling of therapeutic contact in a family based behavioural weight control programme for children. *Behavioural Psychotherapy*, **13**, 265–87.

Thorensen, C.E. & Mahoney, M.J. (1974) *Behavioral self-control.* New York: Holt, Rinehart & Winston.

WHO (1997). Report of the World Health Organization on Obesity, Geneva.

Wilkinson, J. (1984). Varieties of teaching. In *The Art and Craft of Teaching*, ed. M.M. Gullette. Cambridge, MA: Harvard University Press.

Zurlo, F., Ferraro, R.T., Fontvielle, A.M. & Ravussin, E. (1992). Spontaneous physical activity and obesity: cross-sectional and longitudinal studies in Pima Indians. *Americal Journal of Physiology*, **263**, E296–E300.

20

Interdisciplinary residential management

Marie-Laure Frelut

Robert Debré University Hospital, Paris

Severe obesity in childhood is likely to persist throughout life and is known to be associated with increased risks of early death, atherosclerosis and its complications, and some cancers. In the most severe obesity, when outpatient management has proved ineffective and the burden on the child or adolescent becomes overwhelming, inpatient management may sometimes be indicated. One alternative to 'hospital' inpatient management is the residential summer camp.

The idea behind residential management is to help children restore the balance between energy expenditure and energy consumption themselves, helped by psychosocial and educational supports, with the aim of providing an ongoing, long-lasting, and progressive slimming process.

20.1 Historical background and implementation

The history of the development of residential care in the management of obesity is rather vague. After World War II, children and adolescents from European cities, especially France, used to leave their families and join summer camps for 1–2 months of 'healthy holidays'. Medical centres which had developed outside cities when tuberculosis was a highly prevalent disease were reoriented towards treating severe, noncommunicable, chronic diseases because of medical and epidemiological changes. Support from National Insurance or private health-care systems enabled chronically ill children and adolescents to benefit from sustained inpatient care. Countries which provide no residential care or provide it only through summer camps may do so for reasons of economy or because of traditional reluctance to accept state intervention in citizens' private lives.

Inpatient clinics for the management of obesity exist in the Czech Republic, France, Germany, Belgium and Poland. Some countries, such as Italy, provide some short-term (around 2 months stay) residential places. Other countries, such as Austria, Italy, USA and the United Kingdom, rely predominantly on the summer-camp system to support various outpatient approaches. Increasing prevalence of childhood obesity in Europe has led to criticism of long-term residential management on the basis of the small number of children treated and the inadequate number and size of centres when compared with the numbers of children needing help and the severity of these children's obesity. Whilst, at first glance, more centres would seem desirable, careful analysis of what they can achieve might lead to different conclusions. The mid- and long-term outcome of the patients seems quite heterogeneous, some subjects relapsing almost immediately while others maintain long-term benefits, suggesting that biological and behavioural background are still poorly understood phenotypes of a complex disease.

20.2 A comprehensive approach

Inpatient treatment aims to provide a comprehensive, multidisciplinary approach to the management of childhood and adolescent obesity. There are few well-documented and objective reports of the programmes offered in residential centres for obesity. However, apart from summer camps where interventions rely largely on physical and nutritional training, management usually includes simultaneous combinations of medical follow-up, psychological support, physical training, nutritional education, cookery classes and educational support including normal school attendance. The extent of family involvement depends on the distance between children's homes and the centre and the readiness of parents to meet the team in charge of the children and adolescents. Careful screening of potential residents is thus particularly important so as to determine whether children and their families can cope with residential treatment and whether they understand the long-term implications of this type of management.

20.2.1 Screening

Most centres focus on adolescents and preadolescents who are usually mentally and physically capable of active involvement with the centres' programmes and who can tolerate long separation from their families. The duration of stay varies from around 8 weeks in Germany (H. Mayer, personal communication) to over one year in some centres such as in Belgium (De Haan Centre or Claus Vallons Centre). Large differences in programme duration reflect two different goals of treatment. With short stays, the aim is to initiate weight loss which, it is hoped, will then continue under local supervision once children go home. Longer stays are expected to bring children to their desirable weights or body mass index (BMI) ranges (Smith et al., 1997) – usually around the 98th centile for age – and to stabilize body weights before leaving the centres. The main goal after discharge is to maintain the fat reduction achieved at the centres.

In France, where most inpatient treatment centres are sited, national recommendations stress that centres should be only one element in a pre-established individual care and follow-up programme. Medical complications and/or psychosocial problems must be sufficiently severe to justify residential management. By no means all severely obese children and adolescents are either able, or ready, to benefit from inpatient management. Careful screening of possible candidates is absolutely essential.

In the Therapeutic Centre, Margency, the procedure prior to admission is as follows: patients, or their families, who contact the centre, either independently or following the suggestion of their physician, are first screened over the telephone to judge the severity of their obesity and any complications. Further screening takes place in two different half-day sessions at about 1-month intervals. Medical, psychological, dietetic and educational assessments are made. These are then evaluated by different members of the team in order to define, within a peer group, a specific management programme for each individual child. This programme can start even before the beginning of the stay.

Admissions are accepted on the basis of the degree of obesity (BMI $\gg$ 97th centile of national charts) (Rolland-Cachera et al., 1991) and the age of the children (9–16 years, either sex) provided no major exclusion criteria have been detected. The commonest exclusion criteria are children's lack of interest in the treatment process, psychiatric disorders such as depression or psychosis, and marked mental retardation.

Screening also aims at detecting complications such as sleep apnoea (Lecendreux et al., 1998) or slipped femoral capital epiphysis (Dietz, 1998) which might indicate urgent treatment before admission.

About half the adolescents and children admitted to the unit have a history of poor school performance which has no specific explanation. The commonest diagnoses which, in our experience, decrease children's chances of success are pathological anxiety, specific learning disability (e.g. dyslexia), low intellectual efficiency or, in contrast, hyperactivity dampened down by obesity. We try to clarify children's problems and to help them and their parents understand their specific problems before admission, in order to develop an individual management approach both before, and during, inpatient treatment (Isnard et al., 1996, unpublished data). Whenever there is a major social problem, the team social worker gets in touch with the local contact in the area where the child lives, so as to understand the child's situation better and to prepare for the child's stay.

These preadmission meetings help focus on the main goal of residential management, namely to maintain a steady weight/height relationship once it has been reduced as close as possible to the 97th centile BMI for age and sex. The duration of residential stay is estimated roughly on the basis of 3–5 kg weight loss per month, prior to the stabilization phase. Different aspects of management are thoroughly explained to the children and their parents. We usually see divorced/separated parents together since most children in such family set-ups, divide their time between parents.

To our knowledge, most teams follow similar formalized general rules for their management centres.

20.2.2 Interdisciplinary management

The significant role played by genetic make-up in the development of early severe childhood obesity, reinforces the concept that each individual fat child or adult needs to restore his or her own energy balance on a long lasting basis (Bar-Or et al., 1998). Eighty per cent of the children in our series have at least one severely obese parent. Thus, treatment includes: dietetic and nutritional education and counselling; physical training; educational and psychological support; and as much parental commitment as possible, despite separation during their children's stay.

The dietetic approach

Most very obese patients, old or young, under-report their food intakes and eat nutritionally 'unbalanced' diets.

Our nutritional goals are to restore children to eating tasty, balanced diets which will be acceptable to them and their families long term. Because planned weight losses are huge, modest dietary restriction is used throughout the stay, apart from the last 3–5 weeks, so as to enhance rates of weight loss. However, the physical training programme and the usual food preferences of these children make it necessary to continue high starch intakes. Balanced family-like diets of energy content 5800–8400 kJ/day (1400–2000 kcal/day) are used. These are about 20% less than French recommended daily allowances for age and sex (Dupin et al., 1992). Restrictions are at the expense of 'simple' sugars and saturated fats. Vegetables and fruit consumption are increased compared with the previous diets of most of the children (Lloyd et al., 1998). Four meals are provided each day as breakfast, lunch, afternoon snack and dinner. Meals are eaten with the children together in the dining room. During the course of the stay, the dietary energy is gradually increased in 836 kJ (200 kcal) steps, up to a 6700–10 000 kJ/day (1600–2400 kcal/day) range, so that the patients leave the unit with potentially stable weights.

Some centres use slightly different dietary regimens, although all aim for the same goals. Energy intakes may be lower, with maximum intakes of 6300 kJ/day (1500 kcal/day) for example. Sometimes, as in Roscoff, France (J. Le Deunff & C. Revert, personal communication), the quantity but not the quality of the food is left unrestricted provided weight loss occurs at the pre-established rate.

Once every 2 weeks, small groups of children (three to five) participate in 2 hour long sessions for instruction in basic nutrition and cooking. Cookery teaching adapts to the customs of local cooking. Dietetic guidelines include guidance on maintaining weight in special circumstances such as parties and meals taken outside the home from restaurants and fast-food outlets. Occasions for eating, such as school dinners, which will occur once children are back at home, are also discussed between dietician and children before the children go home.

In our unit, parents are given the same dietary advice as their children when the children are admitted to the project and they are then taught twice per term in special parent sessions. They are invited to get in touch with the dietician, at least by phone, whenever they have nutritional or dietary queries or problems. They are also encouraged to discuss traditional home cooking, which remains, fortunately, still deeply rooted amongst families in many parts of Europe. The aim of management is to preserve the positive aspects of the traditional cooking but, nevertheless, to improve what is now too rich and too fattening a style of cooking for the physical activity levels seen in today's cities.

Protein-modified sparing diets are not used much with residential care for child and adolescent obesity (Suskind et al., 1993). Our personal opinion is that these diets do not fit into the remit of our therapeutic programme, which aims to re-establish healthy, well-balanced family lifestyles. Some authors (Rolland-Cachera et al., 1998) are currently trying to assess whether lower protein intakes within balanced diets produce better outcomes. So far, no differences have been observed.

Physical training

Physical training is an important component of the treatment for several reasons. Most patients have almost totally abandoned any sport and physical training, including exercising at school. Other physical activity is reduced to a minimum. This seems to stem more from the negative perception of sport and physical activity due to the shame of being unsuccessful and ridiculous when compared with peers than from reluctance to take exercise. Successful physical training thus becomes another important component of the process of enhancing self-esteem and social life (Saelens & Epstein, 1998). It facilitates energy balance by, sometimes very modestly, enhancing energy expenditure, judging from reference to observations in healthy subjects (Torun et al., 1996), and by reducing the caloric restriction otherwise required to produce the same loss of fat. When obese individuals are restored to adequate physical fitness (Katzmarzyk et al., 1998), activity contributes towards maintaining higher levels of energy expenditure and thus facilitates long-term energy balance. Obese children do not seem to develop increased appetites because of their extra activity, confirming findings in healthy adults undergoing moderate physical training (King, 1998; Spreit & Peters, 1998).

Chosen sporting activities should fulfil several criteria:

- use stored fat as a preferential energy substrate (i.e. be submaximal and last over 20 minutes per session);
- be adapted to unskilled patients with modified body shapes (Bratteby et al., 1997); appeal to children (i.e. be varied);
- take into account potential cardiovascular, orthopaedic and other risks (Ward et al., 1997; Dietz, 1998; Horton, 1998).

Choice of activity, support during activity, and a progressive build-up in activity are important aspects of the programme.

Time spent in the different activities varies according to the time of year. Summer camp programmes may include 3–4 hours of physical activity per day whilst 3–6 hours per week are more typical average duration at other times of year if spontaneous activity and walking to school are excluded. The geographical area in which the treatment centre is located influences the variety of physical activities offered. Most centres offer gymnastics, walking and swimming sessions of about 1 hour each. Other sports are offered depending on local facilities, season and indoor/outdoor facilities. Any spontaneous activity is vigorously encouraged.

In our unit, physical training only starts after careful cardiorespiratory and muscular fitness tests have been carried out in order to identify obesity complications and determine individuals' submaximal heart rates, that is rates just below the anaerobic metabolism threshold. Aerobic metabolism is a necessary condition for mitochondrial oxidation of stored triglyceride fatty acids (Vettor et al., 1997). After testing, children are provided with cardio-testers to help them exercise at the heart rate associated with 70–75% maximal oxygen consumption. We have found that with activity at this submaximal oxygen consumption level, the echocardiographic abnormalities found in two-thirds of our subjects (left atrial and ventricular dilation and septum hypertrophy) diminish (Frelut et al., 1995), lean body mass (measured by dual X-ray absorptiometry), and muscular strength are maintained (Oberlin et al., 1998, Frelut et al., 2000) and cardiorespiratory fitness increases (Savigny, 2000). Physical growth might be making an important contribution to improved physical fitness. Preadolescence and adolescence seem, from the physical point of view, to represent ideal ages to recover from the potentially deleterious consequences of severe obesity.

Physical activity is restored both by decreasing physical inactivity and by increasing physical training. Physical inactivity, however, may be hiding conflicting attitudes such as the avoidance of some negatively perceived choices and a preference for activities such as video games. It is important to try to help children and their families distinguish and differentiate such choices and issues. Confronting both the reluctance to exercise and the greater enjoyment offered by physical inactivity can be combined in treatment support and have proved effective in obesity management (Epstein et al., 1997). Children are encouraged to change their lifestyle progressively during the periods they spend at home whilst residential care is continuing. For example, they have to choose which sport(s) they will practise on a regular basis in addition to their school activities.

Psychological support

Psychological disturbance secondary to the development of obesity is a major component of the complications associated with obesity in childhood and adolescence. When obesity is so severe that inpatient treatment is necessary, most patients have entered a vicious circle. Inactivity and social avoidance are consequences of obesity which further enhance obesity by reducing physical activity and increasing food intake, especially as binge eating. Thus, the first goal of psychological support is to help the obese child or adolescent escape from this vicious circle. Separation from the family for which obesity has often become a source of conflict, educational support from adults who have no negative perceptions of the child and integration into a peer group suffering similar problems are important psychological benefits of inpatient treatment.

The second goal of psychological support is to detect and treat disturbances occurring in association with obesity. Common findings are a high degree of anxiety, which contributes to isolation through poor school performance and failure to make contact outside the home with people who might be able to help them. Specific support in speech and writing or psychomotor sessions is also available (Kazdin & Weizs, 1998). Some teams (Zwiauer & Schmidl, unpublished data) have also introduced relaxation therapy.

The observations made by children or adolescents when away from their families can also help identify and reduce family dysfunction by providing opportunities either to help the family as a group or to help the child understand and cope with family dysfunction. Losing weight contributes to a more positive perception of the child by family and friends through the development of a successful and more autonomous individual.

An informal behavioural approach is by far the most common psychological intervention reported by different teams. Since clinicians rarely have competence in this field as well, the techniques used usually go unreported. Thus, the psychological effectiveness of inpatient treatment has been analysed only rarely. We have shown that depression scores which, before treatment, were significantly higher in obese adolescents than in their lean siblings, returned to normal with therapy, whilst self-esteem increased markedly (Isnard et al., 1996, unpublished data). During summer camps, Gately et al. (1998) found a significant improvement in self-awareness, self-esteem and body image. This is in agreement with data reported by Epstein but underlines the failure to discriminate between the effects of weight reduction and the effects of nonspecific treatment (Epstein et al., 1997, 1998).

Educational support

During residential stays, children and adolescents live together (groups range between 15 and 75 subjects, with mean size around 30) and share daily life except whilst attending their respective schools. In the centre, children are supported by education professionals who are in charge of the organization of daily life for the groups but who also care for individual children in close relationship with other members of the team. These professionals cover broad fields (as parents would) and sometimes include physical training in their activities. They contribute to establishing a balance between choice and control with the children – something to be practised at home as well.

The observations of these professionals are especially important in detecting day-by-day improvement or problems. They help children both adapt to the various changes they face and implement new changes. Children are encouraged to seek their help and advice when required. They, in turn, are supported by a psychologist and a paediatrician and work in close collaboration with dietician and physiotherapist.

The objectives of these education professionals must, on the one hand, be adapted to the individuals in their charge (some centres have developed a referee system) and, on the other hand, allow a pleasant social environment for the whole group. The professionals are continually balancing their activities between individual and group support as well as providing links between teams of therapists and teachers. Their relationships with children's parents depend very much on the way the centres function in relation to their geographical location relative to the children's homes. Major differences are reported between centres. At some centres, children go back home for 1 or 2 weeks holiday, once a term. In other centres, all weekends are spent with the family so as to maintain normal family life and to allow this to evolve progressively towards agreed objectives. In these centres, the education professionals maintain a weekly relationship with the children's families.

Family involvement

Parents, although they accept temporary separation from their children, remain a key element in the effectiveness of residential care. First of all, since they agree to keep in touch with the centre team (twice weekly in our unit), call by phone and welcome their children back home during weekends or holidays, they keep an active role and provide important feedback. Ideally, the professional teams' roles include helping families anticipate and manage changing relationships with their

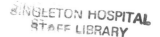

children. In the centres, children face other adults who provide evidence that some rules are necessary in life. Rediscovering a social life makes the children more confident and happier in relationships outside the unit, including those with their parents. Family therapy is not used, as such, to our knowledge during the inpatient stays but may be proposed as a follow-up measure. Assessing the difficulties which prevent the development of improved family relationships requires complicated step-by-step procedures which we use as necessary. As with outpatient management, poorly supported children and adolescents are less likely to be successful. Social workers can be extremely helpful in reinforcing support during and after treatment.

20.3 Results and outcome

Immediate results are reported as very good since most children lose significant amounts of weight, something they have previously failed to do. Since most units do not organize postdischarge follow-up of the children, few long-term results are available.

In the United States, Boeck et al. (1993) achieved significant results in a semi-structured long-term adolescent setting after a mean stay of 8 months. Mean BMI in 21 patients was $47.5\,\mathrm{kg/m^2}$ on admission. Mean decrease in BMI was $11\,\mathrm{kg/m^2}$. Nine patients left the programme prematurely, mainly for social and psychological problems.

We have recently analysed, retrospectively, the outcome for 259 adolescents who were treated between 1990 and 1997 in our obesity unit at Margency, France. Patient outcome has been assessed either by physical examination or by interviewing either the practitioner in charge of follow-up or the one who sent the adolescent to the unit in the first place. Eighteen patients have been excluded from analysis because of immediate (i.e. during the stay) treatment failure. The main reasons for failure were either psychiatric disorder or obesity secondary to the sequelae of a brain tumour. We obtained information on 118 (49%) of the remaining 241 children (156 girls and 85 boys). Mean age at admission was 13.8 ± 2.2 years and 13.3 ± 1.8 years respectively for girls and boys. Mean BMI was $34.9\,\mathrm{kg/m^2}$ at admission, falling to 26.2 at discharge and 29.2 at follow-up. At all points in the follow-up period BMI remained significantly lower than at admission (Frelut et al., 1999).

Comparisons of summer camp interventions (Zwiauer & Schmidl, 1993; Lisá et al., 1997; Di Pietro et al., 1998; Gately et al., 2000), long-term stays, as reported here, and the results of 32 predominantly randomized, controlled studies of the treatment of childhood obesity analysed by Epstein at the request of the American Academy of Pediatrics (Epstein et al., 1998), show that the mean BMIs at the beginning of the treatment in our study are among the highest reported. At the same time, mean reduction in BMI with treatment is amongst the most dramatic. The 1-year follow-up data for the summer camps indicate sustainable effects from this treatment approach also, despite the absence of randomization in these prospective studies. We draw the same conclusion regarding our own data, despite the putative bias of retrospective studies. However, the time and investment required by residential care requires better definition of the procedures used as well as better characterization of the severely obese children who will benefit. Our results need confirmation by other teams using prospective studies.

Inpatient treatment does not differ in its general principles from most reported treatment profiles for the management of childhood and adolescent obesity. A combination of therapeutic methods is always required to decrease the health consequences of obesity (Suskind et al., 1993; Williams et al., 1997; Dietz, 1998; Epstein et al., 1998). However, the duration of the stay and the interaction between the team and the group of adolescents or children can offer a broader range of treatment possibilities than those offered by outpatient management. Inpatient treatment allows a combination of therapeutic approaches for which the impact of each is not yet independently assessed. For us, both theoretically and practically, adolescence seems the best time to intervene with inpatient treatment but even this conclusion needs verifying.

As with all treatment of childhood obesity, no data exist to show the impact on long-term reduction, in adulthood, of obesity-associated risk factors. However, short-term controls have repeatedly established a significant improvement of cardiovascular risk factors (Epstein, 1998).

20.4 Conclusions

Inpatient treatment is an effective way to treat severe obesity in adolescents and children, on a long-term basis, when a comprehensive approach is used and a reasonable target chosen by a skilled team. The evaluation of the apparently high cost-effectiveness ratio of this approach should be compared not only with outpatient treatment but also with the global, social and medical costs of early severe untreated obesity.

20.5 REFERENCES

Bar-Or, O., Foreyt, J., Bouchard, C., Brownell, K.D., Dietz, W.H., Ravussin, E., Salbe, A.D., Schwenger, S., St Jeor, S. & Torun, B. (1998). Physical activity, genetic, and nutritional considerations in childhood weight management. *Medicine and Science in Sport and Exercise*, **30**, 2–10.

Boeck, M., Lubin, K., Loy, I. et al. (1993). Initial experience with long term inpatient treatment in morbidly obese children. *Annals of the New York Academy of Sciences*, **699**, 257–9.

Bratteby, L.E., Sandhagen, B., Lotborn, M. & Samuelson, G. (1997). Daily energy expenditure and physical activity assessed by an activity diary in 374 randomly selected 15-year-old adolescents. *European Journal of Clinical Nutrition*, **51**, 592–600.

Dietz, W.H. (1998). Health consequences of obesity in youth: childhood predictors of adult disease. *Pediatrics*, **101**, 518–24.

Di Pietro, M., De Cristo Faro, P., Campanaro, P. et al. (1998). School-camp: short and long term results. *International Journal of Obesity*, **22** (suppl. 4), S32.

Dupin, H., Abraham, J. & Giachetti, I. (1992). *Apports nutritionnels Conseils pour la Population Française.* Paris: Tec & Doc, Lavoisier.

Epstein, L.H., Saelens, B.E., Myers, M.D. et al. (1997). Effects of decreasing sedentary behavior on activity choice in obese children. *Health Psychology*, **2**, 107–13.

Epstein, L.H., Myers, M.D., Hollie, A.R. et. al. (1998). Treatment of pediatric obesity. *Pediatrics*, **101**, 554–70.

Frelut, M.L., Azancot, A., Boromée, V. et al. (1995). High rate of mild cardiac abnormalities in obese children. Impact of weight loss. *International Journal of Obesity*, **19** (suppl. 2), S122.

Frelut, M.L., Isnard, P., Pérès, G. et al. (1999). Etude retrospective de 259 adolescents obèses traités en centre de moyen séjour entre 1990 et 1997. *Archives de Pédiatrie*, **6** (suppl. 2), S556.

Frelut, M.L., Dao, H.H., Oberlin, F. et al. (2000). Changes in fat free mass and muscular strength in obese adolescents during weight reduction. *International Journal of Obesity*, **24** (suppl. 1), S581.

Gately, P., Cooke, C., Barth, J.H. et al. (2000). Efficacy of a 6 week residential program for children. *International Journal of Obesity*, **24** (suppl. 1), S96.

Gately, P., Knight, C., Butterly, R.J. et al. (1998). The effect of an 8 week diet, exercise and behavioral/educational camp program on obese children. *International Journal of Obesity*, **22** (suppl. 4), S32.

Horton, T.J. (1998). Exercise and obesity. *Proceedings of the Nutrition Society*, **57**, 85–91.

Isnard, P., Frelut, M.L., Naja, W. et al. (1996). Psychopathology in obese adolescents before and after a treatment program in a dietetic center. Proceedings of the International Congress on Eating Disorders, New York.

Katzmarzyk, P.T., Malina, R.M., Song, T.M.K. et al. (1998). Physical activity and health related fitness in youth: a multivariate analysis. *Medicine and Science in Sport and Exercise*, **30**, 709–14.

Kazdin, A.E. & Weizs, J.R. (1998). Identifying and developing empirically supported child and adolescent treatment. *Journal of Consulting and Clinical Psychology*, **66**, 19–36.

King, N.A. (1998). The relationship between physical activity and food intake. *Proceedings of the Nutrition Society*, **57**, 77–84.

Lecendreux, M., Frelut, M.L., Quera-Salva, M.A. et al. (1998). Weight loss reduces sleep associated breathing disorders in obese children. *Journal of Sleep Research*, **7** (suppl. 2), 152.

Lisá, L., Blaha, P. & Srajer, J. (1997). Problems of obese children in the Czech Republic. In *Proceedings of The Round Table Meeting on Obesity Management in Central Europe*, eds. W. Hainer & M. Kunesova, pp. 31–2. Prague: The Czech Society for the Study of Obesity.

Lloyd, T., Chinchilli, V.M., Rollings, N. et al. (1998). Fruit consumption, fitness and cardiovascular health in female adolescents: the Penn State Youth Young Women's Health Study. *American Journal of Clinical Nutrition*, **67**, 624–30.

Oberlin, F., Frelut, M.L., Novo, R. et al. (1998). Body composition and mineralization in obese children. *Bone*, **23** (suppl. 5), S393.

Rolland-Cachera, M.F., Cole, T.J., Sempé, M., Tichet, J., Rossignol, C. & Charraud, A. (1991). Variations of the Wt/Ht^2 index from birth to age 87 years. *European Journal of Clinical Nutrition*, **45**, 839–46.

Rolland-Cachera, M.F., Thibault, H., Soulié, D. et al. (1998). Weight loss in two groups of obese children consuming diets containing different amounts of proteins. *International Journal of Obesity*, **22** (suppl. 4), S32.

Saelens, B. E. & Epstein, L.H. (1998). Behavioral engineering of activity choice in obese children. *International Journal of Obesity*, **22**, 275–7.

Savigny, A. (2000). Evolution des aptitudes physiques chez des adolescents de 9 à 17 ans atteints d'obésité majeure primaire sous traitement multidisciplinaire dont les activités physiques. Thèse de Médecine, Faculté de Médecine Lariboisière-Saint Louis, Université Paris VII.

Smith, J.C., Sorey, W.H., Quebedeau, D. et al. (1997). Use of body mass index to monitor treatment of obese adolescents. *Journal of Adolescent Health*, **20**, 466–9.

Spreit, L.L. & Peters, S.J. (1998). Influence of diet on the metabolic response to exercise. *Proceedings of the Nutrition Society*, **57**, 25–33.

Suskind, R.M., Sothern, M.S. & Farris, R.P. (1993). Recent advances in the treatment of childhood obesity. *Annals of the New York Academy of Sciences*, **699**, 181–99.

Torun, B., Davies, P.S.W., Livingstone, M.B.E. et al. (1996). Energy requirements and dietary energy recommendations for children and adolescents 1 to 18 years old. *European Journal of Clinical Nutrition*, **50** (suppl. 1), S37–S81.

Valverde, M.A., Patin, R.V., Oliveira, F.L.C. et al. (1998). Outcomes of obese children and adolescents enrolled in a multidisciplinary health program. *International Journal of Obesity*, **22**, 513–19.

Vettor, R., Macor, C., Rossi, E. et al. (1997). Impaired counterregulatory hormonal and metabolic response to exhaustive exercise in obese subjects. *Acta Diabetologica*, **34**, 61–6.

Ward, D.S., Trost, S.G., Felton, G. et al. (1997). Physical activity and physical fitness in African-American girls with and without obesity. *American Journal of Clinical Nutrition*, **5**, 572–7.

Williams, C.L., Campanaro, L.A., Squilllace, M. et al. (1997). Management of childhood obesity in pediatric practice. *Annals of the New York Academy of Sciences*, **817**, 225–40.

The future

W. Philip T. James

International Obesity TaskForce, London

21.1 Introduction

The challenge presented to the author was to speculate what might emerge in the field of childhood obesity over the next 20 years. Though this sounds simple, readers will agree that predictions are usually wrong, and the broader the scope of the endeavour the greater the opportunity for error. Nevertheless, this chapter is written in the hope that, by being broad and speculative, it may stimulate efforts to prove at least some of the predictions wrong, thereby closing unproductive blind alleys and encouraging new avenues of research. The predictions range from the molecular and metabolic to the public health and political.

21.2 Assessment of childhood obesity

Clearly, we need a coherent, meaningful and preferably simple method for defining childhood obesity. The recent attempts by the International Obesity TaskForce (IOTF) were based on the idea that we needed coherence between childhood and adult indices of obesity. The choice of the centile of body mass index (BMI) at any age which corresponded, when children attained the age of 18, to BMIs of 25 and 30, was a straightforward, logical step (see Chapter 1). Of course, the choice of the BMI is crude, with groups of short and tall children of similar age and sex showing very different prevalences of overweight when a single BMI cut-off point is used (Franklin, 1999). Thus, Franklin's observations that tall children are more likely to be classified as overweight at the same BMI as short children, emphasizes the crude nature of the BMI based as it is on a height power of two. Given the ease of current computational processes, one prediction is that a new scheme may emerge where the power p of height is adjusted for the ages 6–15 years, as suggested by Franklin. This will at least allow some corrections for obvious problems with the BMI.

Difficulties are also likely to arise because the use of BMI cut-off points will stress the problem of specifying suitable cut-offs in adolescence, when girls and then boys display a growth spurt and a developmental surge at different ages within one community. The discrepancies may be amplified when Chinese and Indian investigators highlight the more delayed puberty in at least half the world's population. Then we have to recognize the conviction that the current World Health Organization (WHO) cut-off point for normal weight in adults, that is a BMI of 25, is too high for Asians (WHO/IASO/IOTF, 2000) so there will be pressure to derive nationally or ethnically appropriate cut-offs for children as well as for adults. It will then be claimed that the current estimates of Third World childhood obesity are exaggerated because of the children's short stature and that new techniques are needed, or a different formulation of weight and height is required. Inevitably, a split will emerge between the technologically driven and those in public health because new measures available in the affluent West will allow the precise determination of the expected body fat for the height, sex and age of the child, once it has been decided what the norm should be for a group of western children. The current large WHO study defining the growth of children breastfed exclusively for 6 months and then followed until they are 5 years of age, could well be extended to potentially become the international norm. The difficulty will be that, if modern techniques, such as impedance or other measures of lean tissue/body fat ratios, are to be used, then they will have to be incorporated into the studies of weight/height relationships in different populations. The WHO breastfeeding study already underway in several Third World as well as Western countries, will, I suspect, identify appreciable differences in body fat in the children from different populations despite the children's common start in life. This will then spark a debate as to the extent of fetal programming and the impact of traditional children's diets in different countries. We already know that obese Indian adults have the smallest proportion of lean tissue, with Chinese adults having intermediate proportions, compared with the supposed Caucasian norm. Yajnik (2000) is now identifying poor fetal accumulation of lean tissue linked to maternal diet and the generation of low-birthweight babies who are still overfat for their size with the children subsequently growing with limited amounts of muscle and other lean tissues. This may well prove to be an environmental effect and not a genetic problem.

The likely differences in lean growth and fat accumulation in different populations will then lead to a repeat of the public-health controversy which raged 30 years ago when so many paediatricians and public-health figures were convinced that the pandemic stunting of children in the Third World reflected their different genetic potential. Only later did it become apparent that environmental factors were far more important than genes. Clearly, this time around we will require the ability to relate technologically sophisticated studies of body fat and its distribution in children to the broader public-health need for crude measures which are reasonable predictors of future well-being. An amplified WHO study could provide the best possible option for resolving some of these problems.

This body-compositional approach to establishing the norm requires the specification of a particular BMI or body fat content as a good predictor of a child's probability of entering adult life at greater risk of handicap from glucose intolerance, lipid abnormalities, hypertension or other risk factors for adult disability. Inevitably, making this decision will depend upon having access to coherent longitudinal studies where, in 6- to 18-year-olds, insulin resistance, lipid profiles, blood pressure and other risk factors are monitored and then related to the adult's risk status. There are a series of marvellous long-term studies already available in countries such as the UK and USA, but there are other opportunities for linking likely outcomes for children of different weights in Third World studies, for example in The Gambia, Mexico and China. The problem will inevitably arise, however, of trying to establish a super-reference base for optimum health.

21.3 Ethnic differences in children's anthropometry

It has long been recognized that children in the developing world display fat distributions which differ from US or UK reference values. Thus, not only are children subject to stunting but, despite having a normal weight for height, they also have a surprisingly small triceps skinfold thickness when this is compared with their subscapular value. This was considered a feature of non-Caucasian children living in the developing world and of ethnic, that is genetic, origin. What now seems to be emerging, however, is a different perspective, that is that the difference in fat distribution is associated with a propensity to truncal adiposity and an increased likelihood of developing abdominal obesity in later life. This is vividly shown by the remarkable features of, for example, Chinese, Mexican or Indian middle-aged women who are positively android in their accumulation of fat. My guess is that we are going to have to re-evaluate completely the acceptance that the low triceps values in Third World children are genetic and link them to the dominant abdominal obesity in Third World adults. Already, Japanese and Chinese investigators are highlighting the marked risks of glucose intolerance, hypertension and abnormal lipids in both men and women at surprisingly low waist circumferences and with BMIs of only 23 or 24. This implies an extraordinary propensity to pathophysiological changes accompanying the abdominal obesity.

One reasonable hypothesis, based on Björntorp's work (Björntorp & Rosmond, 2000) and the proposal that low maternal protein intakes induce hypertension in the offspring by the excessive transfer of maternal cortisol to the fetal circulation, is that we are dealing with a pandemic resetting of the control of corticosteroid and, indeed, hypothalamic metabolism in Third World subjects. Obesity now affects the poor and deprived and mothers in these communities may well be on a suboptimal diet which now seems increasingly related to the child's future propensity to disease. If on a poor maternal diet there is excessive fetal cortisol and this leads to a resetting of the control for corticosteroids so that excessive secretion is the norm, then this hormonal shift will actually have been fetally generated and is not a genetic feature. Björntorp's work has now been duplicated in several parts of the world showing that people with truncal and visceral obesity have hyperresponsive adrenals with lower growth hormone levels and a reduction in testosterone levels in men. It is remarkable to see escalating obesity in China displaying itself in children, and now in adult women, in a form which, in my endocrinological days, we would immediately have investigated as potential Cushing's disease. The distribution of fat, the paucity of lean tissues, the thin arms and the moon-shaped features with a surprising frequency of skin striae analogous to that seen in Cushing's disease is accompanied by a high incidence of glucose intolerance and hypertension. My hunch is that the thin triceps skinfold thickness observed in children over the last 40 years in the developing world will be seen, in due course, as one of the earliest physical manifestations of the hypercorticoidism and early resetting of the corticosteroid control system.

The implications of these observations and speculations are profound. They imply that the catastrophic problems of abdominal obesity, diabetes and hypertension now becoming rampant throughout the Third World are preventable. This prevention need, however, relates not only to events in late childhood and adult life, but to maternal well-being and environmental factors during infancy. Yajnik's work amplifies evidence from Jamaica and South Africa showing that there is a relationship between crude indices of poor fetal growth, such as weight and length at birth, and later insulin resistance and a propensity to high blood pressure by the age of 4 years in Jamaica, at 4 and 8 years of age in India with a persisting link into adolescence as now observed in South Africa (Yajnik, 2000). Even more worrying is Yajnik's finding that the risks are markedly increased if there is a combination of a poor fetal outcome – displayed crudely by birthweight – combined with rapid catch-up growth in the first few years of life. Paediatricians have spent their time emphasizing the value of catch-up growth and this is clearly of extraordinary value in stunted children in relation to their mental development – see Grantham-McGregor's data on the importance of mental stimulus plus good nutrition in promoting intellectual development (Grantham-McGregor et al., 1999). Yet if we continue to emphasize the importance of catch-up growth to achieve appropriate heights and weights in relation to the WHO reference, then we may be putting children at greater risk of diabetes and hypertension by having them grow fast following a disadvantaged early life. Clearly we will need to establish the interventions needed in pregnancy to avoid children already showing insulin resistance and a propensity to high blood pressure at an early age.

Experimental data on the pregnancy programming of fetal metabolism, for example by Jackson and his colleagues (Gardner et al., 1998), and Yajnik's data suggest that one carbon pool metabolism needed for nucleic acid synthesis and new tissue growth may be acutely limited. Whether this is helped by more glycine in pregnancy, or a different balance of methionine with other amino acids, or is profoundly related to folate input is unclear. The problems of how the alterations in amino acid metabolism induce the propensity to hypertension and whether there are distinguishing features between the corticosteroid shift, with its likely impact on the subsequent propensity to insulin resistance, and the mechanisms relating to blood-pressure control, highlight the value of coherent experimental work. Hales's work (Petry & Hales, 2000) suggesting alterations in pancreatic capacity and liver structure, cell selection and metabolism may also be of profound significance and in due course we may require the development of crude clinical indices of fetally redesigned livers and pancreases.

21.4 The Thrifty Genotype

Neel's original hypothesis that some populations have selectively acquired the Thrifty Genotype is re-emerging strongly (Neel, 1999). There are a host of opportunities for using modern molecular techniques to establish whether there are genetic differences in various ethnic groups which promote both their selective accretion of energy, the fractionation of energy to protein or fat gain or their likelihood of having a high corticosteroid response with central adiposity by virtue, for example, of differences in the promoter region of the hypothalamic glucocorticoid receptors. Solomons & Kumanyika (2000) have recently taken on board the politically sensitive question of whether there are genuine differences between the races: this issue is clearly of key importance and needs to be resolved. My bias has been to emphasize the environmental factors. The efforts to have nationally based growth charts in the 1950s and 1960s in order to mollify Third World investigators who were appalled by the remarkable deficits in growth in their children ended with a recognition that environmental factors were of overwhelming importance. It is now important to ensure that the modern obsession with gene-probing does not divert funds from crucial issues relating to environmental hazards in obesity to a wonderful world of expensive studies on different genes in different societies without regard to the environmental influences. This does not deny the importance of population differences in gene prevalence. Nutritionists are now happy to accept, for instance, differences across the globe in lipoprotein E_4 prevalences (Simopoulos, 1997), the supposed reduced risk of coronary heart disease because of the relative infrequency of lipoprotein $Lp_{(a)}$ in people of Hispanic origin (Haffner et al., 1992), and the differences in handling alcohol or lactose in different ethnic groups. It will be relatively simple to identify, for example, a single glutamine for glutamate change in the β_2 receptor which produces higher average BMIs and triples the obesity rates in French men and women, but only if they are inactive. This is a clue to a truly physiologically important enhancement of the efficiency of energy conservation. Whether or not this preliminary observation in France can be applied to the Thrifty Genotype hypothesis remains to be seen, but it is a single base change affecting a third of the population and links to both obesity and one of its environmental promoters. To find direct evidence of energy efficiency is, however, very difficult. Our errors in dietary assessment are huge, and locking people in calorimeter chambers or using D_2O^{18} in free-living people still presents problems if we are looking for 2% to 3% differences in the capacity to control energy balance. The hunt for genes which affect appetite, energy metabolism or, indeed, behaviour in terms of spontaneous eating or physical activity will doubtless be funded substantially over the next 10 years. Nevertheless, there will need to be consistent results from several different investigators in different parts of the world with detailed studies of the environmental circumstances before one can feel confident that the Thrifty Genotype really does account for the extraordinary rapidity of the obesity epidemic now underway.

21.5 The prevalence of childhood obesity

If, for the present, we take the IOTF approach to defining prevalence rates, recognizing that this corresponds roughly to the 85th National Center for Health Statistics (NCHS) centile, then we are dealing with a definition very different from the two standard deviation (SD) limit still used for defining malnourished, stunted or underweight children. Gurney's original attempt to use $+2$ SDs has internal consistency in paediatric terms, but does not have the long-term implications and coherence with the adult BMI cut-off points. It seems clear that we should not be too troubled by data on children under 5 years of age from an obesity point of view except in relation to the fetal programming issues previously discussed. Therefore, we need essentially to think about the obesity rates observed around the globe in 5- to 9-year-old children, that is before the pubertal spurt starts. As yet, we have only limited data on global prevalences, but a quick perusal of different data sets reveals overweight prevalences based on the 85th NCHS centile which are disturbing. Thus the prevalence of overweight in Mexican children is now reported as already 24%.

I think we can confidently predict that, except perhaps in the war-torn and AIDS (acquired immunodeficiency syndrome)-ridden sub-Saharan African region, we will see a rate of obesity increasing perhaps by 1% per year on average throughout the globe. On this basis, one might predict that 30–50% of children will be overweight by the year 2020 and, as one looks at the social forces currently underway, there seems no reason to modify this seemingly outrageous projection. Whether one is dealing with the 'Little Emperors' of the single-child family in China or the manifestly obese children of the Middle East, there seem to be the same forces under way, as are readily observed in Europe and in North and South America.

21.6 Weaning practices and early eating habits

One can argue that the process of establishing healthy eating habits starts with weaning. Recently, a battle regarding the appropriate length of time for exclusive breastfeeding has surfaced with WHO, UNICEF (United Nations Children's Fund) and the food industry as major protagonists. For some time, WHO, which was instrumental in establishing a Code of Practice for companies producing infant formulae, has specified that breastfeeding should continue exclusively for 4–6 months. Although there was international agreement to comply with this Code, in practice, implementation at a local level has not only been imperfect, but in some countries it has been routinely flouted. Recently, UNICEF and a number of governments have specified that exclusive breastfeeding should continue for 'about 6 months', in an attempt to prevent companies from interpreting the 4- to 6-month rule as indicating infants should start the weaning process from 12 weeks onwards. It is rare for any national group of women to have a good record for exclusive breastfeeding and certainly few can claim the astonishing rates which seem to be emerging in Norway where it is reported that about 95% of women breastfeed exclusively for at least 4 months and over 90% of the women in the breastfeeding study were still exclusively breastfeeding at 6 months. In India, it is often claimed that most mothers establish exclusive breastfeeding but this, in practice, includes providing a baby from a few days of age onwards with additional water, teas and other herbal infusions which may account for their intercurrent infections, despite supposedly breastfeeding exclusively.

It is becoming clear that the same difficulties that apply to establishing and maintaining breastfeeding also apply to the clear recommendation that fruits and vegetables, rather than cereals, should be the first novel foods used as a routine for weaning. When the majority of women in the world are now moving into an urban environment where breastfeeding can be a handicap, given the mother's need to return to work, it is not surprising that snack foods, confectionery and even soft drinks are introduced as a routine to many children before they are 1 year of age. The WHO Baby Friendly Hospital movement is almost unknown in many countries such as the UK and, with such intense food-industry promotion of alternative feeding systems for any child over a few months of age, it is understandable if mothers fear that breast milk alone is not sufficient for their baby. The simplicity of providing snacks rich in enticing sugar, salt and fat means that mothers inadvertently acquiesce in establishing precisely the type of eating behaviour which is so conducive to excess weight gain and so difficult to change once established.

21.7 The 'obesogenic' environment

With falling fertility rates and lengthening life expectancy almost everywhere except in Africa and Russia, and with rapidly changing attitudes to marriage and divorce, the social structure of families is changing dramatically. Throughout the world there is explosive urban development with a concomitant decline in agricultural employment, a situation which can lead to the bread-winner or the whole family moving to urban areas to find work, and children growing up without the support of an extended family. More and more women need to work simply to maintain the basic family income so that spending hours in the preparation of traditional foods for family meals is no longer a practical option. Cooking skills are being squeezed out of the curriculum, on the basis of both lack of time and cost factors just as the opportunity to learn by example in the home is also declining. Many children are allowed to 'graze' from the refrigerator or food store, often eating easily prepared ready meals high in fat, salt or sugar, unsupervised by an adult. A pervasive westernization of cultures is spreading at an astonishing pace, facilitated by global television networks. We have the strange anomaly of a plethora of television cooks demonstrating a wide range of culinary skills, yet a marked diminution in the preparation of food in the home. Eating out is a frequent occurrence for many, encouraging the consumption of large portions of unknown calorific content.

Vast numbers of children spend their lives in town and city environments where there are few public play areas. The intensity of poorly planned urban development and a universal fear for children's safety mean that pupils are increasingly bussed or taken to school. In the holidays or after school hours they may be confined to their homes with easy access to snack foods while watching television or videos, or playing computer games. This makes them ever more vulnerable to a sedentary lifestyle and completely inappropriate dietary habits. There is little opportunity or incentive in this environment for physical activity, and poor eating habits are constantly reinforced by exposure to untrammelled advertising. It would seem that the traditional family environment, where the principles of appropriate eating and behavioural patterns could be taught by example, are becoming a rarity.

Five years ago, I was asked by the then UK Minister of Public Health to put forward suggestions on how to combat the increasing problem of obesity, paying particular attention to children. I and colleagues had already provided a set of guidelines for preventing adult obesity for the previous government, but these had been fraught with controversy because of opposition from the food industry, and in particular the snack foods and soft drinks producers, who were unhappy with the emphasis on diet. Their preferred approach, predictably, was the desirability of increased physical activity with little or no reference to dietary issues.

There is little evidence that the governmental/industrial approach to food and health will change despite the current valiant attempts to reintroduce dietary guidelines for school meals. When we examined the diet of UK children from preschool age up to adulthood, we found alarming evidence of confectionery, snack foods and soft drinks dominating their eating patterns. We discovered that schools were often dependent on profits from soft drink and confectionery sales to generate funds for items which were previously considered essential, such as writing materials and books. Profit-making was also dominating the provision of school meals, encouraging caterers to use fat- and sugar-enriched options which would be most popular with their 'customers', who were expected to make 'informed choices' from the age of 4 years upwards. In fact, discussions with child psychologists and experts in education and child development revealed it was unlikely that children below the age of 12 years, even when of high intelligence and brought up in an appropriate environment, could make wise food choices. This requires balancing the pros and cons relating to different food options at a time when children are exposed to a barrage of inappropriate food advertising. Children were also spending about £130 million per year purchasing soft drinks, snacks, sweets and chocolate on their way to and from school. Inevitably companies with direct access to ministers were concerned when policies were suggested which would threaten this revenue. This raises a fundamental issue as to how we are going to promote public health in an environment where the free market and business lobbying of governments dominate.

21.8 Can policy initiatives work?

We might do well in the future to learn from the experience of some Scandinavian countries where stringent regulations have been introduced regarding the advertising of foods to children, difficult though this might be in a free-market economy where interference from the government in a citizen's right to choose is considered to be a manifestation of the dreaded 'nanny state' approach. In some Scandinavian countries school meals and an active, healthy school environment have been established on the basis of recognizing that children need to be educated gradually over a substantial period of time without being bombarded, or indeed manipulated, by companies selling their products. This is particularly relevant to the consumption of vegetables and fruits. The Bangor studies (Horne et al., 1995) have shown that in older children these foods have to be introduced many times, with frequent reinforcing techniques. It seems much easier to establish appropriate food patterns if children have been introduced to a variety of vegetables and fruits at an early age. On a broader front, Finland promoted a policy in restaurants and canteens of always providing salads or vegetables as an intrinsic component of the meal, rather than charging separately for these items. This has encouraged the reluctant individuals to increase their intake.

From a public-health point of view, the drive by most governments to encourage medical and scientific investigators to seek funding from industrial groups is worrying and likely to increase as this approach has even spread to some United Nations agencies. Those of us who are closely involved with policy-making at a national, regional, for example European Union, and global level are now all too aware that some components of the food industry are brilliantly organized in their political lobbying and marketing schemes. They resemble the tobacco industry in their unwillingness to contemplate any independent view which highlights issues that might interfere with their business. In fact, the major tobacco companies in the US have now purchased food businesses, despite their often low profit margins and growth opportunities; this ploy is a mechanism whereby these companies can gain access to lobbying groups in Congress, since tobacco interests are no longer considered legitimate areas for lobbying activities.

Counteracting the pressures of food advertising is a much more difficult proposition than dealing with tobacco because the scientific evidence on fat, sugar and salt, for example, or the worrying impact of acidic soft drinks on the newly recognized epidemic of dental erosion (Dental Practice Board for England and Wales, unpublished data) is more difficult to prove. All these factors involve judgement and the integration of data sets where other, less obvious factors are also important. It is not feasible to undertake experiments analogous to quitting smoking where fat, sugar or salt, or other specific food products, are excluded. The tobacco industry's habit of paying willing scientists to promote, endorse or simply accept their views is now spreading to important components of the food industry. We are moving into a world where a substantial proportion of the nutritional, paediatric and general medical community knows that their prominence, acceptability to governments and research funding depends upon tacit or even overt support of views which are not in keeping with the public-health imperative.

When sectors such as the sugar industry manage to persuade the US government to change the wording in relation to sugar in the latest US dietary guidelines, and where they can pay full-time lobbyists to serve as officials of national nutrition societies, our ability to introduce new public-health initiatives to limit escalating obesity in either children or adults is, indeed, a challenge.

21.9 Devising and implementing new policies

This gloomy picture calls for innovative strategies to combat the insidious and almost universal trend towards unchecked weight gain. The response of the professional civil servant or Minister of Health to adult obesity is still to lay the blame at the door of the victim and fall back on the mantra of the need for self-control, because the issues are too great and too long-term for any immediate solution to be found. To be challenged with the fact that 6-year-olds are now displaying the problem of serious overweight and obesity is likely, however, to challenge the glib assertion that it is all the problem of the individual. This is particularly true as the prevalence of overweight increases.

Those health-care professionals involved in childhood obesity therefore have a responsibility to highlight the big issues associated with this epidemic and not fall into the routine approach so common in the US and increasingly elsewhere of blaming the mother or the family in general for not having dealt with the problem. Policy-makers usually come up with the standard refrain that mothers should be better educated. The 'educational' approach to health promotion is now clearly seen to be one of the least effective approaches, although general health education is a necessary component of an integrated health strategy. Few doctors understand that they are inadvertent reinforcers of the problems associated with obesity because they are unwilling to confront the broader societal issues. They also endorse the common emphasis on individual responsibility and the need for education without recognizing the intense pressures which run counter to public health needs.

We need to learn how some societies have achieved much better feeding and physical activity practices. Whether one is dealing with improving general health and reducing the risk of chronic disease, as in Scandinavia, or attempting to eliminate malnutrition in countries such as Thailand and Costa Rica, the need for strong advocacy by highly qualified doctors, nutritionists, physical-activity specialists and public-health personnel is clearly crucial. This has to be brought together at a national level in a coherent manner and gain access to the political processes at parliamentary and ministerial level. Then these policy-makers who must be independent can set out clear goals and take on the big industrial pressures. This only works if the scientists and doctors are not constantly criticized by their colleagues who emphasize the uncertainty of one or more components of the proposals for public-health initiatives. The Norwegians managed this difficult process by establishing a Nutrition Council to which physical activity has now been added. An account of how this emerged shows how complicated it is to achieve political initiatives and to sustain appropriate nutritional policies at the highest political levels. Part of this process involved a very public debate on the issues by outstanding doctors and nutritionists. In Finland, huge changes also occurred in terms of chronic disease by virtue of the community becoming outraged by the remarkable death rates amongst middle-aged men and women and the failure of doctors to take the initiative. The people themselves forced the specialists to take up the cudgels. Subsequently the National Institute of Public Health in Finland became pre-eminent in devising strategies for breastfeeding initiatives, exclusive control of preschool and school feeding policies with doctors and dieticians being set guidelines about appropriate practice that can then be monitored. Publicly funded canteens were set precise nutritional goals for changing their practices. Restaurants were persuaded to include vegetables or salads in the price of main meals. As a result of the marked dietary changes affecting the whole population the health profile of Finland was transformed over 20 years without the need for draconian laws. Nevertheless, the Scandinavian assumption that the government has a fundamentally important role in establishing children's and adults' behavioural practices is being dramatically challenged by the rejection of this as left wing social engineering and the imposition of a 'nanny state'. The responsibility of society to create an environment conducive to the well-being of the vast majority is a disappearing concept. Only the affluent, educated and intelligent can cope with the consequences of this philosophy based as it is on individual action and initiative. The challenge for those of us in public health is how to highlight the need for government and multisectoral action with health education as a useful adjunct, but not the primary activity.

We need to transform the obstetric and paediatric services with nursing input to support a modern view of appropriate care of the mother and her child. The development of novel local government sponsored arrangements for ensuring that children are cared for in an appropriate environment when mothers return to work is also required. In both preschool and early childhood there should be quite rigid control of what foods are provided for children and the nature of the physical skills that they learn. The WHO Healthy School Initiative needs to become routine with the playing fields and the school environment becoming a focus for good nutritional and activity practices. Girls in most societies do not readily take to competitive sports and need to have a range of individual skills taught to them so that they avoid, as at present, becoming sedentary from the age of 8 years onwards. This is developing in societies where there is every inducement for girls to eat energy-dense snacks which make it difficult for normal appetite control systems to regulate their energy balance and match the low energy outputs. It is little wonder that so many girls take up smoking as an aid to restricting their food intake. The involvement of parents and the rest of the community in changing the environment of schools, in establishing safe walkways and bicycle tracks for children to make their own way to school, and the development of strategies to make the school a community centre for lifelong learning is only now being recognized as important.

Looking to the future will require much more unorthodox thinking and a recognition that we as health professionals need to look beyond our specialist areas. For example, town planning fundamentally affects childhood behaviour: if the planning of new estates allows the possibility of the streets being used as short cuts for traffic in congested areas, then children are not allowed out to play. Generating traffic-calmed and pedestrian-only areas is fundamental to changing children's behaviour. This is but one example of how the paediatric world is going to have to think in new dimensions if it is going to do anything useful to combat the growing epidemic of childhood obesity.

21.10 REFERENCES

Björntorp, P. & Rosmond, R. (2000). Obesity and cortisol. *Nutrition*, **16**, 924–36.

Franklin, M.F. (1999). Comparison of weight and height relations in boys from 4 countries. *American Journal of Clinical Nutrition*, **70**, 157–62S.

Gardner, D.S., Jackson, A.A. & Langley-Evans, S.C. (1998). The effect of prenatal diet and glucocorticoids on growth and systolic blood pressure in the rat. *Proceedings of the Nutrition Society*, **57**, 235–40.

Grantham-McGregor, S.M., Fernald, L.C. & Sethuraman, K. (1999). Effects of health and nutrition on cognitive and behavioural development in children in the first three years of life. *Food and Nutrition Bulletin*, **20**, 53–99.

Haffner, S.M., Gruber, K.K., Morales, P.A., Hazuda, H.P., Valdez, R.A., Mitchell, B.D. & Stern, M.P. (1992). Lipoprotein(a) concentrations in Mexican Americans and non-Hispanic whites: the San Antonio Heart Study. *American Journal of Epidemiology*, **136**, 1060–8.

Horne, P.J., Lowe, C.F., Fleming, P.F. & Dowey, A.J. (1995). An effective procedure for changing food preferences in 5–7-year-old children. *Proceedings of the Nutrition Society*, **54**, 441–52.

Neel, J.V. (1999). The 'thrifty genotype' in 1998. *Nutrition Reviews*, **57**, S2–9.

Petry, C.J. & Hales, C.N. (2000). Long-term effects on offspring of intrauterine exposure to deficits in nutrition. *Human Reproduction Update*, **6**, 578–86.

Simopoulos, A.P. (1997). Genetic variation: nutrients, physical activity and gene expression. *World Review of Nutrition and Dietetics*, **81**, 61–71.

Solomons, N.W. & Kumanyika, S. (2000). Implications of racial distinctions for body composition and its diagnostic assessment. *American Journal of Clinical Nutrition*, **71**, 1387–9.

WHO/IASO/IOTF (2000). The Asia-Pacific perspective: redefining obesity and its treatment. February 2000. Full document available from: http://www.idi.org.au/obesity_report.htm

Yajnik, C. (2000). Interactions of perturbations in intrauterine growth and growth during childhood on the risk of adult-onset disease. *Proceedings of the Nutrition Society*, **59**, 1–9.

Index

abdomen, pendulous 135
abdominal fat *see* intra-abdominal (visceral) fat
abdominal obesity *see* central obesity
abdominoplasty 355
abstract thinking 161, 162
acanthosis nigricans (AN) 135, 141, 202–3
acne 135
acrocephalo-polysyndactyly type II 183
adenosine antagonists 348–9
adipocytes 55
  differentiation 60, 61
    hormonal and nutritional regulation 62–5,
      198
    methods of study 62–3
    in PPARγ-2 deficiency 54
    stimulation by human serum 61–2
  lipogenesis 58–9
  lipolysis 59
  number 4, 5, 56, 57–8
    protein intake and 78
  secretory function 65–6
  size (volume) 4, 5, 57–8
adipose tissue
  development
    changes during 55–7
    critical periods 56, 57–8, 61, 66
    hormonal/nutritional factors regulating
      62–5, 198
    methods of study 62–3
  hyperplasia/hypertrophy 58
  lipid storage 58–9
  preadipocytes in human 60
  regulation of energy stores 55
  surgical resection 355
  see also body fat
adiposity
  definition 3
  food intake behaviour and 79–83, 85
  lifestyle and 83–5
  measurement 3, 4–14
  natural history 4
  nutritional intake and 74–9, 85
  predicting morbidity and mortality 14–15
  pubertal changes 155
  reduced physical activity predicting 99–100
  tracking (persistence) 14, 143, 155, 234

weight/height^p and 9
  see also body fat; fat mass
adiposity rebound, age at 56
  nutritional determinants 76–7, 78
  predicting adult obesity 14, 42–4
adolescence
  as critical period for developing obesity 44, 155
  definition of obesity 390
  eating disorders *see* eating disorders
  promoting physical activity 253
  psyche 161–2
  socioeconomic status and obesity development
    110
  see also puberty
adolescents, obese 154–66
  with additional problems 163–4
  bariatric surgery 357–8
  biophysical factors 154–60
  body composition and energy expenditure
    155–6
  cardiovascular risk factors 157–8
  complications of obesity 159–60
  day-care programmes 164–5
  dieting 272, 299–301, 365
  eating patterns 272
  endocrine disorders and contraception 158–9
  psychological aspects 160–6
    approach to 162–3
    important issues for 162
    self-esteem 116, 117
  psychotherapy 334, 339–40
  risk of becoming obese adults 143, 155
  vitamin and mineral status 159
adoption studies 39
adrenarche 191
adrenocorticotrophin (ACTH) 54, 62, 191
adult life
  morbidity and mortality 15, 145, 146, 157,
    234–5
  persistence of obesity 14, 143, 155, 234
  psychosocial problems 122–3, 143–4
adults, definition of obesity/overweight 16
adverse effects of obesity
  in adolescence 159–60
  immediate 131–42
  intermediate 142–4

adverse effects of obesity (*cont.*)
   long-term 145, 146
advertising
   food 251–2, 261, 262–3, 397–8
   indirect 262–3
   to promote physical activity 256
aerobic capacity (VO_{2max}) 101–2, 312, 313
aerobic exercise 309, 314, 316, 382
aerobics 318
age
   anthropometric indices and 8–9
   of menarche 134, 192, 208
alanine aminotransferase, serum 137, 157–8
Alstrom syndrome 182
amino acid metabolism 393
aminophylline 351
amphetamines 282, 345–6
amylobarbital 282
anaerobic threshold 309
androgens
   adrenal 191, 192
   leptin interactions 156, 207
   in overweight girls 136, 192–4
   in polycystic ovary syndrome 136, 158
android fat pattern *see* central obesity
anorexia nervosa 165, 248
   as complication of obesity 273, 298
   leptin levels 207
anthropometry 6–14
   circumferences and diameters 13
   ethnic differences 391–3
   indices based on weight/height centiles 10–12
   measurement technique 6–7
   percent of median, centiles and Z-scores 7
   see also body mass index; height; skinfold
     thickness; weight; weight/height^p
anxiety 118, 142, 383
aortic atherosclerosis 157
apnoea–hypopnoea syndrome 177
apolipoproteins 291–2
appearance, physical
   discontent with 115–16, 117–18
   peer-group appraisal 117
appetite
   excessive, in Prader–Willi syndrome 176, 177
   postexercise 309
   regulation 50, 51–2
appetite suppressants 345–8
arthritis 145, 146, 160
assertiveness training 368–9
asthma 138, 333
atherosclerosis 145, 146, 157, 221
attitudes
   helpful, in obese children 276
   to obesity 111–15, 123
attractiveness, peer-group appraisal 117
attributions of health 112–14
authoritarian attitudes 362–3

balanced low-calorie diet (BLCD) 284–6
   guidelines for use 300, 301
   negative effects 293–9
   positive effects 288, 290–3
   in residential programmes 380
balanced normal-calorie diet 284
Bardet–Biedl syndrome (BBS) 180, 181
bariatric surgery 355
   in adolescence 357–8
   complications 356–7
   techniques 355–6
basal metabolic rate (BMR) 95–6, 195
behaviour therapy 329–31, 338
   in outpatient programmes 366–7
   in residential programmes 383
   school-based 332
behavioural change 361–3
behavioural problems, in Prader–Willi syndrome
   175, 177, 178
benzphetamine 346
β_3 receptor agonists 346, 349
Biemond syndrome 182
biliary–pancreatic diversion (BPD) 356, 357
binge eating 81
   as complication of dieting 298
   day-care programmes 164–5
   see also bulimia nervosa
binge-eating disorder (BED) 165–6
bioelectrical impedance analysis (BIA) 5–6
biological factors 50–66
blood pressure
   association with obesity/overweight 144, 157,
     224–5, 228
   benefits of dieting 292–3
Blount's disease 136
BMI *see* body mass index
body composition
   in Prader–Willi syndrome 178
   pubertal changes 155–6
   see also body fat; fat mass; lean body mass
body fat
   amount *see* adiposity
   balance, fat oxidation and 102–3, 104
   distribution 3
     after dietary therapy 290–1
     assessment 12
     cardiovascular risk factors and 141–2, 230–3
     changes during development 57
     in definition of obesity 390–1
     ethnic differences 391–2
     gender differences 57, 156
     in insulin resistance 200
     leptin and 206
     macronutrient intake and 78–9
     see also body shape; central obesity
   measurement 3, 4–14
     anthropometry 6–14
     research methods 4–6
   see also adipose tissue; fat mass
body image, disturbed 142
body mass index (BMI) 9–10, 56, 222
   adiposity rebound point *see* adiposity rebound,
     age at
   cardiovascular risk factors and 225, 226
   centiles 10, 16–17, 18–22

definition of obesity 3, 16–22
    cut-offs 16–17, 30, 222, 223, 389–90
    in epidemiological studies 28, 29–30
    IOTF 18–22, 389
    WHO 17–18
    distribution 35–9
    indicating bariatric surgery 357, 358
    mean values 31
    natural history 4, 5, 10
    North–South gradient 31, 34
    as predictor of morbidity and mortality 15
    reference populations 16, 20
    secular trends 223
    self-worth and 116, 117
    tracking 14, 234
    Z-score 11–12
body shape
    attitudes to 111–12, 113
    attributions of health and 112–14
    discontent 115–16, 118
    see also body fat, distribution
body weight see weight
Bogalusa Heart Study 141, 221, 223–4, 226
bone age 134, 191
bone mass, peak 159
bone mineral content 159
Borjeson–Forssman–Lehmann syndrome (BFLS)
    182
bread 278, 279
breakfast 79–80, 257–8
breast cancer 157
breast milk, leptin in 209
breastfeeding 390, 395–6
breathing exercises 318–19
bronchial hyper-reactivity 138
bulimia nervosa 165
    as complication of obesity 118, 331
    day-care programmes 164–5
    as side effect of prevention 248
    see also binge eating
bullying 121–2
butabindide 350

C-peptide, serum 199
C/EBP family proteins 63
caffeine 346, 348–9, 351
callisthenics 318
Candida infections 135
carbohydrate intake
    adiposity and 75, 76, 77, 85
    in diets 284, 285, 286, 287
    physical activity and 85, 86
    secular trends 70, 71, 72
carbohydrate oxidation 103
carboxypeptidase E (CPE) 53–4
cardiac abnormalities 160, 181
cardiac failure, in Prader–Willi syndrome 177
cardiovascular disease (CVD)
    in adult life 145, 146, 234–5
    see also coronary heart disease; hypertension
cardiovascular risk factors 140, 144, 221–35
    associations of obesity/overweight 224–30

body fat distribution and 141–2, 230–3
clustering 227–8, 229
longitudinal analyses 234–5
in obese adolescents 157–8
Carpenter syndrome 183
catecholamines 59
centiles 7
central obesity (trunk, android fat pattern) 3, 156
    cardiovascular risk 141–2, 230–3
    effects of dieting 290–1
    effects of exercise 312–13
    ethnic differences 391–2
    in insulin resistance 200
    protein intake and 78–9
    reproductive function and 192, 194
    role of cortisol 191
    see also intra-abdominal (visceral) fat
cereals 279
chest circumference, cardiovascular risk and 230
child abuse 370
childhood obesity
    assessment 389–91
    definition 15–22, 28, 29–30, 389–90
    persistence into adult life 14, 143, 155, 234
    psychotherapy 338–9
children
    degree of responsibility 249–50
    perception of obesity 111–12
cholecystokinin (CCK) 350
cholelithiasis (gallstones) 137–8, 298–9
cholesterol, serum total (TC) 141
    association with obesity/overweight 225, 226,
        227, 228
    effects of dieting 291
    parental, as screening guide 229–30
chromosomal disorders 171, 172
    see also Prader–Willi syndrome
chylomicrons 58
circadian patterns, food intake 79–80, 85
circumferences 7, 13
clinical examination 131, 133
clinical features of obesity 131–42
clinical history 132
clothing 6, 162
cognitive behavioural therapy 330–1, 339
cognitive therapy 329–31, 337
    binge-eating disorder 165
Cohen syndrome 183
colorectal cancer 145, 146, 157
community programmes 256, 263
competition 253
compliance
    dietary therapy 301
    physical activity programmes 320–1, 366
complications of obesity see adverse effects of
        obesity
computer games 257, 275, 277, 314, 396
computer tomography 4
contraception 158–9
cooking
    methods 278, 279, 396
    teaching 257, 381

Cooley, Charles 116–17
coronary heart disease (CHD) 146, 157, 234–5
  risk factors *see* cardiovascular risk factors
cortisol 173–4, 190–1, 391–2
cosmetic problems 135
counselling, simple nutritional (SNC) 284, 299,
  300
craniopharyngioma 174
critical periods
  adipose tissue development 56, 57–8, 61, 66
  for development of obesity 42–4, 156
cryptorchidism, in Prader–Willi syndrome 176,
  180
Cushing's syndrome 64, 173–4, 392
  vs. simple obesity 189
cycling
  benefits 311, 318
  to prevent obesity 254, 255, 256
  in slimming programmes 276

dancing 311, 317–18
day-care programmes
  obese adolescents 164–5
  recommended use 339, 340
deafness 182
dehydroepiandrosterone (DHEA) 156, 191
Department of Health and Human Services (US)
  255
depression 118, 383
developing countries
  anthropometry 391–3
  defining obesity 390–1
  prevalence of obesity 33, 34
  socioeconomic status and obesity 40, 109
dexedrine sulphate 282
dexfenfluramine 346, 347–8, 351
diabetes mellitus
  body fat patterning and 230
  non-insulin-dependent *see* non-insulin-
    dependent diabetes mellitus
diacylglycerol 59
diameters 13
diet
  balanced normal-calorie 284
  healthy *see* healthy eating
  low-calorie *see* low-calorie diet
  as risk factor for obesity 245
  in slimming programmes 277–80
  traffic light 285, 365
  very-low-calorie *see* very-low-calorie diets
  see also eating; food intake; nutrition
dietary reference values (DRV) 284
dietary surveys 69
dietary treatment (slimming) 282–302
  approaches 284–7
  eating disorders as complication 118, 273, 298,
    365
  family therapy with 333–4, 338
  goals 270–1, 274, 283
  guidelines 299–301
  history 282–3
  home-based 270–80

imposed 84
in interdisciplinary outpatient programmes
  365
modifying lifestyle to encourage 273–5
negative effects 273, 293–9
parental 119, 120
physiological 271
positive effects 290–3
programmes
  aims 274–5
  benefits of formal 271
recommendations 275–80
in residential programmes 380–1
role of family 272–3, 276–7
simple nutritional counselling (SNC) 284
see also weight reduction
diethylpropion 346
dietician, primary health care 338
digestive inhibitors 346, 349–50
dinitrophenol 345, 348
diurnal patterns, food intake 79–80, 85
DNA methylation test 178
domestic activities 276–7, 308
doubly labelled water technique ($^{2}H_{2}^{18}O$) 93–4,
  95, 97, 98, 100
Down's syndrome 173, 245
drinks 278–9, 397
drug therapy 282, 345–52
dual energy X-ray absorptiometry (DEXA) 4
dyslipidaemia 141–2, 198
  see also lipids, serum profiles

eating
  habits, early 395–6
  healthy *see* healthy eating
  parental control 84, 86, 119–20, 249–50, 363
  patterns 79–82, 85
    adolescents 272
    to aid slimming 277–8
    behaviour therapy and 329
  speed 82
  see also diet; food intake; meals
eating disorders 154, 165–6, 327
  cognitive therapy and 331
  as complication of dieting 118, 273, 298, 365
  day-care programmes 164–5
  not otherwise specified 165
  parental 119, 370
  psychotherapy 165–6, 339, 340
  as side effect of prevention 248
  weight-related teasing and 122
  see also anorexia nervosa; binge eating; bulimia
    nervosa
educational level 41, 143–4
educational support, in residential programmes
  384
elevators (lifts) 254, 276, 308
endocrine disorders
  monogenetic, causing obesity 52–4
  in obesity 136, 158–9, 189–209
  in Prader–Willi syndrome 179
  secondary obesity 171–4

endogenous (secondary) obesity 171–84
endurance training 312–13
energy balance
    fat oxidation and 102–3
    lifestyle influences 84–5
    in prevention strategies 245–6
    regulation 50, 66
    in slimming programmes 274
energy expenditure
    activity-related 97–8
    increasing
        in obese children 276–7, 308–9
        to prevent obesity 245–6
        see also physical activity
    lean body mass and 310
    lifestyle influences 84–5
    low
        impact of television 100
        as predictor of weight gain 99–100
        vs. excess energy intake 98–100
    physical activity 97–8, 310–12
    in Prader–Willi syndrome 178
    pubertal changes 155–6
    regulation 52
    resting/basal (REE/BEE) 95–6, 310, 311
        after exercise training 312
        during television viewing 100
    total (TEE)
        assessment 93–4
        components 95–8, 308
        in obese children 95, 104
        to REE ratio 97–8
        vs. energy intake 94–5, 274
energy intake
    adiposity and 75
    assessment 94–5
    in balanced low-calorie diets 284, 285, 380
    excess, vs. low energy expenditure 98–100
    reducing
        to prevent obesity 245–7
        in slimming programmes 277–80
    secular trends 70–4, 85
    self-regulation in children 84, 86, 120
    in very-low-calorie diets 286, 287
    vs. energy expenditure 94–5, 274
    see also food intake
energy stores, regulation 55
enjoyment, physical activity 252–3
environmental therapy 338
ephedrine 345, 346, 348–9, 351
epidemiology 28–45
    methods 28–30
    risk factors for obesity 39–44
    see also prevalence of obesity
epidermal growth factor (EGF) 65
erythrocyte sedimentation rate (ESR) 140
ethnic differences
    anthropometry 391–3
    definition of obesity and 390
    insulin sensitivity 199–200
    risk of obesity 40, 41–2
    thrifty genotype hypothesis 393

European Childhood Obesity Group (ECOG) 18, 29
examination, clinical 131, 133
exercise
    aerobic 309, 314, 316, 382
    definition 307
    food intake after 309, 310
    in outpatient management 365–6
    postural 316–17, 318–20
    recommendations 309–10
    training 102, 314–20
        effects on fat mass 310–13
        in residential programmes 381–3
    traumatic side effects 310
    see also physical activity
exogenous (simple) obesity 131, 171

'faddy' children 278
family
    changing structure 396–7
    diet, changing 278
    dynamics, during slimming 275
    dysfunction 120–1, 329
    influences on physical activity 252–3
    interaction 120–1
    meals 246, 257, 277
    obese adolescents 160–1
    physical activity programmes and 316, 321–2
    prevention of obesity 249–50
    promotion of healthy eating 257–9, 272
    in psychotherapeutic approaches 331
    residential management and 378, 384–5
    role in slimming 272–3, 276–7
    see also parents
Family Environment Scale 120
family therapy 160–1, 331, 333–5
    definition 337
    in outpatient programmes 370
    questions 335–7
    recommendations for use 338–40
farming policies 261
fat
    body *see* body fat
    cells *see* adipocytes
    substitutes 350
    see also lipids
fat-free mass *see* lean body mass
fat intake
    adiposity and 75, 76–7, 85
    in diets 279, 284, 285, 286, 287
    obese children 82, 95
    secular trends 70–4
fat mass 3
    age-related trends 4, 5
    changes during development 55–7
    fat oxidation and 103
    pubertal development and 156
    reduction, dietary therapy 290–1
    see also adiposity
fat oxidation
    fat balance and 102–3, 104
    physical activity and 307, 313

fat oxidation (*cont.*)
   rate, in obese children 103, 104
fat/fat-mouse 54
fatty acids 64
   free 58, 59, 200, 286
fatty foods 82, 85–6, 95, 262
fatty liver 137, 157–8
feeding *see* eating
femoral epiphysis, slipped capital (SCFE) 136,
     137, 159–60, 379
fenfluramine 346, 347, 351
fetus
   adipose tissue development 55
   leptin function 208, 209
   metabolic programming 391–2, 393
fidgeting 276, 334
'filling periods' 55–7
films, advertising in 262–3
fitness *see* physical fitness
flats, high-rise 254
fluorescent in situ hybridization (FISH) 178
fluoxetine 346, 348
fluvoxamine 348
food
   advertising 251–2, 261, 262–3, 397–8
   availability 261
   exchange systems 365
   good quality 258–9
   policy 261
   preferences 82–6
   as reward 83, 280
   sheets (diaries) 365
   in slimming programmes 277–8, 279
food-(guide) pyramid 262, 285
food industry 395–6, 397, 398–9
   promoting healthy eating 262, 263
   role in prevention 251–2
food intake
   assessment 69, 94–5
   behaviour 79–83, 85
   circadian distribution 79–80, 85
   external control 84
   impact of television 100
   postexercise 309, 310
   secular trends 69–74, 85
   self-regulation 84, 86, 119–20
   see also eating; energy intake; meals
foster homes 164
friends 142, 161
   see also peer group
fruit 260, 279, 380, 395–6, 398

gallstones 137–8, 298–9
gardening 277
gastric banding (GB) 355–6
   laparoscopic 356, 357
gastrointestinal bariatric surgery *see* bariatric
     surgery
gastrointestinal problems 137–8, 176
gastroplasty, vertical (VGP) 356
gender differences
   adipose tissue development 55–6

attitudes to obesity 111, 112
   body fat distribution 57, 156
   family functioning 121
   insulin sensitivity 201
   leptin and 206–7
   long-term effects of obesity 145, 146, 234–5
   parental control of eating 120
   psychosocial consequences 123, 143–4
   pubertal changes in body composition 155–6
   risk of obesity 42
   secular trends in nutrition 70
   socioeconomic status and obesity development
     40–1, 109
genetic disorders
   with secondary obesity 171, 172, 180–4
   see also monogenetic forms of obesity
genetic factors
   in body weight regulation 52
   in obesity 39–40, 156
genitalia
   apparent hypoplasia 135
   hypoplasia, in Prader–Willi syndrome 179
genu valgum 318
GH *see* growth hormone
glucagon-like peptide (GLP)-1 54
'gluco-stat' hypothesis 51
glucocorticoids
   in adipose tissue development 62, 63, 64
   leptin interactions 208
   in lipogenesis 59
   in obesity 190–1
   see also cortisol
glucose
   intolerance 200
     benefits of dieting 291–2
     ethnic differences 392
   in lipogenesis 59, 102
   metabolism, in Prader–Willi syndrome 177
   transport 54, 199
GLUT 4 glucose transporter 59, 199
glycogen depletion 293–7, 309
gonadal function 190, 192–4
gout 145, 146
government
   breastfeeding policies 395
   devising and implementing new policies
     399–401
   health promotion 254–6, 261, 397–401
   role in prevention 251
group activities, participation in 162
group therapy 331–2, 370, 372
growth
   catch-up, in early life 392–3
   dietary restriction and 198, 297
   monitoring 264
   obese children 133–4, 196
growth hormone (GH)
   in adipose tissue development 63–4, 65, 198
   body fat distribution and 79
   deficiency 63–4, 174, 198
     in Prader–Willi syndrome 179
   leptin interactions 196, 198, 207

in lipogenesis/lipolysis 59
metabolic syndrome and 142
nutrition and 77–8
in obese children 195–8
treatment, Prader–Willi syndrome 180, 351
growth hormone-binding protein (GHBP) 195–6, 198
growth hormone–insulin-like growth factor (GH–IGF) axis 190, 195–8
gynaecomastia, benign pubertal 135
gynoid fat pattern 3

'halo effect' 115
handicap 163–4, 245
see also intellectual impairment
HDL *see* high-density-lipoprotein
head circumference 13
health, attributions 112–14
health education 255
Health Education Authority 255
health professionals
health promotion role 253–4, 260–1, 399–400
role in prevention 250–1
health promotion 397–401
by government 254–6, 261, 397
by health professionals 253–4, 260–1, 399–400
by industry 256, 262
new policies 399–401
in schools 250, 253, 259–60, 397, 400–1
on television 257
health services 256
health visitors 253–4
healthy eating 246–7
promoting 250, 257–63
in slimming programmes 277–80
within family 257–9, 272
healthy lifestyle
as goal of slimming 270–1
promotion 250, 255, 260–1, 272
psychotherapeutic approaches 328–9, 331
in slimming programmes 272, 275–80
heart rate monitoring 94, 382
heating levels, home 277
height
centiles 10–12
children on weight-reducing diets 198
measurement 6
obese children 133–4, 195
secular trends 70, 74
self-reported 6
short *see* short stature
velocity 134
weight/height^p and 8–9
heritability of obesity 39–40
high-density-lipoprotein (HDL) cholesterol
association with obesity/overweight 141, 157, 225, 228
body fat distribution and 231–2, 233
in metabolic syndrome 200
hip circumference 13
hirsutism 135, 136, 192
history, clinical 132

hobbies 277
home
-based management 270–80
heating levels 277
hormone replacement therapy, in Prader–Willi syndrome 180
hormone sensitive lipase (HSL) 59
hormones
analogues/antagonists 346, 350–1
changes in obesity 136, 158–9, 189–209
regulating adipose differentiation 62–5
see also endocrine disorders; *specific hormones*
housing quality 110
hunger *see* appetite
hydroxyacyl-coenzyme A (HOAD) 313
17-hydroxysteroids 191
25-hydroxyvitamin D (25OH vitamin D) 159
hyperadrenocorticism 173–4
hyperandrogenism 192–4
hyperinsulinaemia 140–1, 189–90, 198–203
benefits of dieting 291–2
body fat distribution and 231
immune function and 140
in obese adolescents 157
ovarian function and 192
relative weight and 224–5, 226, 227, 228
hyperphagia
in Prader–Willi syndrome 176, 177
in single gene defects 53, 54
hypertension
in adult life 146
ethnic differences 391–3
in metabolic syndrome 200
in obesity/overweight 144, 157, 224–5, 228
in pregnancy 146
hyperuricaemia 298
hypogonadism
in Bardet–Biedl syndrome 181
hypogonadotrophic, in massively obese men 194
in Prader–Willi syndrome 175, 179
pseudo, in simple obesity 135, 189
hypopnoea 160
hypothalamic–pituitary–adrenal (HPA) axis 190–1
hypothalamus 50
body weight regulation 51, 205
dysfunction, in Prader–Willi syndrome 176, 179
hypothyroidism 63, 171–3, 195
slipped capital femoral epiphysis 137
hypotonia, neonatal 174–6

IGF *see* insulin-like growth factor
immunological problems 139–40
industry 398–9
promoting healthy eating 262
promoting physical activity 256
role in prevention 251–2
see also food industry
infants
adipose tissue development 55, 56

infants (*cont.*)
    feeding, parental control 119
    food intake 70, 72–4, 76–7
    weaning practices 395–6
infections 139
infertility 146, 193
inpatient management 340, 377–8
    see also residential management
insulin 350
    in adipose tissue development 63, 64
    leptin interactions 208
    in lipid metabolism 58, 59
    mechanism of action 199
    ovarian effects 192
    plasma
        benefits of dieting 291–2
        high *see* hyperinsulinaemia
        relative weight and 224–5, 226, 227, 228
    protein-sparing modified fast and 286
    resistance 103, 140–1, 198–203
        acanthosis nigricans (AN) 135
        ethnic differences 392, 393
        in obese adolescents 157
    sensitivity 103, 199–200, 292
insulin-like growth factor binding protein
        (IGFBP)-1 196
insulin-like growth factor binding protein
        (IGFBP)-3 62, 196, 197
insulin-like growth factor binding proteins
        (IGFBP) 192, 195, 196, 197–8
insulin-like growth factor (IGF)-1
    in adipose tissue development 62, 64, 198
    leptin interactions 207
    nutrition and 77–8
    in obese children 196–8
    treatment 198
insulin-like growth factor (IGF)-1 receptors 64
insulin-like growth factor (IGF)-2 196
insulin-like growth factors (IGFs) 195–8
insulin receptor 199
insulinoma 164
intellectual impairment (mental retardation) 245
    in obese adolescents 163–4
    in other obesity syndromes 181, 183
    in Prader–Willi syndrome 177
    psychotherapeutic approaches 339, 340
interdisciplinary outpatient management 361–74
    goal and general philosophy 361–4
    organization 370–3
        collaboration problems 373–4
        individually tailored approach 371
        integrated approach 372–3
        standardized treatment 371–2
    treatment programmes 364–70
interdisciplinary residential management 380–5
interdisciplinary team approach 361
International Obesity TaskForce (IOTF),
        definition of obesity 18–22, 389
intertrigo 135
intestinal bypass operations 355, 356
intra-abdominal (visceral) fat
    cardiovascular risk and 230–3

dyslipidaemia and 141–2
in insulin resistance 200
measurement 12, 13
NIDDM risk 141
see also central obesity
iris coloboma 182
iron deficiency 159

James, William 116–17
'junk' food 81, 262

ketosis, starvation 286
kyphosis 320

lactate 59
laparoscopic gastric banding (GB) 356, 357
Laron's syndrome 198
latitudinal gradient, BMI 31, 34
Laurence–Moon syndrome 180–1, 182
lawn mowing 277
LDL *see* low-density-lipoprotein
lean body mass (LBM, fat-free mass)
    energy expenditure and 310, 312
    loss, caused by dieting 293–7
    in obese children 96, 134
    pubertal changes 155
    see also muscle mass
learning, food likes and dislikes 83–4
left atrial enlargement 160
leisure time, physical activity programmes 314–15
length, measurement 6
leptin 203–9
    body fat distribution and 206
    body weight regulation 51–2, 204–6
    gene mutations (deficiency) 52–3, 156, 206
    GH–IGF axis interactions 196, 198, 207
    immune function and 140
    lipolytic effect 59
    obesity and 204–6
    other functions 208–9
    in Prader–Willi syndrome 179
    in pubertal development 57, 134, 156, 207–8
    regulation of secretion 65–6
    resistance 205
    sexual dimorphism and 206–7
    single-gene defects affecting 39, 52–4, 172, 184
    treatment 205, 206, 350–1
leptin receptors (ObR) 203–4, 205
    gene mutations (deficiency) 53, 156, 205, 208
lifestyle 83–5
    healthy *see* healthy lifestyle
    modification principles 273–5
lifts (elevators) 254, 276, 308
lipase inhibitor (orlistat) 346, 349–50, 351–2
lipids
    mobilization 59
    oxidation *see* fat oxidation
    serum profiles 141–2, 157
        body fat distribution and 231–3
        effects of dieting 291–2
        in metabolic syndrome 200
        relative weight and 224–6, 227

role of GH 198
    screening guidelines 229–30
  storage in adipose tissue 58–9
lipogenesis 58–9, 102
lipolysis 59
lipoprotein lipase 58, 59
liposuction 355, 356
liver, fatty 137, 157–8
liver enzymes (aminotransferases) 137, 157–8
LMS method 19, 20
local government
  health promotion 254, 261, 400–1
  role in prevention 251
lordosis 320
low-calorie diet (LCD) 282–3, 365
  balanced *see* balanced low-calorie diet
  positive effects 288, 290–3
  see also dietary treatment
low-density-lipoprotein (LDL) cholesterol
  association with obesity/overweight 141, 225,
      226, 228
  benefits of dieting 291
  body fat distribution and 231–2
  screening 230
lower extremity exercises 319–20
lung disease, obstructive 138
lung function 138
luteal phase deficiency 193–4

macrosomic babies 44
magnetic resonance imaging (MRI) 4
margarines 279
mastoplasty 355
mazindol 346
meal-induced thermogenesis (MIT) 96
meals
  family 246, 257, 277
  number per day 80–1
  regular, to prevent obesity 246–7, 257–8
  in residential programmes 380
  school 260, 279, 397
  skipping 80, 257–8
  in slimming programmes 277
  see also diet; eating; food intake
measurement techniques 6–7
median, percent of 7
melanocortin-4 receptor 54
  defect 54
α-melanocyte-stimulating hormone (α-MSH) 54
menarche, age of 134, 192, 208
menstrual cycles, anovulatory 192
menstrual problems
  in adult life 145, 146, 192, 193
  in obese girls 136, 158
metabolic changes in obesity 140–2, 189–209
metabolic rate
  basal (BMR) 95–6, 195
  during television watching 256
  resting, regulation 52
  while playing computer games 257
metabolic syndrome (multi-metabolic syndrome)
      142, 200, 201, 208

metamphetamine 345–6
micronutrient supplements 286–7
mid-upper arm circumference 13
milk 70, 259, 279
minerals 159, 286–7
molecular factors 50–66
monogenetic forms of obesity 39, 52–4, 172, 184
morbid obesity, bariatric surgery 357–8
morbidity
  in adult life 15, 145, 146, 157, 234–5
  in childhood/adolescence 14–15
mortality
  in adult life 15, 145, 146, 234–5
  in childhood/adolescence 14–15
mothers *see* parents
Motivation Enhancement Therapy 368
multidisciplinary approach 361
muscle mass
  effects of exercise 312
  obese children 70, 134
  see also lean body mass

naloxone 351
National Center for Health Statistics (NCHS) 17,
      18
National Health and Nutrition Examination
      Surveys (NHANES) 32, 34, 224
neglect, parental 44, 110, 249, 370
neonates
  fat metabolism 59
  leptin levels 208, 209
  Prader–Willi syndrome 174–6
nesidioblastosis 164
neurological problems 139
neuropeptide Y (NPY) 205, 207
  inhibitors 350
neutropenia 183
'night eating syndrome' 80
nitrogen balance 293–7
non-insulin-dependent diabetes mellitus
      (NIDDM)
  in Bardet–Biedl syndrome 181
  ethnic differences 392–3
  in obese children/adolescents 140–1, 157,
      202–3, 224
  pathogenesis 201–2
  in Prader–Willi syndrome 177
nonpathological (simple) obesity 131, 171
noradrenergic agents 345–6
noradrenergic/serotoninergic agents 348
North–South gradient, BMI 31, 34
nutrient intakes *see* carbohydrate (CHO) intake;
      energy intake; fat intake; protein intake
nutrition 69–86
  adipose differentiation and 62–5
  adiposity and 74–9
    cross-sectional studies 74–5
    retrospective/longitudinal studies 76–8
  assessment of intake behaviour 79–83
  body fat distribution and 78–9
  data collection 69
  documentation of status 254

nutrition (*cont.*)
  education 259, 261, 381
  lifestyle factors 83–5
  secular trends 69–74
  see also food intake
Nutrition Council 400
nutritional counselling, simple (SNC) 284, 299,
    300

ob-17 cells 62–3
ob/ob mice 51, 203, 205
obesity
  in adults 16
  childhood *see* childhood obesity
  definition 3, 15–22, 28, 29–30, 222, 389–90
  prevalence *see* prevalence of obesity/overweight
  risk factors for 39–44, 245
obesity syndromes 164, 171–84
'obesogenic' environment 396–7
obstructive sleep apnoea 138–9, 160, 357–8, 379
oestrogens 156, 158, 194
Olestra 346, 350
oral contraceptive pill 158
orlistat 346, 349–50, 351–2
orthopaedic problems
  exercise training and 315–16, 320
  in obesity 136–7, 159–60
  in Prader–Willi syndrome 176
osteoarthritis 145, 146, 160
outpatient programmes 340, 361–74
  cognitive behavioural therapy 330–1
  interdisciplinary *see* interdisciplinary outpatient
      management
ovarian function 192–4
overweight
  in adults 16
  definition 15–22, 28, 222
  prevalence *see* prevalence of obesity/overweight
oxygen uptake, maximal (VO_{2max}) 101–2, 312,
    313

pancreas, endocrine 190
  see also insulin
parabiotic experiments 51
parents 118–22
  control of eating 84, 86, 119–20, 249–50, 363
  eating disorders 119, 370
  influence on food preferences 83–4
  neglect by 44, 110, 249, 370
  obese 249
    adult obesity risk 155
    childhood obesity risk 39
    infant feeding 119
    nutrition and 83
    physical activity and 98
  obese adolescents 160–1, 162
  physical activity programmes and 316
  prevention of obesity 249
  promotion of physical activity 252, 255
  residential management and 378, 381, 384–5
  restriction of television viewing 256–7
  role in child's slimming 272–3, 276–7

total cholesterol (TC), as screening guide
    229–30
  training 367–8
  see also family
pathological (secondary) obesity 171–84
peer group
  attitudes to obesity/overweight 117, 142
  behaviour 121–2
  importance 162
  influence on food choices 83, 249–50
  relationship problems 142, 161
Pepper syndrome 183
percent of median 7
peroxisome-proliferator-activated receptor
    (PPAR) 63
  γ-2 (PPARγ-2) defect 54
persistence (tracking) of obesity 14, 143, 155, 234
pharmacotherapy 282, 345–52
phenmetrazine 345–6
phentermine 346, 347
phenylpropanolamine 346
photographs, measurements using 13
physical activity 93–104, 245
  assessment 94
  definition 307
  energy costs 97–8, 310–12
  family therapy approaches 334
  guidelines 255
  impact of television 100
  increasing
    in obese children 275–6
    to prevent obesity 245–6, 252–7
  nutrition and 84–5, 86
  political initiatives 400
  as proportion of day 98
  reduced, predicting weight gain 99–100
  in residential programmes 381–3
  treatment programmes 307–23, 365–6
    aims 308–10
    choice of exercise 315–18
    efficacy in lowering fat mass 310–13
    factors affecting outcome 309
    general principles 313
    improving compliance 320–1
    leisure time 314–15
    in practice 314–20
    progressive postural exercises 318–20
    role of family 321–2
  see also exercise; sedentary lifestyle
Physical Activity Level (PAL) 98, 99–100
physical appearance *see* appearance, physical
Physical Appearance Related Teasing Scale
    (PARTS) 122
physical education 255, 315–16
physical fitness
  definition 307
  improving 321
  obese children 101–2
Pickwick syndrome 139, 177
picture-rating task 111
Pima Indians 201–2, 365
pituitary–adrenal axis 190–1

pituitary–gonadal axis 190, 192–4
pituitary–thyroid axis 190, 194–5
placenta, leptin secretion 208–9
plastic surgery 355
plate model 259
platelet derived growth factor (PDGF) 65
play therapy 370
playing outside 254, 275, 308, 396
polycystic ovary syndrome (PCOS) 136, 158, 194
polydactyly 181, 183
popularity, peer-nominated 117
population-based prevention 244–5
populations, reference 16, 20, 30
postural exercises 316–17, 318–20
potassium loss 293–7
Prader–Willi syndrome (PWS) 174–80, 245
    adolescence 163, 164
    clinical features 174–8
        childhood 176–8
        perinatal 174–6
    diagnosis 178, 183
    endocrine abnormalities 179
    management 179–80, 340, 351
preadipocyte factor-1 63
preadipocytes 60
    cell lines 62–3
    differentiation *see* adipocytes, differentiation
    proliferation 61
pregnancy
    fetal metabolic programming 391–2, 393
    hypertension in 146
    leptin in 208–9
prevalence of obesity/overweight 34–9
    BMI distribution and 35–9
    current data 32–3, 34
    factors affecting 39–44
    methodological issues 29–30
    predictions of future 394–5
    secular trends 35, 36–7, 223–4
        role of nutrition 69–74
    in super-obesity 38, 39
prevention 243–65
    monitoring and evaluation 264
    primary 243–4
    programmes 263
    reasons for 243
    by reducing poor dietary habits 257–63
    by reducing sedentary activity 252–7
    responsibilities for 248–52
    secondary 244
    side effects 248
    strategy 245–8
    target population 244–5
    target risk factors 245
    tertiary 244
principal components analysis 232
problem-solving training 368
progesterone 193–4
progestogens 158
proglucagon 54
prohormone convertase 1 (PC 1) defect 53–4
pro-opiomelanocortin (POMC) 54

deficiency 54
protein intake
    adiposity and 75, 76–8, 85
    animal vs. vegetable 72
    body fat distribution and 78–9
    in diets 284, 285, 286, 287
    GH and IGF-1 levels and 78
    obese children 83
    in pregnancy 391–2
    secular trends 70, 71, 72–4
protein nutritional status (PNS) 293–7
protein-sparing modified fast (PSMF) 286–7, 381
pseudo-gynaecomastia 135
pseudo-hypogenitalism 135, 189
pseudotumor cerebri (PTC) 139
psychodynamic therapy 166, 329, 338
psychoeducation 364–5
psychological problems
    management 369–70, 383
    obese children 118, 142
psychosocial factors 109–23, 245
psychosocial problems
    in adult life 143–4
    management approaches 368–9, 379
    obese adolescents 160–6
    obese children 142, 325–6
    see also psychological problems; socioeconomic
        status
psychotherapy 327–41
    approaches 329–35
    early 333
    eating disorders 165–6, 339, 340
    in outpatient programmes 368, 369–70
    perspectives 337–40
    questioning techniques 335–7
    rationale for 328–9
    in residential programmes 383
    see also family therapy
puberty 155
    age of 134
    body composition and energy expenditure
        155–6
    dieting at time of 299–301
    growth spurt 57
    IGF-1 and 197
    insulin sensitivity changes 200–1
    leptin and 57, 134, 156, 207–8
    in Prader–Willi syndrome 179
    precocious 134, 207–8
    see also adolescence
pubic hair development 156
pulmonary hypertension 160
punishment 367

questions 335–7
    circular 163, 336
    linear 162, 335–6
    reflexive 163, 337
    strategic 337
Quetelet's index *see* body mass index

racial differences *see* ethnic differences

recommended dietary allowances (RDA) 284
reference populations 16, 20, 30
renal anomalies 181
reproductive function
    leptin and 207–8, 209
    in Prader–Willi syndrome 179
    in simple obesity 192–4
research funding 398
residential management 377–86
    comprehensive approach 378–85
    duration of stay 378, 379–80
    historical background 377–8
    interdisciplinary approach 380–5
    physical activity and exercise programmes 314
    results and outcome 385–6
    screening 378–80
    see also summer camps
respiratory problems 138–9, 177–8
retinitis pigmentosa 181, 182
retinoids 64
rewards, food 83, 280
risk factors
    cardiovascular *see* cardiovascular risk factors
    for obesity 39–44, 245
Rohrer's index *see* weight/height³
role models 321
Roux-en-Y gastric bypass (RYGP) 356
running 311

satiety 82, 84
    regulation 50, 51–2
scapegoating 335
scapulae, winging of 320
schizophrenia 333
school
    behavioural therapy in 332
    breakfast programmes 258
    health promotion 250, 253, 259–60, 397, 400–1
    meals 260, 279, 397
    performance, poor 41, 143–4, 379
    in residential programmes 384
    special 340
    sports 253, 276
school nurse 338, 339
scoliosis 320
screening
    for obesity 264
    for residential management 378–80
    serum lipids 229–30
secondary obesity 171–84
secular trends in obesity/overweight *see*
        prevalence of obesity/overweight, secular
        trends
sedentary lifestyle 396–7
    obese children 98
    as predictor of weight gain 99–100
    reducing
        to prevent obesity 246, 252–7
        to promote slimming 276–7
    see also physical activity
selective serotonin reuptake inhibitors 348
self-control 362–3

self-efficacy 252
self-esteem
    assessment/conceptualization 116–18
    enhancing 363, 383
    obese children 115–16, 117–18, 142, 327–8
self-monitoring 366–7
self-perception 115–16
Self-Perception Profile for Children 117
self-regulatory skills, acquisition 84, 86, 119–20
self-worth 115–18
sensitive periods *see* critical periods
serotonin 350
serotoninergic agents 346, 347–8
sertraline 348
serum, adipogenic activity of human 61–2
sex differences *see* gender differences
sex-hormone binding globulin 158, 192, 194
sex steroids
    adrenal 191, 192
    gonadal 192–4
    see also androgens; oestrogens; testosterone
sexual activity 158–9
sexual dimorphism
    leptin and 206–7
    see also gender differences
short stature
    in Bardet–Biedl syndrome 181
    in Cushing's syndrome 173, 189
    definition of obesity and 390–1
    in GH deficiency 174
    in hypothyroidism 171–2, 195
sibutramine 346, 348, 351–2
silhouettes, body shape 111–12, 113
simple obesity 131, 171
single gene defects 39, 52–4, 172, 184
skating 318
skeletal abnormalities 183
skiing 311, 318
skinfold thickness 12, 14
    cardiovascular risk and 230–3
    in definition of obesity 17–18, 29–30
    ethnic differences 391
    measurement 7
    secular trends 223, 224
    tracking 14
    trunk/extremity ratio 12, 13
skipping rope 320
sleep apnoea, obstructive 138–9, 160, 357–8, 379
sleep disorders 138–9
slimming *see* dietary treatment
slipped capital femoral epiphysis (SCFE) 136, 137,
    159–60, 379
smoking 157, 248
snacking 81, 247, 396
    in early life 395–6
    recommendations 279
    role of television 262
snoring 138
social class *see* socioeconomic status
social disadvantage
    obese adolescents 164
    as risk factor for obesity 40–1, 110–11

social factors
  in obesity risk 40–1, 109–11, 245
  in prevention of obesity 253
  see also socioeconomic status
social problems *see* psychosocial problems
social relationships 118–22
  see also parents; peer group
social-skills training 368–9
social workers 379, 385
socioeconomic status (SES)
  attitudes to obesity and 112–14
  effects of obesity on 122–3, 143–4
  as risk factor for obesity 40–1, 109–11
sodium intake 292
soft drinks 278–9, 397
speech delay, in Prader–Willi syndrome 177
spine, exercises 319
sports
  energy costs 311
  participation by obese children 275–6, 317, 381
  in prevention of obesity 253, 254, 255–6
  in residential treatment programmes 381–3
stadiometers 6
stairs 254, 276, 308
starvation 207, 286
stature *see* height
steatomastia 134
Stein–Leventhal (polycystic ovary) syndrome 136,
    158, 194
stereotyping 112, 114–15
street, playing in 254, 275, 401
'stretching periods' 55–7
striae 135
subfertility 146, 193
subscapular skinfold thickness 12
  age-related trends 4, 5
  in WHO definition of obesity 17
substrate balance 102–3
  see also energy balance
substrate oxidation 102–3
sucrose consumption 72, 82
summer camps 377
  cognitive behavioural therapy 330–1
  physical activity programmes 314, 317–18,
    320–1
  see also residential management
super-obesity
  definition 30
  prevalence 38, 39
surgical treatment 355–8
  complications 356–7
  techniques 355–6
sweet foods 82, 85–6
sweets 83, 397
swimming 254, 311, 316, 318
sympathetic nervous system 208
syndactyly 183
syndrome X *see* metabolic syndrome

teasing 121–2
television viewing 84, 275, 314, 396–7
  effects on diet 262–3

impact on physical activity 100
  reducing
    to prevent obesity 247–8, 256–7
    to promote slimming 277
testis 194
testosterone 194
  leptin interaction 156, 207
  in polycystic ovary syndrome 158
thermodynamics 51
thermogenesis, meal-induced 96
thermogenic agents 346, 348–9
thermoregulatory disturbances 176
Third World countries *see* developing countries
3T3 cells 62
'thrifty genotype' hypothesis 201–2, 393–4
thymidine, radioactive-labelled 62
thymidine kinase 57–8
thyroid function 137, 194–5
thyroid hormones 63, 345, 348
tobacco companies 398
town planning 401
tracking (persistence) of obesity 14, 143, 155, 234
traffic light diet 285, 365
transforming growth factor (TGF)β 64–5
transport
  policies, national 254–5
  public 276
travel industry 256
triceps skinfold thickness 12
  cardiovascular risk factors and 226–7
  ethnic differences 391
  in WHO definition of obesity 17–18
triglycerides (TG) 55
  breakdown 59
  formation 58–9
  serum 141, 157, 200
    association with obesity/overweight 225, 226,
      228
    body fat distribution and 231
    effects of dieting 291
triiodothyronine (T3) 63, 194–5
trisomy 21 (Down's syndrome) 173, 245
trunk fat pattern *see* central obesity
trunk skinfold thickness *see* subscapular skinfold
    thickness
trunk/extremity skinfold ratio 12, 13
tuck shops 259–60
tumour necrosis factor (TNF)α 64–5
twin studies 39

underwater weighing 4
UNICEF 395
upper extremity exercises 320
uric acid, raised serum 298

vegetables 260, 380, 395–6, 398
very-low-calorie diets (VLCD) 83, 283, 286–7
  guidelines on use 300, 301
  negative effects 293–9
  positive effects 289, 290–3
very-low-density lipoproteins (VLDL) 58, 102,
    200

videos, watching 257, 275, 277, 396
visceral fat *see* intra-abdominal (visceral) fat
visual impairments 181, 182, 183
vitamin D 159
vitamins 159, 286–7

waist circumference 13
  cardiovascular risk and 230–3
  insulin resistance and 200
waist/hip ratio (WHR) 13
  cardiovascular risk and 230–3
  insulin resistance and 200
  tracking 14
walking
  benefits 308, 310–11, 314
  decrease in 275
  promoting 254, 255
weaning practices 395–6
weighing
  frequency 274–5
  technique 6
  underwater 4
weight 8
  activity-related energy expenditure and 97, 98
  centiles 10–12
  goals, dietary therapy 299–301
  maintenance, as goal of dieting 274, 299–301
  regulation 51–2, 204–6
  relative 8–9, 222
    cardiovascular risk factors and 224–6, 227
    secular trends 223–4
    see also body mass index; weight/height³
  secular trends 223
  self-reported 6
weight-centile-adjusted for height-centile, Z-score
  of 11
weight-control programmes *see* dietary treatment
weight-for-age 8
weight-for-height 8
  to define obesity 29–30
  Z-score 11

weight reduction
  bariatric surgery 356
  effects of exercise 312
  GH–IGF axis changes 195, 197–8
  as goal of dieting 274, 283, 300, 301
  leptin levels 204, 205
  negative effects 293–9
  positive effects 141, 202, 290–3
  in published studies 282, 288–9, 290
  residential management 378–9, 385
  see also dietary treatment
weight training 312
weight/height² *see* body mass index
weight/height³ (Rohrer's index) 8, 9
  cardiovascular risk factors and 226, 227
  to define obesity 29–30, 222
  secular trends 223–4
weight/height^p 222
  correlated with adiposity 9
  as predictor of morbidity and mortality 14–15
  uncorrelated with height 8–9
  see also body mass index (BMI); weight/
    height³
weight/ideal weight 29–30
wholefoods 278, 279
will-power 362
working women 261, 396
World Health Organization (WHO)
  Baby Friendly Hospital movement 396
  breastfeeding and 390, 395
  definition of obesity 17–18
  Healthy School Initiative 400–1

xanthines 348–9

yellow obese mouse 54
'yo-yo' syndrome 301
yoga 318
yoghurts 279

Z-scores 7, 11–12